Health and health care in the Third World

David R. Phillips

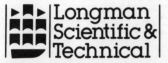

Longman Scientific & Technical

Copublished in the United States with
John Wiley & Sons, Inc., New York

Longman Scientific & Technical,
Longman Group UK Ltd,
Longman House, Burnt Mill, Harlow,
Essex CM20 2JE, England
and Associated Companies throughout the world.

Copublished in the United States with
John Wiley & Sons, Inc., 605 Third Avenue, New York, NY 10158

First published 1990

British Library Cataloguing in Publication Data
Phillips, David R. (David Rosser), _1953_ –
  Health and health care in the Third World. – (Longman developmental studies).
  1. Developing countries. Health services
  I. Title
  362.1′09172′4

ISBN 0-582-01418-2

Library of Congress Cataloging-in-Publication Data
Phillips, David R.
  Health and health care in the Third World/David R. Phillips.
      p.   cm. — (Longman development studies)
  "Copublished in the United States with John Wiley & Sons, Inc., New York."
  Includes bibliographical references.
  ISBN 0-470-21658-1 (Wiley)
  1. Public health — Developing countries.   2. Medical care — Developing
countries.   I. Title   II. Series.
  RA441.5.P45   1990
  362.1′09172′4 — dc20   89-49720
                                                                                        CIP

Set in 10/11 Plantin

Produced by Longman Group (FE) Limited
Printed in Hong Kong

Contents

List of Plates

Foreword

This book grew from my teaching and research interests in health and health care. These have been particularly concerned with spatial aspects of health and development and the availability and use of health services. I consider myself fortunate to have been able to research health and health-service related issues in many developing countries in Asia, Africa and the Caribbean over the past decade or more, and to have been able to relate such research – academic and applied – to my teaching responsibilities.

In terms of health and health care in the so-called 'Third World' (I readily acknowledge the limitations of this epithet), there are numerous excellent books and articles covering specific aspects of disease, disease ecology, epidemiology, traditional and modern health services, fertility, demographic change and the like. However, I have for some time felt that there is a lack of any text that considers many of these topics together, and that tries to point out some of their interrelations and their associations with modernization, socioeconomic and political change. I have therefore attempted in this book a synthesis of writings and research from numerous academic disciplines; and from bodies such as the World Health Organization, United Nations Children's Fund and the World Bank. This has proved to be a major undertaking, but in spite of inevitable limitations, I hope that a coherent framework has been provided in the chapters of this book both for students and researchers in various disciplines who wish to enter this field. I also hope that researchers and professionals already working in some parts of it might find this book useful as a broad-based source text.

The complex question of health and how (or if) it relates to development is increasingly being recognized as crucial, especially in the poorer countries of the Third World. There is, of course, a continuing debate as to how far 'health' can be measured and quantified, and also whether the term 'development' has any definable meaning. The nature of health care has also been discussed at length: whether it means purely medical care, or includes support services for health, or whether it should be broadened to include many other services such as housing, education and community care. Evidence is growing to suggest that direct medical interventions can only achieve a limited and probably often impermanent improvement in people's health. Their more general well-being has to be addressed; and to sustain and enhance health requires social, economic, environmental and political improvements.

The diversity of experience between Third World countries and the massive diversities within specific countries are almost sufficient to dispel any notions that the 'Third World' is a realistic categorization, especially in health or health care. This is discussed in some detail in Chapters 1 and 2, and subsequent chapters illustrate the great range in types of health services (public, private, traditional) and in their availability, accessibility and utilization. I have tried to emphasize that stereotypical 'Third World' problems do not have uniform existence. For example, some countries (many in Africa) are still struggling to contain high fertility and battling with infectious disease. Other countries, principally in East and South-East Asia and Latin America, are starting to face the problem of providing for ageing populations whilst sometimes concomitantly dealing with infectious diseases and the needs of young populations. Some countries have relatively well-to-do, stable economies, some are bankrupt and others are sadly engaged in prolonged and very damaging internal or external conflicts. The potential for, and reality of, health improvements and health care provision varies enormously among them.

I have tried to illustrate many important, often unresolved, debates and issues in Third World health care, although many are not confined to developing countries. The most notable debate is perhaps between those who suggest that only broad-based, comprehensive primary health care should be sought, and the more pragmatic supporters of selective, targeted interventions, which often only deal with common conditions for which known cost-effective preventions or cures currently exist. Another, often parallel, debate surrounds the imposition of top-down strategies versus grass-roots, broad, horizontal programmes, often heavily reliant on community participation. Yet other related discussions focus on the relative strengths and roles of highly trained technocratic medical professionals, primary level and community workers, and traditional practitioners. The debates are very much open, and the relative advantages of most approaches can only be weighed in the light of realistically available international, national and community resources, the cultural acceptability of programmes, and local circumstances and responses.

Writing this book has been very much a one-man task but one that has, nevertheless, been eased by advice and assistance from many people. In particular, in the Institute of Population Studies at the University of Exeter, Dr Nick Ford provided useful comments on the first two chapters and Dr Ian Askew provided suggestions for the sections of Chapter 7 on family planning issues. The Series Editor, Professor D. J. Dwyer, gave extremely helpful comments on the final draft of this book. I am also pleased to acknowledge the advice and help of many other academics who discussed ideas on the text with me. Mrs Jane Hayman, on this occasion as on many others, carefully read and checked the typescript and proofs of the book. Mrs Judy Gorton and Miss Jane Skinner diligently prepared numerous drafts of the text and are heartily relieved that it is now completed. Terry Bacon, of the University of Exeter Geography Department Drawing Office, provided superb cartographic help and prepared all the diagrams in the book. Andrew Teed, in the same Department, applied his usual high standard of skills to preparing photographs and copies of the diagrams.

David R. Phillips
Department of Geography,
and Institute of Population Studies,
University of Exeter.

Abbreviations

CHW	Community Health Worker
DPT	Diphtheria–Pertussis–Tetanus (vaccine)
EDP	Essential Drugs Programme
EPI	Expanded Programme on Immunization
ESCAP	Economic and Social Commission for Asia and the Pacific (UN)
FP	Family Planning
GNP	Gross National Product
GOBI/FFF	Growth monitoring, Oral rehydration therapy, Breast-feeding and Immunization/Family spacing, Food supplementation and Female literacy
IPPF	International Planned Parenthood Federation
IUD	Intra-uterine device
LGA	Local Government Area
MCH	Maternal and Child Health
MOH	Ministry Of Health
NIC	Newly Industrializing Country
NGO	Non-Governmental Organization
ORS	Oral Rehydration Salts
ORT	Oral Rehydration Therapy
PEI	Predisposing, Enabling, Illness (model)
PHC	Primary Health Care
SPHC	Selective Primary Health Care
TBA	Traditional Birth Attendant
TMP	Traditional Medical Practitioner
U5MR	Under-5 Mortality Rate (number of children who die before 5 per 1 000 born alive)
UN	United Nations
UNFPA	United Nations Fund for Population Activities
UNICEF	United Nations Children's Fund
USAID	United States Agency for International Development
VHW	Village/Volunteer Health Worker
WFS	World Fertility Survey
WHO	World Health Organization

Acknowledgements

We are grateful to the following for permission to reproduce copyright material:

The editor, Prof. R. Akhtar for fig. 4.7 from fig. 18.2 (Okafor, 1987); the author, Prof. J. Akin for fig. 6.6 from fig. 3.1, p. 56 (Akin *et al.*, 1985); Baywood Publishing Co., Inc. for fig. 6.2 from fig. 1 (Gross, 1972) © 1972 Baywood Publishing Co., Inc.; Basil Blackwell Ltd. for fig. 4.3 from fig. 1 (Fosu, 1986); Centre of Asian Studies (University of Hong Kong) for figs. 2.1 & 2.2 from figs. 1 & 3, pp. 19–20 & 33 and table 2.1 from table 2, p. 18 (Phillips, 1988a); Christian Medical Commission for fig. 1.1 from a figure (Werner, 1980); Croom Helm Ltd. for fig. 4.4 from a figure (Werner, 1978); Economic and Social Commission for Asia and the Pacific for fig. 7.12 from fig. A, p. 4 (ESCAP, 1986); Evaluation and Planning Centre for Health Care (London School of Hygiene and Tropical Medicine) for fig. 1.2 from fig. 11.3 (Harpham *et al.*, 1988); The Guildford Press and the author, C. Good for figs. 3.1, 3.3, 3.4 and 6.1 from figs. 1.1, 2.4, 10.1 & 4.2, pp. 24, 61, & 313 (Good, 1987a); Institute for Population and Social Research (Mahidol University) for fig. 2.3 from fig. 10, p. 107 (Institute for Population & Social Research, 1988) and table 6.4 from table 7, p. 19 (Porapakkham, 1982); the editor, International Journal of Epidemiology for figs. 2.6 from fig. 1 (Hakulinen *et al.*, 1986), 6.7 from figs. 2 & 3 (Habib & Vaughan, 1986); Macmillan Accounts and Administration Ltd. for figs. 1.4 & 8.4 from figs. 88 & 124, pp. 154 & 228 (Morley & Lovel, 1986); the editor, Dr. J. Morgan for fig. 3.2 from Illustration No.1 (Simpson, 1983); The New England Journal of Medicine for table 5.1 from table 3 (Walsh & Warren, 1979); Parkes Foundation and the author, Dr. K. Singh for fig. 7.8 from fig. 5 (Singh *et al.*, 1988); Pergamon Press PLC. for figs. 4.2 from fig. 1 (Paul, 1983), 4.8 from fig. 9 (Akhtar & Izhar, 1986b), 4.10 from fig. 2 (Okafor, 1984), 4.11, 4.12, 6.10 & 6.11 from figures (Bailey & Phillips, 1990), 5.2 from figs. 1 & 2 (Smith & Bryant, 1988), 6.4 from fig. 1 (Dutton, 1986), 6.12 from fig. 5 (Stock, 1983) and tables 4.1 from table 11 (Akhtar & Izhar, 1986b), 4.2 from table 8 (Mesa-Lago, 1985), 4.3 from table 4 (Zaidi, 1985), 4.4 from table 1 (Annis, 1981), 6.1 & 6.2 from tables

1 & 10 (Wolffers, 1988), 6.3 from table 3 (Chernichovsky & Meesook, 1986) © 1981, 1983, 1984, 1985, 1986, 1988 & 1990 Pergamon Press PLC; Royal College of General Practitioners for fig. 4.1 from a figure (Fry, 1979); the author, G. Salem for figs. 4.13 & 4.14 from figures (Laloe *et al.*, 1986); Unicef for figs. 7.1 & 7.11 from figs. 7 & 9 (Wilson *et al.*, 1986), 7.2, 7.3, 7.4, 7.5, 7.6 & 7.10 from figs. 13, 4, 3, 5, 12 & 10, pp. 50, 15, 13, 19, 49 & 35 (UNICEF, 1988) and table 1.1 from tables 1 & 2, p. 42 (Antoine & Manou-Savina, 1988); The World Bank for fig. 7.7 from fig. 7.1, p. 130 (World Bank, 1984); World Health Organization for figs. 5.1 from fig. 4, p. 21 (WHO, 1987d), 7.16 from a figure on p. 203 (Foster & Drager, 1988) and tables 3.2 & 3.3 from tables 1 & 3 (Chiwuzie *et al.*, 1987).

Whilst every effort has been made to trace the owners of copyright material, in a few cases this has proved impossible and we take this opportunity to offer our apologies to any copyright holders whose rights we may have unwittingly infringed.

Chapter 1

Health, development and health care

What is health care in the Third World? This apparently simple question defies a neat, simple answer. In developed countries, health care, whilst still distinguishable by its orientation to technology and medicine, has evolved as part of a wide network of social and welfare improvements, including public infrastructure, housing, education and the like. It is almost impossible to detach 'health care' except in its very limited sense (of 'illness care' and disease intervention) from general processes in society. The Third World is, to an extent, no different, in that considerable social and welfare change is occurring but, whilst some conditions are improving, other are deteriorating and there is excessive pressure on resources related to population numbers and age structure.

Even in its limited technical sense, however, the nature of health care in the Third World is more varied than it is in most developed nations. It is as varied as are the countries comprising the nebulous categorization Third World, which, indeed, many authors question both as a concept and as a shorthand classification (Harris 1987; Naipaul 1986; Toye 1987). The Third World has been taken to include very different countries. At one extreme of the categorization are the East Asian newly industrializing countries (NICs), the 'four tigers': Hong Kong, Singapore, Korea and Taiwan. After unpromising starts in industrialization and modernization, these economies have grown strongly; their governments have intervened to establish a variety of social programmes, with realistic policies for compulsory education and often extensive public housing and welfare schemes. They have also provided a range of preventive and curative health programmes, often with public and private involvement, although with variations in detail (Conyers 1982; MacPherson 1987; MacPherson and Midgley 1987; Midgley 1984, 1986). At the other extreme of the Third World categorization is a large group of much poorer countries in which the reality of official welfare policies is that they are non-existent except, sometimes, on paper. In between are countries of many varying levels of economic and social development. Whilst health programmes often have high political priority, the health care systems to implement them are in reality varied and under pressure, especially in the poorer Third World.

In addition to the formal, recognizable modern health care sector, comprising hospitals, clinics, doctors' surgeries and the like, in many Third World countries, traditional systems of various sorts may in fact coexist and serve the majority of people: the phenomenon known as 'medical pluralism' (Bannerman *et al*. 1983; Good 1987a; Leslie 1976). Indeed, it is widely noted that relatively few people, especially in the poorer Third World countries, have any access to, or contact with, a modern 'Western' health sector. A commonly cited figure is that up to 70 per cent of the populations of the poorer Third World nations do not have basic access to modern medicines or health care; in some countries this rises to above 80 per cent. It is widely assumed that most health care in such countries must be either from traditional sources or by self-treatment. In Chapters 3 and 6, the importance of pluralistic and holistic health care systems in the Third World is therefore stressed. So, too, are the many differences in availability of health care of various sorts for different socioeconomic, ethnic, urban–rural and intra-urban groups. To many rural dwellers, modern health care may be effectively unavailable because of distance. For many of the urban poor, modern health care may be quantitatively, qualitatively or economically unavailable (Harpham *et al*. 1988).

Definitions of health

A technocratic view of health is 'the absence of disease' (generally organic but possibly also mental). This definition implies that medical intervention can often restore health and places emphasis on medical diagnosis, treatment and cure along standardized lines. However, illness and disease are to some extent relative matters and, to sociologists, they are social constructs in which different societies view symptoms and appropriate treatments differently. Health therefore becomes a complex notion to define (Learmonth 1988). For instance, the World Health Organization (WHO) indicates that health encompasses 'a state of complete physical, mental and social well-being, not merely the absence of infirmity' in an individual. Clearly, much more than the absence of diagnosed disease is involved; 'basic human needs' will, by implication, be satisfied in a healthy individual. Thus, it is today widely agreed that the concept of health as a technical measure, the absence of diagnosed illness, is insufficient for most purposes (Feachem *et al*. 1989). Rather more useful, perhaps, is the objective of basic needs approaches to provide for a 'full life' in which healthy individuals live in caring, well-provided and intellectually stimulating communities (Lachenmann 1982; Stewart 1985). This is a more comprehensive perspective but its achievement will obviously require involvement of far more than the medical sector alone.

Many efforts to quantify health have nevertheless been made; quantification tends largely to be based on epidemiological characteristics referring to morbidity, disability and mortality in populations. It might appear reasonable to attempt to measure individual health by the WHO criteria noted above, but how does one assess the notion of 'complete' well-being? Is a physically handicapped but mobile and otherwise fit person 'unhealthy', when compared to, say, a person who has at the moment no detected disease or infirmity (Audy 1971)? What factors indicate social well-being? The quantitative expression of this nebulous ideal has long eluded social scientists. The debate over the quantitative definition of 'health' bears considerable conceptual and philosophical similarities to that concerning the definition of 'development', which, as discussed below, also has quantitative elements and much wider and more qualitative components.

Even in the use of apparently simple statistics such as birth or death rates, major problems arise in the quantitative expression of 'health' in many Third World individuals and communities, because of the lack of reliable data. Many births and deaths go unrecorded or are registered without any detail. Nevertheless, some attempts at quantification are important and the different conceptions of health noted above are of relevance in so far as they influence the 'nature' of restorative or promotive activities embarked upon. For example, the medical technician might feel able to restore someone to 'health' by curing organic or parasitic disease, or at least by treating symptoms. By contrast, the achievement of physical, mental and social well-being must imply a broader-based approach, involving the improvement and upgrading of the social and physical environment as well as of bodies and minds. This demands a much greater total involvement than medical intervention alone. Such a realization has great implications for the nature of nations' health care, as to whether 'top-down' intervention and programmes are imposed, whether 'total packages' are adopted or whether selective medical care is sought. This also will partly determine the extent to which people can become involved in, and take responsibility for, their own health and welfare.

Health and development

There appears to be a reciprocal relationship between 'development', broadly defined, and health, equally broadly defined. Traditionally, a 'healthy' population and workforce have been assumed to favour economic development, whilst an unhealthy population has been associated with poverty and underdevelopment. Until recently, considerable discussion focused on the ways in which changes in health of populations might or might not be associated with changes in economic indicators such as per capita income or gross national product (GNP), and on whether investment in health, for example, might be recouped or at least justified in economic terms (Grosse and Harkavy 1980). Today, it is recognized that there is not a simple, one-way relationship between 'health' and development. Indeed, even in 1958, in the book, *World health*, Brockington pointed out that 'development' affects health both favourably and unfavourably, although the balance of advantage clearly lies with the developed countries and greater modernization. However, for the poor particularly in the Third World, post-war development has often brought very little advantage (Abel-Smith and Leiserson 1978). Furthermore, overall, whilst development generally brings improved diets, housing, social change and reductions in infectious diseases, it is also usually associated with rises in degenerative diseases, mainly apparently of non- infectious aetiology (often called 'Western' diseases) (Hutt and Burkitt 1986; Trowell and Burkitt 1981). Changes in age structure, adverse aspects of industrialization, stress, and exposure to harmful substances can all be side-effects of modernization detrimental to health. In addition, ideas have also modified considerably as to what development is, how it should be measured and, indeed, sometimes questioning whether it is even desirable. Its supposed relationships with health have likewise been modified.

One problem of analysing relationships between health and development is that development is a rather vague notion. Some organizations are reasonably content to identify development in terms of changes in certain economic or socioeconomic indicators. For example, an increase in per capita income is taken by some as a proxy for development. 'Orthodox' development is assumed to be along Western lines, usually involving industrialization, often on increasing scales, and associated with economic growth measured via increased GNP. However, others are less happy with this rather narrow view of development. For example, various populist and neo-populist views hold that development implies some sort of small-scale, localized improvement and just or relatively equal distribution of income or wealth. Kitching (1982) provides an overview placing this type of discussion in historical perspective. In addition to the economic productivity aspects of development, broader issues may involve national development that enhances the power and independence of nation–states. Such notions of development often relate either to improved distribution or to increased economic efficiency of industrialization, but the necessity for Western-style industrialization is often questioned.

Modernization theory, when pre-eminent in development studies, identified change as occurring in a progression from traditional societies to modern, economic, industrial ones. However, its Eurocentric bias and assumptions of international uniformity have rendered modernization theory largely unacceptable in its original form, although in Chapter 7, for example, the recognition of cultural and societal diversity in modifying the impacts of modernization is discussed (in the context of changing attitudes to the care of elderly people in the Third World). It is, however, important to realize from the standpoint of health that modernization theory initially did not consider adequately or explicitly the possible detrimental effects of Western innovation (Stock 1986) or the widespread emergence of Western diseases. Whilst it appears that many so-called 'Western' diseases did actually exist in traditional societies, modernization with increased expectation of life has brought epidemiological change and such conditions are growing in importance. Health-care needs change and new health resource problems both replace and stand alongside the old.

In conceptual and practical terms, populist and 'small is beautiful' ideologies have their counterparts in health care as in economic development. Enormous improvements in health can and should be gained without the use of high technology, and Illich (1976) provides a critique of modern medical care in Third World settings. However, broader-based development for health demands considerable intersectoral collaboration, which is often difficult to achieve. Globally, there has been something of a shift in philosophy – if not always in practice – from favouring large-scale, top-down (vertical), technology-oriented development projects to smaller-scale, bottom-up or 'grass-roots' approaches to development and provision of human services such as health care. Nevertheless, top-down, 'vertical' approaches remain commonplace in health care provision, particularly in selective disease-oriented programmes, even if broader-based, horizontal, 'community' approaches in primary health care (PHC) have for some years been gaining prominence. In addition, basic needs provision and a basic needs approach to development have become widely appreciated (Stewart 1985). Small-scale approaches to development are frequently regarded as more human, more satisfactory, less externally imposed and generally less prone to many of the adverse side-effects that have often accompanied large-scale modernization projects. For probably the majority of poorer Third World residents, the benefits of many neo-modernization strategies have been elusive and the measures possibly even counterproductive. This remains as true today as when suggested by Gish in 1979. Certainly, the effects of large-scale, expensive strategies in terms of health and quality of life have often been ambiguous at best and lethal at worst, as the environmental degradation and dangers to health in places such as

Cubatao in Brazil and Bhopal in India sadly illustrate. Large-scale, largely uncontrolled modernization along Western lines may be highly damaging to health in the Third World.

The term 'development' thus has many meanings, which are not always clearly specified in practice or in research. These can include general improvement or progress; economic growth; increased labour productivity; satisfaction of basic human needs; modernization, including education and social change; and infrastructure provision. Social indicators such as the changing place of women or of particular social groups often feature in definitions of 'development'. Seers' well-known distinction between growth and development is of interest in the context of health since his work criticizes the obsession of many economists with quantifiable economic characteristics such as per capita income and the like. Such measures of an economy's performance must be seen in relation to overall goals and values in forming definitions of development (Seers, 1969, 1979). This requirement is set in the context of the conditions necessary to fulfil what he feels should be a 'universally acceptable' aim: the realization of human potential. In other words, how does development measured by changing economic indicators have impact on the lives of people?

Development is inevitably a normative concept and, to Seers (1979), almost a synonym for improvement. He sees the existence of at least three conditions as necessary for 'development': the capacity to buy food and physical necessities; a job (paid or otherwise); and equalization of income distribution (this he suggests because gross inequalities in the distribution of income not only indicate the existence of mass poverty but also are correlated with many other manifestations of inequality). To these three necessary conditions may be added others such as adequate education levels and political participation (Bernstein 1983). Indices of national income are not totally meaningless, it is argued, but have greater utility as indicators of development potential than as measures of development. It is therefore as important in the development process to achieve change (improvements) in non-economic indicators as it is to obtain economic growth. Indices of health would be among such non-economic indicators but improvements in health are also crucial in themselves. Clearly, however, much Third World modernization has not led to development in Seers' sense.

Other paradigms of development and underdevelopment also impinge to some extent on views of health and the nature of health programmes, particularly those externally funded. Dependency theorists such as Frank (1966, 1971) have viewed the relationship between the industrial core and the Third World periphery as a grossly unequal one in which the periphery is reduced to dependent subservience in a global capitalist system. European colonialism and neo-colonialism, it is alleged, brought dependency and under-development rather than development. The Third World can thus become dependent on developed areas for health care, as for other improvements. A national bourgeoisie with foreign links can often continue to control the distribution of economic and social re-sources, including health resources (Navarro 1974). However, critics claim dependency theory inverts modernization theory and ascribes little of a positive role to the periphery, and some feel it has become an explanatory cul-de-sac. It is useful, nevertheless, to remind us that health as an indicator has often been ignored in classic modernization theory. Marxist theories of underdevelopment have focused on modes of production and the ways in which the colonial state assisted the growth and strengthening of capitalist economies. The Marxist paradigm finds favour among those who feel it addresses significant questions concerning the control of the means of production and its potential for integrating explanations at scales ranging from global to local. However, whilst providing an essential view on underlying circumstances for health, its value is more limited in terms of practical solutions to contemporary health problems.

Seers' (1979) 'meaning of development' emphasizes the satis-faction of human needs and social justice, which are widely shared concerns, but there are still limits to what normative debates and definitions can achieve. Similar group concerns or assumptions may be shared, but theorists often disagree on the causes of poverty, inequality and injustice, and hence disagree as to ameliorative measures. As a result, very different solutions will often be proposed. The analysis of underlying causes of health problems, in particular, tends to be clouded by pressing practical requirements to satisfy normative demand, often perforce ignoring or failing to research root causes of the problems. To the researcher, the choice of a developmental perspective or underdevelopment paradigm is instrumental in the selection of research questions, choice of methodology and conclusions (or explanations) drawn (Stock 1986). Unfortunately, many studies of health problems related to develop-ment have made little explicit reference to the contexts in which they arose. Many health problems, Stock considers, should be viewed as integral to the expansion of capitalism, rather than as unanticipated side-effects of development initiatives. Whilst this recognition may be fundamental in reorientating policy recommen-dations, it is still important for researchers to be aware of many of the empirical 'side-effects' that were, and are, associated with accelerated development.

Today, the debate has moved on. In the 1970s and early 1980s, ideas of dependency had come to the fore, particularly with the suggestion that Third World development was being prevented and underdevelopment even being exacerbated by dependent relations with industrial countries. The publication in 1980 of the Brandt Report argued the need for common action at a global scale based on the recognition of mutual interests. Whilst this is still widely accepted, the means of achieving common goals are now questioned. In simple terms, there has been a theoretical and political shift in the debate, in which conviction is growing among some that market liberalization can mutually benefit the Third World and First World and bring about development. The debate tends to be between dependency and free-market thinkers (Elson *et al.* 1989). Whilst this juxtaposition of two schools of thought inevitably over-simplifies a deep and complex issue, it is nevertheless important since, if the free marketeers come to the fore, it will have major implications for health and health provision in much of the Third World (in particular, for the future perception of state responsibility for health care and, perhaps, how this might be minimized).

Trends in the philosophy and foci of health provision

The debates about the causes of underdevelopment and the relationships between development and health have progressed considerably in recent years although they are probably no nearer resolution than in the 1960s. However, within the field of health care, important philosophical and practical issues have been emerging. These have concerned the people served, the services provided, the coverage and the sponsorship of programmes. It is useful to consider such trends in a broad summary diagram (Fig. 1.1), which illustrates how the philosophy, content and spatial coverage of health care have evolved over the past two decades in the Third World.

There has been a clear movement towards attempting to make health and related services universally accessible in Third World countries. Historically, élites and the lucky few living in accessible areas have tended to have been favoured with modern, Western-style health care provision (for a discussion of this in historical contexts, see Abel-Smith and Leiserson 1978; Leng 1982; Manderson 1987). The majority of people have had to rely on self-care or traditional medicine. Today, whilst modern health care is by no means universally available, at least there is a trend towards serving all populations, if starting perhaps with the majority living in the more accessible areas.

Similar trends have occurred in the nature of health care and the location or venues of services provided. Previously, a

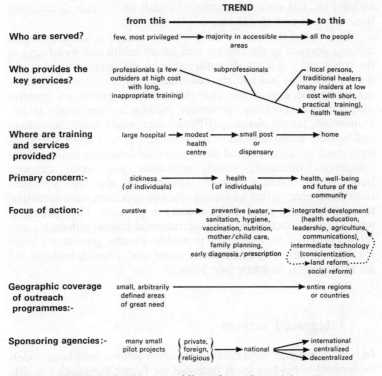

Fig. 1.1   Trends in health care philosophy and provision (from Werner 1980)

professional-centred philosophy prevailed; today, the use of ancillary workers (subprofessionals) and local volunteers (particularly village health workers, VHWs), sometimes incorporating traditional healers, is common. This trend, of course, is not confined to the Third World; as in most developed countries, ancillary, paramedical and support personnel are nowadays incorporated in PHC 'teams'. Allied to this trend is a movement from a large-scale, facility-oriented health care system (usually top-heavy, hospital-based) to the provision of smaller-scale units and home care. This trend may be facilitated by the ability to reduce the size of some diagnostic devices and to provide certain treatments locally, but it is sometimes hampered by a professional orientation towards hospital care and diagnosis. Many mixed systems have naturally evolved, recognizing the need for some specialized health care. Within horizontal, community-based systems, many elements of top-down, vertical programmes thus remain. Some maternal and child health (MCH) programmes and disease-eradication programmes allegedly within PHC fall within this group (Fendall 1987). This is discussed further below and in Chapter 5.

In terms of the orientation of programmes, increasing attention is being devoted to the current and future health and well-being of the community as a whole, rather than to the sickness and cure of individuals. This has had the concomitant requirement of developing integrated approaches that do not focus purely on curative medicine but encourage *preventive* medical actions (such as immunization, family planning (FP) and community health screening) and broader-based activities that nevertheless have *direct* health effects (such as sanitation and clean water) or *subsequent* health effects (education, nutrition, health education and social change). Geographical coverage of many schemes has also been extended from small areas (often in capital cities or specimen rural localities) to reach as many parts of the country as possible. The funding of health care has moved into the international league, although many related activities such as water provision, income generation, housing and education do not directly come out of health budgets but are intersectoral in scope (see below).

Integrated actions

In both urban and rural areas, integrative actions have been widely recognized as holding great potential for future community health. Harpham *et al.* (1988) provide the example of a holistic approach to community health in one of the poorest and most congested parts of Addis Ababa, Ethiopia: the *Kebele 41* urban dwellers' association. The major focus is on environmental upgrading as a way to improve community health, with the three main components being health, physical upgrading and community development (Fig. 1.2). The health component was initially supported by some six government offices and nineteen non-governmental organizations (NGOs). An integrated development programme was started in the early 1980s, but with ultimate responsibility to be taken over by the *Kebele*. The project is in keeping with the trend towards integrated action as it has emphasized, for example, that preventive health cannot be isolated from factors such as water supply, sanitation, income generation, education, training and house building. The activities undertaken by the project are as diverse as the people involved locally.

Whilst initial capital costs of this and other similar programmes have been criticized as high, the recurring costs of the health component are not expensive and the future role of the *Kebele* project is to make good use of the resources that have been developed

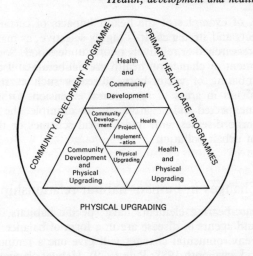

Fig. 1.2 Holistic approaches to community health adapted in an urban dwellers' association in Addis Ababa (after Harpham et al. 1988)

within the project to serve the wider community. Harpham *et al.* (1988) emphasize that the complexity of factors affecting health, especially in poor urban environments, makes integrated programmes particularly attractive and arguably essential for long-term development. As discussed further in Chapters 4 and 5, if dependence on curative health elements (hospitals, doctors and drugs) becomes established, popular participation and support might diminish and an integrated preventive programme might be difficult to sustain. A community may, by contrast, feel the need to focus on improving its environment rather than its health services *per se*. When a community is fully involved, collaboration between sectors leading to integrated action may be much enhanced.

Impact of selected development projects and strategies on the health of groups and areas

Development along modern, Western lines may bring benefits but it also often has associated costs. Whatever underlying explanation is accepted of the reasons for, and nature of, development, many side-effects can impinge directly on health, so the health implications of change become important. Below is a list, by no means

exhaustive, of examples of the health impacts of certain development projects and strategies. It is highly selective, as many impacts
are still unresearched or relatively poorly understood. Some impacts
of development or change on health are deliberate and positive, as
in the combating of vector-borne diseases such as malaria and
trypanosomiasis in areas of agricultural extension. Others are accidental, unexpected and negative, as, for example, the emergence
of water-borne diseases with hydrological schemes or the dangers
to health of urban pollution.

1. Changes in human–habitat relationships

Many disease-bearing elements have specific habitats. Sometimes
the hosts and agents of disease are in a form of balance but, often,
habitat or environmental changes will give one a temporary boost
(Last 1987; Learmonth 1988; Pyle 1979). Habitat changes often follow people working in new environments, or under different
geographical or ecological conditions, and these may have long-
term health implications. Urbanization of rural dwellers and the
extension of settlements into previously uninhabited areas may
bring people into contact with new or unfamiliar ailments (Halberstein 1985). It may also put them into less favourable
circumstances in which to resist or cure ailments if work is exhaust-
ing or health care provision insufficient.

2. Population movements and concentration

Urbanization and migrations for work, social reasons or as a result
of wars or famine can have very important implications for health.
They can assist the spread of various infectious diseases and underlie psychological problems of readjustment. They can also remove
people from traditional resources or family support. Reasons for,
and timing of, movements may be very varied, as may be resulting
health effects (Chapman and Prothero 1983; Prothero and Chapman
1984). Different types and sizes of settlements can be linked with
variations in rates and causes of mortality and morbidity, and
urban–rural differentials in these can also be high (as discussed in
Chapter 2 and illustrated in Table 1.1). The concentration of people
into large settlements has been well recognized as increasing the
possibilities of spread of disease; today in the Third World, urbanization is often on an unprecedented scale and resources for
public health provision are severely stretched or non-existent. Indeed, many Third World cities appear to be reaching or to have
passed the reasonable limits of being able to provide housing,
employment, transport and health services for their citizens.

Table 1.1 Infant mortality and juvenile mortality according to settlement size and environment in selected African countries (after Antoine and Manou-Savina 1988)

	Cameroon 1977	Ghana 1979	Kenya 1977	Benin 1982	Ivory Coast 1979	Senegal 1978	Lesotho 1977
Infant mortality (per 1 000)							
Rural	136	81	104	138	121	146	120
Small town	106	77	88	105	127	81	134
Large town	86	48	85	70	70	71	103
Juvenile mortality (1 to 5 years; per 1 000)							
Rural	80	59	64	147	69	222	
Small town	50	46	30	138	71	116	
Large town	50	60	41	90	50	94	

3. Micro-environmental changes, including housing

Changes in housing conditions, sanitation, drinking-water availability, transport availability and family support may all have direct health impacts. The range of variables under this heading can only briefly be touched upon here and sociospatial differentiation within settlements means that different groups often live in different worlds from the point of view of the risks they face to health. As discussed in Chapter 2, residents in the slum areas of many Third World cities and villages may be at risk from numerous infectious diseases and infestations, whereas changed diets and lifestyles may render their richer neighbours increasingly subject to degenerative, 'Western' diseases. However, the extent of such sociospatial differences in specific Third World cities has rarely been measured. Reliable data and detailed surveys at local levels are often needed to identify specific environmental risks in various urban sub-areas to enable priority to be assigned to improvement in public utilities and housing, but they are rarely available in most Third World countries.

The paucity of data and inadequacy of medical records on morbidity and mortality, and their lack of locational details, make research into disease and specific environments in Third World cities very difficult. To overcome this problem, the use of relatively simple environmental indicators, often visual, in the risk assessment of disease may be possible. What have sometimes been called 'environmental risk containers' have occasionally been used to identify specific sites that might be hazardous to human health.

A simple method for analysing housing and local environmental conditions in Third World cities has been suggested by Tipple and Hellen (1986), who have tried to identify the areas of the city of Kumasi in Ghana that score badly on health-related environmental conditions. The indicators chosen were: percentage of households with access to water supply and sanitation; residential density; occupancy rates; percentage of households occupying one room; and per capita income. These indices, gathered from neighbourhood surveys, were mapped on the 330-m grid-squares map of the city for twenty-eight residential areas, and scores and rankings on the six variables were converted to one map. The overall performance of each area was assessed, and areas with highest priority for local environmental improvements were identified. Such data are difficult to gather but can at least provide basic indicators to allow priority to be assigned to areas for improvement of housing, sanitation and services, particularly where resources are scarce in Third World cities.

Housing patterns and the domestic environment are important elements in health and disease, and the numerous links between health and various aspects of the physical environment (including housing, crowding and siting) are clearly identified by the International Institute for Environment and Development (1983). Geographically based, ecological (aggregate) scale projects can help to identify areas and micro-environments that are injurious to health. However, on the whole, there is relatively little published work that has explicitly examined the relationship between housing and health in the developing world and more detailed research is needed. Initial studies in Sri Lanka (Patel 1980), Costa Rica (Haines and Avery 1982) and in the rural Philippines (Johnson and Nelson 1984) have all indicated positive correlations between increased child death rates and poorer housing or sanitation.

The link between housing conditions and health has thus frequently been noted but less successfully measured. Nevertheless, the study in the rural Philippines found that children from better quality housing were more likely to live to age 5 than were children from poorer quality housing. Likewise, life expectancy at birth was 63.4 years for children from poorer housing compared with 69.9 years for children from better quality housing (Johnson and Nelson 1984). This has obvious implications for health needs but, more significantly, indicates the importance of developments in housing rather than purely in health care to increase survival rates (as well as quality of life).

4. Water availability and water flow

Agricultural development in general and water-regime alterations more specifically have created many 'new' or renewed health hazards or have exacerbated existing ones (Verhasselt 1987). Improved availability of clean drinking water can be a major influence in enhancing health and, particularly among children, in reducing deaths and illness from diarrhoeal disease. Poor urban dwellers attach high priority to water for drinking and cooking, as research in Manila indicates (Hollnsteiner 1979), and this has obvious health implications. However, citing schemes in Ethiopia, Malaysia and Liberia, Roundy (1985) fears that projects to provide safe water have often failed or are in jeopardy (see Chapter 8).

Even where clean drinking water is available, domestic storage conditions may repollute it. In terms of the increase in disease-causing organisms, incorrect storage of water may have very much more serious effects in a hot, tropical climate than it would in a temperate zone. On a larger scale, irrigation schemes and flood control measures can have the positive effects of increasing the amount of usable agricultural land and raising food availability and farm incomes, giving rise to better diets and the reduction of undernutrition and malnutrition (and deficiency diseases). However, it is increasingly recognized that such schemes may also have adverse side-effects. Water, for example, can act as a medium for transmission of harmful chemical pollutants or human diseases. It can allow disease-carrying organisms to breed, and can carry them near to homes or to other sites where humans may come into contact with them. People resettled in large-scale irrigation schemes, in particular, may have little experience of, or immunity to, certain water-borne or water-related diseases. Barrow (1987) lists some seventeen diseases and disease vectors associated with irrigation development, and Worthington (1977) reminds us that careful monitoring and appropriate health measures should be included in all such schemes. The literature on irrigation, and on hydrological schemes more generally, identifies side-effects, some quite serious, although it is important to maintain a balanced view of the overall benefits of schemes versus health risks.

Two common Third World health problems are often associated with hydroagricultural and irrigation schemes – malaria and the schistosomiases (bilharzia); other mosquito-transmitted and helminthic diseases may also occur. As Learmonth (1988) notes, WHO workers well over a decade ago issued a little-regarded warning on the relationship between man-made lakes and the spread of diseases including schistosomiasis (Brown and Deom 1973). Indeed, by the early 1970s, many adverse effects of large-scale water improvements were becoming evident in Africa and also elsewhere in Asia and Latin America. The schistosomiases, for example, a group of severe, often serious, debilitating, water-related diseases, currently affect some 500 million people, of whom perhaps only 1 to 2 per cent receive treatment. In Egypt, the schistosomiases are thought to have been responsible for a high number of deaths in connection with the Aswan High Dam and associated irrigation. Nevertheless, for many reasons, in spite of the resurgence or new appearance of water-related diseases, water-extension schemes have to continue.

Whilst some diseases cannot be attributed solely to water-extension schemes, they may be related to them. For instance, severe outbreaks of malaria can occur following the irrigation of warm, arid environments where previously most mosquito vectors were unable to survive. The use of anti-malarial drugs and pesticides, apart from the cost, can lead to rapid build-up of resistance, and any water spraying or ingestion of toxic drugs is, of course, undesirable. Malaria is widely recognized as an increasing problem in the tropics and as an impact of irrigation in particular and of agricultural development in general. Ebéné (1987) discusses a range of risks to the health of the population directly and indirectly associated with the irrigation of cotton fields in the Gezira in Sudan. The government of Sudan wishes to expand cash-crop production for economic reasons, in spite of numerous health side-effects, including malaria, schistosomiasis and cotton-dust lung disease (byssinosis). However, data are generally not available in Third World countries to allow the investigation of the late chronic effects of industrial-related diseases such as byssinosis.

Of course, it would be nonsensical to say that all water-extension schemes should be abandoned on health grounds alone, since most have many positive economic benefits as well as some positive health effects such as the provision of potable water and improved nutrition if food crops are grown. Malaria, schistosomiasis and many other irrigation-related diseases must be dealt with using an integrated approach involving chemotherapy, prophylaxis, health education, improved sanitation and disease-avoidance engineering, with clear knowledge of the nature of the diseases. Careful advanced planning for health-related matters must be incorporated into water-extension schemes if their disadvantages are not to outweigh possible benefits.

5. Socioeconomic changes accompanying development

Development often involves changes in individual or family activities, in work, income, nutrition and housing. It is, of course, widely recognized that health problems and socioeconomic problems are intimately linked (WHO 1981, 1986; Hill 1985; Hill and Roberts 1989). There are considerable socioeconomic differentials in the availability and use of health care, especially in the Third World, where social change is often particularly rapid and frequently outruns service provision (Morgan 1983). Not only is the current health and socioeconomic picture unsatisfactory in many developing countries but the future is also bleak. The increasing proportion of poor in the population, growing disparities in income and opportunities, and frequently worsening living conditions have sometimes been aggravated by 'development' strategies. For example, some development projects may favour certain sectors of the population and disadvantage others, or merely exacerbate existing imbalances. Green Revolution policies in India, for example, have increased social stratification in many villages, enabling the better-off peasant households to become wealthier and better housed and fed; poorer peasant households have often been reduced to the status of landless labourers (Crow et al. 1988). The health opportunities of the poorer strata have often suffered as a result.

'Marginalization' may also be considered in this context. It may be physical – forced movement into areas where living conditions are harsher (in rural or urban settings) – but also socioeconomic, as certain sectors of the population can become marginalized by being increasingly unable to exert pressure for public goods and services, and suffering a reduction in political power. Income-generating schemes may benefit those with skills or resources to participate and disadvantage those who cannot, marginalizing them further.

In many Third World countries, women in poor households are often expected to do 'double work', both inside and outside the home. They often have greater exposure to health problems than do males in that they are subject to the dangers of (multiple) pregnancy and childbirth as well as to the other conditions that threaten all the population. Ferguson (1986) provides data to illustrate that, in a physically marginal area of Kenya, women are subject to a particularly high degree of stress and accompanying ill health, and are less strong and healthy than males, or females from environmentally more favoured areas. Within specific settings, marginalized households or groups at high risk from the point of view of health can be identified by using various composite indices, including economic status, nutrition, access to water, housing, family size and age. Methodologies for doing so have been refined in Kenya by Ferguson *et al.* (1986), and findings of surveys within communities can help to identify households at risk, especially those who may be socially and physically marginalized. Knowledgeable local VHWs may also assist in identifying specific disadvantaged households.

6. War, disturbance and political upheavals as influences on health

A potent influence on health status and the need for health care comes in another man-created form, from war and smaller-scale upheavals. Political violence, in particular, appears to be increasing in much of the Third World; it may be extensive like war, or intensive, involving assassinations, disappearances and torture (Zwi and Ugalde 1989). Whilst not confined to Third World countries, political violence has considerable effects on health, both directly, through injury to military personnel and civilians, and indirectly, by increasing the need for health care while decreasing the ability to provide it. There are unfortunately many current examples of the health effects of armed conflicts in developing countries and numerous others from the recent past. Formally ceased conflicts in Korea, South Asia and South-East Asia still leave their marks on the health of the population injured in them or at risk from unexploded munitions and chemicals in the environment. The anti-Somoza insurrection in Nicaragua in 1978 to 1979, whilst leading to the ascendancy of a Sandinista regime with notable health care policies, is itself thought to have cost the country 40 000 lives and 100 000 injured (Donahue 1986a, 1986b). The conflict rumbles on today, further disrupting the economy and people's health.

Nevertheless, revolutions can also help to establish more just and equitable regimes, in spite of their initial physical and human costs. The Sandinistas, for example, attach high priority to health care and, whilst their ability to sustain this has been reduced in the late 1980s, the initial increases in popular access to health care were considerable, as Fig. 1.3 shows (Garfield and Taboada 1984). During the first 5 years of the Sandinista regime, the proportion of the population with access to modern health care grew from 28 per cent to more than 80 per cent (Garfield 1985). Particular attention has been paid to child health and oral rehydration therapy (ORT) for infant diarrhoea (Halpern and Garfield 1982). However, attacks on health care providers by Contras (enemies of the regime) and the disruption in the country because of the continuation of hostilities have reduced the impact of health care and have permitted the re-emergence of endemic diseases such as malaria. Malaria epidemics typically occur in those areas of Nicaragua subject to Contra attacks, but the war has, ironically, made community involvement in the building of health centres all the more popular (Garfield 1985).

The low-intensity war against Nicaragua (with external support from the United States) had wide-ranging impacts on health between 1983 and 1987. Destruction and embargo have cost the health system almost the equivalent of 2 years' entire health budget.

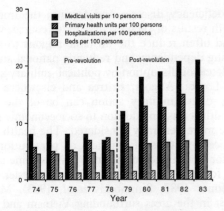

Fig. 1.3 Nicaragua: changing provision of health services and facilities after revolutionary political change (based on information from Garfield and Taboada 1984)

According to Garfield (1989), the continuation of war has decreased accessibility and availability of services, and 10 per cent of the population now have no access to modern health facilities. In addition, perhaps 10 per cent of the demand for acute care services is generated by the war, which has also created extensive need for long-term psychiatric and rehabilitation services.

During the 1980s, armed conflicts have developed in other countries such as Angola and Mozambique in which peoples' regimes have attached great importance to health care. However, war-ravaged economies have found the continued costs of care hard to sustain, and unstable conditions have made health infrastructures vulnerable. Opposing factions in Angola, for example, frequently raid hospitals and clinics. By late 1988, there were estimated to be over 40 000 amputees as a result of war wounds, including many civilians. These people require not only immediate medical care but often long periods of after-care (which is frequently unavailable). Many thousands of children have been injured or orphaned in Third World struggles, at great cost in human suffering and lost opportunities (Ressler *et al.* 1988). Large tracts of countryside in South-East Asia and Afghanistan have been rendered dangerous by unexploded bombs and mines, which continue to maim and kill people long after hostilities have ceased.

We must bear in mind the profound direct and lasting indirect health and health care effects of such man-created war incidents. In addition, disruption to food cultivation, harvests and to food distribution networks can underlie famine or deficiency diseases in areas of political or military strife (Dando 1980). This can exacerbate existing deficiency diseases and famine; the immediate and long-term health results of such events are, of course, very difficult to quantify and often reduce the unstable regions to aid-recipient status, increasing dependency and reducing national autonomy and esteem. The effects of disruption by political–military strife (for example, in Sri Lanka, Angola, Eritrea and elsewhere, in the late 1980s) and by direct military action can be of the utmost significance in health terms, in addition to socioeconomic and political factors that are more generally considered. The health of refugees, often the innocent victims of conflicts or persecution, and their special needs for health and social care, have become an important contemporary focus of concern and research (Ressler et al. 1988; Sandler and Jones 1987; Simmonds *et al.* 1983). Many refugee camps still exist in the areas surrounding Vietnam and Kampuchea (Cambodia). In Malawi, refugees from Mozambique place significant burdens on the existing health infrastructure; they need temporary or even long-term assistance, which is beyond the capability of the host government and requires inputs from international organizations.

Major characteristics of health care in the Third World

It is essential to review health care provision in the Third World in as widely defined terms as possible and not merely focus on its modern, technical components. It is important to examine expenditure on, and provision of, not only direct health care facilities, but also facilities in many related sectors. In addition, the extent of community resources in general requires assessment. This is particularly important with regard to the issue of 'vertical' or 'horizontal' links in health services and the debate relating to comprehensive PHC and selective PHC (SPHC), which targets only certain conditions and groups (see Chapter 5).

There is a fear, for example, that SPHC might involve the establishment of parallel, vertical health delivery systems for the implementation of specific, selective interventions (such as immunization or malaria control) that would divert attention from basic underlying health needs. Whilst Smith and Bryant (1988) feel there is probably little evidence to date for this happening on a large scale, and that variants on 'integrated' vertical programmes may be achieved, others are less hopeful. They continue to see 'planning without people' as a major danger; the converse risk, of course, is a broad level of popular participation but with little practical progress.

It has often been felt that there is little direct relationship between conventional medical inputs and traditionally defined health outputs. It appears that prevention of disease by social improvements and environmental management is a more promising avenue for enhancing health than merely increasing expenditure on medical technology (see, for instance, McKeown 1965, 1976; McKinlay 1979). Indeed, it is often argued that the principal determinants of health in any society are basically nutritional status and environment (Ruzicka 1986). McKeown and Record (1962) were probably the first to express serious doubts about the impact of medical science and technology on the early stages of mortality transition (see Chapter 2) and to stress the importance to mortality reduction of hygienic and nutritional improvements associated with socioeconomic change. Whilst crucial in the early stages of mortality decline, such a broad view is probably even more critical in today's Third World.

Therefore, breadth of vision with respect to issues addressed and broad participation are important because many aspects of health are inseparable from wider economic and social factors. Social and environmental action (of a public health type) often has beneficial effects that are not specific to a single disease. For example, attention to a population's nutrition not only may alleviate specific deficiency diseases and malnutrition but also may reduce the incidence of tuberculosis, infantile diarrhoea and possibly some cancers, and perhaps have a beneficial influence on coronary heart disease. Similarly, the provision of clean drinking water will have wider effects on health than only preventing childhood dysenteries.

Nevertheless, there is still something of a tendency in the Third World, as elsewhere, to regard health care in a rather narrow, technical light, although this has now largely been challenged by the WHO and in many other quarters. The provision of comprehensive PHC has become an important thrust in the 1980s in Third World health care and this will no doubt continue in the 1990s. However, as Rifkin and Walt (1988) note, it is not difficult to reduce even theoretically comprehensive PHC itself to a technocratic strategy that ignores the wide role of the state (in distribution of resources, for example), and regards 'health' as something determined by (or created by) the delivery of health services rather than by overall development (Barker and Turshen 1986). In part, modern medical paraphernalia and state-of-the-art health services may be espoused for prestige reasons in individual countries that wish to have modern hospital or high-technology equipment as symbols of modern development. An imbalance in use of the resources available for health care can therefore be perpetuated and a neglect of social–environmental management can occur, which may remain the poor relation of 'high-tech' medicine. The interest

of many institutions, training systems and technology and pharmaceutical companies continues to be served by the 'Asclepian cult'
favouring medical intervention. McKinlay (1979) identifies this as
the medical/health care distinction ('why medicine rather than
health?'). Illich (1976) has raised the debate to a different plane in
suggesting that many of the ills of the world can be traced to unnecessary,   excessive   or   over-potent   medical–technological
intervention. Collier (1989) attributes the excessive use of medication and multiplication of useless drugs to the extensive influence
of multinational pharmaceutical companies. Others seek to explain
health more abstractly as being largely a function of rational living
and personal lifestyles. Clearly, some balance needs to be achieved.

How does this discussion relate to 'health care' in its broadest
sense in today's Third World? Health care is regarded by most
governments (at least in theory) as a productive investment, increasing labour productivity, reducing waste of life and enhancing
quality of life. Nevertheless, resources for health in the 'South' continue to be minimal (Fig. 1.4) and many countries have consistently
failed, for various reasons, including poverty, administrative inability and political instability, to achieve significant gains in the
health field. Some general assessments about Third World health
care can be made; many seem critical or even pejorative; fortunately, not all apply fully in many countries. Sadly, however,
hindrances to rational health care and environmental improvement
have persisted for some decades; in 1966, King identified scarcity
of resources, manpower, equipment, education and housing as criti-

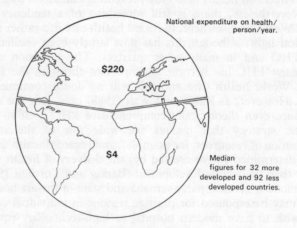

National expenditure on health/
person/year.

$220

$4

Median
figures for 32 more
developed and 92 less
developed countries.

In the South $4 is spent for each person each year.
This is only 2% of the amount spent in the North

**Fig. 1.4   North-South differences in expenditure for health (from
Morley and Lovel 1986)**

cal. In some aspects and in some areas, improvements have been seen, whilst in others, conditions have even deteriorated. It may be that the most promising hope of achieving a 'middle way' in health will be by the decision of international agencies largely to abandon 'top-down', superimposed and selective vertical programmes, which many agencies have promoted, in favour of longer-term development strategies (Rifkin and Walt 1988). If wider development in Seers' (1979) sense may be achieved, then children cured by medical intervention of infectious ailments, for example, will not be returned to squalid, reinfecting environments in which undernutrition and socioeconomic disadvantage continue to threaten their health.

These crucial wider issues of health and development aside, the World Bank (1980) has identified a number of features that tend to characterize health and health care in the Third World. To some extent, these characteristics can be grouped, although some straddle categorizations; in addition, not all are wholly undesirable or negative.

Some specific features of health care in the Third World

Availability and accessibility

- Health facilities, especially Western facilities, are often geographically inaccessible to the majority of populations. Women and children in particular may experience difficulties in reaching a source of care.
- Urban and rural differences and inequalities frequently persist in health and health care.
- The availability of services and treatment (such as drugs or X-rays) is often erratic, not only in rural areas but also in some parts of towns.
- Official health facilities sometimes fail to provide the necessary medicines, whereas the private black market may do so.
- Economic barriers as well as physical barriers exclude many people from formal health services; transport costs and time lost from work may prove too great for poor people to be able to use services.
- Imbalances therefore characterize health care: imbalances between individuals and communities (rich versus poor; favoured versus unfavoured), between regions, between urban and rural areas, and between countries.

Systematic factors and training

- Curative medicine is often emphasized, whilst prevention and early treatment, which need an effective system, are frequently neglected.
- Related to this, hospital facilities are often excessive in relation to primary and community provision; they are also often accessible only to a small proportion of national populations.
- The 'cost explosion' in health care often has disproportionately serious effects for Third World countries, which have limited financial resources and, frequently, debt burdens.
- Education of physicians is rarely geared to conditions in the country.
- Common health problems are often neglected, as are appropriate technologies, whilst relatively unusual diseases and high-technology equipment may be emphasized in professional training and facility provision.
- By contrast, an extensive 'appropriate' system of traditional medicine often coexists with the modern, but its degree of integration, official recognition or support is extremely varied.
- Health workers, especially in rural areas, are frequently insufficiently trained, supported and supervised.
- There is often heavy, sometimes excessive, reliance on paramedics or community workers without wholesale community participation.

Intersectoral and coordination features

- Referral and advisory support systems are often weak or non-existent.
- Community participation in health is sometimes weak, and intersectoral integration of health (with housing, education and infrastructure) is often underdeveloped.
- Integrated approaches are increasingly recognized as a major vehicle for improving health at the wider level, but political jealousies and intersectoral rivalries have frequently hindered effective coordination.

Political and social importance

- Considerable political importance is often attached to health development although practical activity and assistance is often inadequate. Unattainable statements of intent can be promulgated; 'slogan-led' health care is frequently apparent.

- The state often assumes responsibility for health care but it is rarely equal to the task. This can be particularly true in the poorest countries and/or revolutionary regimes where conditions are unstable.
- Development of selective health care programmes (with limited objectives) is sometimes promoted whilst citizens remain exposed to other, continuing hazards.
- Social security systems are at best partial and at worst non-existent, so families and individuals are often reliant on their own financial resources to support care.

Environmental conditions

- The socioeconomic environment is often injurious to health; housing, working and travel conditions may pose hazards and create extra health burdens. This may be exacerbated by a lack environmental controls, and weak industrial or labour legislation.
- Natural environmental disasters such as flooding, drought, hurricanes and fires may drain financial and other resources, as well as creating greater pressures on existing health provision.

Significance of these features

Virtually all agencies and individuals involved in Third World health care provision, administration, research and related social programmes (including famine and disaster relief) are aware of the above characteristics. The World Bank, as well as the WHO, recognizes that the most persistent problems in improving health and welfare do not necessarily stem solely from the complexity or expense of medical technology and the scarcity of financial resources. Rather, problems tend to derive from design deficiencies or from practical difficulties of policy implementation and management. As a result, firmer programmes are stressed; the WHO strongly advocates, in particular, improving access to low-cost PHC (discussed further in Chapters 4 and 5). The World Bank (1980), whilst only since the early 1980s directly involved in lending for health projects, notes that the most frequently encountered obstacles in lending for health components tend to relate to lack of planning, coordination and capacity to implement new programmes rather than to the unavailability of international funds, although this is possibly an excuse for low support. Other obstacles include shortages of trained technical and administrative staff, and poor transport and distribution systems, which hamper the logistics of programmes in terms of procurement and availability of supplies.

In addition, existing laws and regulations often provide inflexible structural impediments to the implementation of programmes.

It may be justifiable and, to an extent, realistic to blame institutional weaknesses and impedimenta for poor health levels and bad provision in many Third World countries, yet this is only one side of the equation. The majority of rural and urban residents in Third World countries are relatively or absolutely poor, and Harpham *et al.* (1988) and others have recognized at least three groups of factors that operate against the urban poor. The first includes the direct correlates of poverty (low income, limited education and bad diet); the second, the conditions of the urban environments to which the poor are exposed (overcrowding, bad housing, pollution, traffic, insanitary conditions and disease); and the third group relates to social and psychological conditions of insecurity, and related health problems and reduced quality of life. Similar, if not identical, conditions face the rural poor (many of whom become the migratory urban poor). Until the difficulties of meeting the life and health needs of such poor people are addressed squarely, the higher-level plans for action may rarely be expected to succeed.

Intersectoral action for health: integrated components?

Recently, a major concern has become the health and well-being of communities as a whole, as opposed to simply the technical cure of varieties of sickness; so, too, has the focus of action shifted to integrated development among many inseparable sectors impinging on health. Agencies, ministries and organizations responsible for health and health care have increasingly recognized that these topics cannot be solely a responsibility of one group of professionals. Indeed, since the WHOs declarations on PHC in 1978 (WHO 1978a), intersectoral cooperation has become accepted as one of the guiding principles in health strategy, even if this is yet to be coherently adopted in most countries. The intersectoral strategy recognizes that the improvement of health will require contributions from many sectors of the economy and society.

As well as the adoption of intersectoral approaches as national policies in some if not all countries, at a rather more localized level, integration of specific activities is increasingly recognized as crucial in promotion of health and healthy conditions. However, until recently, notably in the mid to late 1980s, the integrated 'community development' approach has had little impact on policy-makers, urban or rural. It is common sense to recognize that specific campaigns are valuable: health education, sanitation, immunization, nutrition, FP; but as a rule they have relatively little effect and durability in isolation if not related to the provision of potable water, shelter, income generation, security and a good, clean environment. Harpham *et al.* (1988: 162) suggest that 'when the community is fully involved, collaboration between sectors for integrated action is often greatly simplified'. They provide two case studies in Bombay and Addis Ababa (noted above) in which, with greater or lesser success, integrated approaches to community development were adopted, with improved living conditions and health status as direct and indirect product. These two case studies illustrate the importance of involving a wide range of health-related activities and basic services provision although, in Bombay, the developments lost credibility when they turned to more specialized curative health services. Nevertheless, these examples and many others indicate the vast potential of the population for improving their own living conditions and health levels. The contribution of community health workers (CHWs) in the context of such projects is discussed further in Chapter 5.

Intersectoral action

To enhance the chances of success of integrated actions at the local level, it is imperative that high-level blessing is given and the avenues and mechanisms for intersectoral collaboration are established. The WHO (1986) indicates that linkages are essential between the sectors that control and influence factors determining health – in particular, agriculture, food and nutrition, education and information, environment and physical infrastructure. The health sector should cooperate in the management of these sectors for health promotion.

It is hardly novel to recognize the significance of the linkages between the major sectors of health, agriculture, education and environment. Indeed, in a few instances, in widely varying political systems, the relationships have already been used to pursue health-promoting goals. However, the WHO stresses the need for more initiative by the health sector in enhancing intersectoral collaboration; health issues are of crucial significance in many other sectors and they may provide a valuable motive force for collaborative action. Indeed, community involvement has sometimes started in PHC and subsequently moved into other sectors; some prefer the term 'community involvement in health development' (CIH) to 'community participation' because of its wider implications (Oakley 1989). Space does not permit a full discussion here, but a few examples from agriculture and education will illustrate intersectoral relations with health and, in particular, PHC. They show that the effectiveness of health care is much reduced if general living conditions of the community are not improved.

In *agriculture*, output, production, land ownership, technology and decision-making have crucial health impacts. For example, the choice of whether to grow cash crops as opposed to staple foods can influence food availability, costs and access for vulnerable groups. Sen's (1981) discussion of the concept of food entitlement is relevant. The income from cash-crop sales rarely accrues in sufficient proportion to those growing and tending the crops. In the modern agricultural sector, high-yielding varieties of crops, sometimes susceptible to disease and drought, are often substituted for the more reliable and robust varieties that can sustain regular, if lesser, local food availability. In addition, labour-saving technology can often reduce the opportunities for income earning in rural areas, further impoverishing vulnerable groups. Changes in land holdings and lack of access to credit can reduce small-scale farmers to landless labourers. This group is often identified as most at risk, and its members are sometimes seen as the victims of Green Revolution strategies. At a macro-scale, economic policies that influence food prices, distribution and availability can have immense impact on the nutritional status of the population, with concomitant correlations with health levels. Examples of intersectoral action to strengthen existing agriculture–health institutional effectiveness are given by the WHO (1986) and Ebrahim and Ranken (1988). Nepal provides a notable case in which a fully fledged food and nutrition programme is being gradually elaborated.

Education can have a similar critical role in health improvement. Formal education is generally felt to be decisive in improving health and reducing mortality (especially among infants) in developing countries (Cleland and Van Ginneken 1989). A few years' basic schooling can make a crucial difference to an individual's ability to cope with the living environment and use services effectively and to his or her awareness of nutrition and hygiene requirements. Universal primary education is intrinsically linked to the 'health for all' goal, and basic education is the foundation for health education (see Chapter 8). The health sector therefore has great interest in promoting equity-oriented education policies that allocate priority to primary education and especially to the health-related needs of women. Reduction of female illiteracy rates is regarded as particularly important, as women so often play the major role in child rearing, the determination of family size, nutrition, and health care utilization. As the mutual support of health and education can probably best take place in school, intersectoral collaboration between health and education must be strengthened, to help teachers become trained in, and oriented towards, health activities. This also requires the incorporation of health information in the curriculum and allocation of resources to school health programmes. The involvement of primary school children in the monitoring and promotion of their own families' health in activities such as the *Doktor Kecil* ('little doctor') programme in Indonesia, the teaching of sanitation in some rural schools in Paraguay, learning about nutrition and health in Jamaica, and the development of a school textbook on health in the home environment in the ex-Portuguese areas of Africa, all provide good examples of the range of activities for health that can be encouraged at the primary level. At higher education levels, the health–education link in university education, for example, should be reoriented into a progressive interdisciplinary direction. Many universities in Third World countries are now recognizing the need for local medical, paramedical and related training to be relevant to local requirements, necessitating links with many related disciplines knowledgeable about national health and environmental conditions.

Other, but by no means less important, sectors that should be involved in collaboration are those of water, sanitation and housing development. The linkages between water, sanitation, housing and health are many. Frequently, water and sanitation projects do not give sufficient attention to the socioeconomic and sociocultural conditions of the communities served. Basic personal hygiene, for example, needs to be maintained even with improved sanitation. The message of boiling drinking water is now widely accepted, but boiled water is often reinfected on storage by use of dirty receptacles and by dipping unclean hands into it, negating the benefits of boiling (Lindskog 1987). A byproduct of this apparent failure of the relatively expensive boiling to prevent infections may be to make people sceptical of other health-promotion messages.

'Health byproducts' of industrialization

A rapid and often poorly planned industrialization process can expose many folk to new hazards that require a different set of intersectoral activities to safeguard them. Unorganized labour is often only poorly protected from industrial and pollution hazards, and casual workers, garbage pickers and others in informal activities are constantly exposed to many health hazards (Bromley and Gerry 1979). Little advice, guidance or safety equipment is currently available to help these workers. Many Third World industries also pose dangers to the community as a whole. Whilst examples of industrial pollution can be seen today in developed countries, severe industrial pollution disasters, such as the leak of toxic chemicals from the plant at Bhopal in India in 1985, seem to be more frequent occurrences in the Third World, where environmental legislation may be weak and maintenance of equipment sometimes lax. Toxic pollutants often affect much broader areas than their immediate locality. Traffic fumes, vehicles, noise and other factors all impinge on the wider environment. However, to encourage investment and economic growth, many of the poorer and middle-income Third World countries are ignoring (or are unaware of) health hazards from numerous industrial or related processes. By contrast, the first wave of NICs, especially those in South-East and East Asia such as Hong Kong, Singapore and Korea, have been developing environmental controls and considerable industrial health legislation over the past decade. Ironically, their effect may only be to encourage polluting or dangerous industrial processes to relocate in countries where controls are laxer.

Intersectoral action at an official level is increasingly crucial for the rapidly growing urban populations of the Third World. Never before have such large numbers of people in so many settings been exposed to and potentially at risk from the direct and indirect effects of industrialization. The health sector should be strengthened so that a dialogue can grow about the health-related aspects of other activities. Importantly, knowledgeable and authoritative health workers at all levels will need to be trained to contribute to the fostering of major intersectoral linkages with health. Community medicine, industrial medicine and environmental health will all have to be enhanced or, more usually, initiated in many Third World countries, so that the health-promoting (and health-damaging) aspects of the activities of other sectors can be identified, regulated and improved.

The preceding discussion illustrates that intersectoral action for health is wide-ranging, almost boundless. The WHO recognizes that prioritization will have to be allocated among tasks that are essential and those less so. Yet long-term goals must urgently be set, as the environment for tomorrow's health and facilities for improving health are established today. Long- and short-term objectives and policies therefore must receive official and practical support if many of the local and other initiatives that will be mentioned in following chapters are to have any hope of success.

Epidemiological transition: the range of Third World experience

Health indicators in the Third World

As a background for subsequent discussion, it is helpful to outline briefly some demographic, epidemiological and health terms used in this and subsequent chapters. A basic distinction needs to be drawn between the terms *mortality* and *morbidity*; the former relates to causes of death and rates of death; the latter to prevalence of illness in the community (Last 1983). Crude death rates as indicators of mortality are usually expressed as a number of deaths per thousand population in a calendar year, either from all causes or from specific causes of death; crude birth rates are likewise expressed per thousand population. However, more satisfactory from comparative and planning viewpoints are mortality and birth rates that reflect the age structure of the population in question, i.e. age-specific birth or death rates (or standardized mortality rates). This is because a high crude death rate, for example, would be more serious if found in a population with a young age structure than it would in an older population. Age-adjusted or standardized death rates can take account of these demographic differences and they can therefore be used with more confidence to compare mortality between various communities.

In many developing countries, however, even crude death rates are unsatisfactory, as they are often estimated inaccurately. Sometimes age-adjusted rates are simply not available because of paucity of data, or they are very unreliable. In addition, recording of causes of death, for example, may be deficient. In most developed countries, deaths are certified by qualified medical practitioners but, even in these circumstances, death certificates can be inadequate or ambiguous for research purposes. In many Third World countries, a considerable proportion of deaths may never be properly certified or causes of death may only be guessed at by unqualified practitioners. This is particularly true of rural and poor urban areas. This means that very important data can be missing and that official mortality statistics are at best guesstimates.

When morbidity (disease prevalence) is considered, statistics are even vaguer in virtually all countries and especially in the Third World. Most developed countries have a system of routine reporting by medical practitioners of a range of notifiable diseases (usually the more important communicable diseases) and some other conditions such as cancers. However, this relies heavily on correct diagnoses being established and scrupulous reporting to administrative authorities. In many Third World countries, such arrangements simply do not exist and many serious, and the vast majority of minor, illnesses are not attended by practitioners qualified in the Western sense. In addition, especially in the poorest countries, health reporting systems are simply inadequate to the task of morbidity surveillance. Therefore, whilst the total burden of morbidity from most notifiable diseases can be assessed in many developed countries, in the Third World this is very rarely the case. At best, a *sample* of morbidity prevalence may be available; at worst, no statistics at all exist. This has proved to be a problem in establishing the true extent of some important diseases such as malaria and tuberculosis. It is even more problematic where generally self-limiting (if potentially dangerous) diseases are concerned. The true burden of disease in the Third World is therefore just not known. As a rule, it cannot be established, as is conventional elsewhere, in terms of numbers of persons ill, duration of illness, or days lost to work through illness. Third World health research therefore is often hampered and the dimensions of, and solutions to, many problems are less readily defined than in other countries. Indeed, a case is made by Timaeus *et al.* (1988) for a single, round-world health survey to collect epidemiological information for developing countries, although this would meet with formidable methodological and logistical problems.

Other vital indicators

The major additional indicators of health are those associated with life expectancy, population increase and infant mortality. Others that have strong associations with health in communities are indices such as adult and female literacy, education, nutrition and employment.

Life expectancy, a hypothetical measure, is conventionally expressed as the average number of years an individual might be expected to live if current mortality trends continue; expectation of life at birth refers to the number of years a newborn baby can be expected to live, whilst expectations of life can be expressed for persons of any given age (Last 1983). As living and health conditions often vary for males and females, life expectancy is often given separately for each. It is a measure of considerable value to those interested in Third World health conditions, and changes in life expectancy can indicate improvement (or deterioration) in health care and basic needs provision.

Population increase is usually expressed as a rate (percentage annual growth) and it may refer to 'natural' increase (the excess of surviving births over deaths) or may include migration (see, for example, Jones 1981). Population projections are sometimes given that estimate the future year at which population growth might become stationary, referring to future fertility and mortality and thus making certain assumptions about health conditions, acceptance of FP and the like. Birth rates may sometimes be expressed as 'age specific', relating to the number of births to women of reproductive years (15 to 44), a more useful figure, demographically speaking, on which to base health care policies.

For Third World countries, in particular, one of the most useful indicators of health in a community is infant mortality. This is a measure of the yearly ratio of deaths of children less than 1 year old relative to the number of live births in any year. Sometimes the neonatal mortality rate is also given, which refers to deaths among children of 4 weeks or younger. A high neonatal mortality rate may suggest a wide range of poor conditions, including malnourished mothers, insufficient child health care facilities or outbreaks of infections afflicting newborn infants. The state of health and mortality rates among young children, the group most vulnerable by and large both to infectious and deficiency diseases, provide very important indicators to health planners and doctors. In many Third World countries in the past, infant mortality rates of possibly 40 to 50 per cent were not unusual. Even today, as noted below, it is still possible to see infant mortality rates in excess of 10 per cent although, thankfully, improved child health services, sanitation, nutrition and social conditions have helped to reduce rates considerably in recent years.

Mortality as an indicator

It appears perhaps paradoxical to start discussing or comparing levels of 'health' by reference to causes of mortality. Often, it seems, the underlying levels of health or ill health (morbidity) that people experience during their lifetime may not be directly related to the causes from which they die. Nevertheless, an examination of mortality causes and their changing patterns can indicate important things about change in society (in a demographic sense, as well as in terms of levels of living and public health). In addition, it will also generally highlight important features such as changes in longevity and population structure in different countries, since these are closely related to the causes from which people die (older people being more likely to succumb eventually from chronic degenerative conditions, younger persons to suffer acute conditions and accidents; however, these general observations will often not be supported in specific cases).

Death certification may be only an unsatisfactory indicator in many poor countries and it does not always reflect accurately the burden of ill health in a community. Only for a relatively limited range of diseases with high case–fatality rates can it be intuitively accepted that mortality rates might be suitable indicators of morbidity (and therefore useful for the purposes of planning the distribution of resources, for example). In fact, it is suggested that only cancer of the lung and acute myocardial infarction fit the bill in this respect, in some ways reflecting the lack of progress in effective treatment for these conditions. The outcome of many other, usually fatal, conditions can be varied to some extent by early diagnosis and treatment (Ashley and McLachlan 1985). Such factors in turn tend to reflect the distribution and availability of health care resources and thus mortality may not reflect accurately community levels of morbidity. In particular, long-term debilitating conditions such as malnutrition, malaria and tuberculosis may not always be fatal or feature as main causes of death, so their impact in human and economic terms might be underestimated by reliance on death-rate statistics. This should remind us that mortality rates are at best only a surrogate measure of ill health in any given locality or country.

Over the past 30 to 35 years, death rates in virtually all Third World countries (including the poorest countries) have been reduced directly through health care interventions and, perhaps more importantly, indirectly through improvements in living standards. Precise data to support this statement are, of course, often only fragmentary. There have also been important differences in the levels and pace of morbidity and mortality change between and within countries through this period. Today, in some places there is evidence of stagnation or even reversal of some of the gains of the past, suggesting that the maximum benefits have already been achieved from purely technical health care intervention separate from sustained economic and social development. This seems particularly true in some of the poorest countries, in which drought, famine and economic collapse have meant that a reversal of earlier improvements in mortality has occurred. McKeown's (1976) statement that most health improvements in the community stem mainly from public health and standards of living gains is pertinent. It is particularly relevant to Third World countries, which may seek health improvements (or have them imposed by external agencies) through technical medical intervention such as SPHC and thus reduce the emphasis on improving community health and housing conditions (see Chapter 5).

Nevertheless, mortality decline generally has occurred. More important, however, is the fact that in most countries mortality decline has been accompanied by significant changes in the causes of death and disease: so-called 'diseases of affluence' or 'Western' diseases have become much more common in many countries of the Third World over the past few decades (Trowell and Burkitt 1981). This epidemiological change is of the utmost significance and will be discussed in more detail below. In brief, what the structural changes in the composition of mortality in many developed nations may mean is that, whereas in the past, public health measures and medical intervention could often reduce the burden of acute infections causing ill health, today these are of much less effectiveness and relevance. To keep populations healthy, investment in far broader spheres is necessary.

Infectious and non-infectious diseases

It has become conventional to distinguish between infectious and parasitic diseases on the one hand and chronic or degenerative diseases on the other. This distinction is important, as the balance of morbidity and mortality from the two major categories has changed in the developed world and appears to be changing today in the Third World. The two major categories of disease have very different causes, treatment and implications for health and health care. The degenerative disease group includes circulatory diseases (heart and cerebrovascular), neoplasms (cancers), certain congenital or acquired handicaps, and certain diseases of the digestive system, some of which have been termed 'Western' diseases (Trowell and Burkitt 1981). They are assumed at present mainly to be of non-infective and almost certainly multifactorial aetiology (Hutt and Burkitt 1986). By contrast, for most infectious diseases, a specific bacterial, rickettsial or viral cause is generally known or suspected, even if complex social and environmental factors are involved in its spread. Many of these infectious diseases are today generally thought of as 'tropical' diseases (see, for example, Parry 1979), although Learmonth (1978, 1988) reminds us that, until relatively recently, some were a cause of problems in the developed world, where many, including leprosy, malaria and plague, were once common or even endemic. Indeed, as Vélimirovic (1984) points out, many infectious diseases still provide a huge burden today in Europe. A significant number of infectious diseases may be preventable or curable sometimes at considerable personal and economic cost but, as recent trends show, a significant number of old killers still exist and new ones such as AIDS sometimes emerge.

Infectious diseases are a major cause of mortality (and morbidity) in the Third World but are by no means the only health problem. Degenerative Western diseases are making their presence increasingly felt, and have considerable implications for future health care planning. In addition, many people in Third World countries experience *malnutrition* (bad feeding); in its extreme form this can lead to a range of deficiency diseases depending on which vitamins or elements in diets are lacking. *Undernutrition* follows from a lack of sufficient quantities of food and does not always occur in association with malnutrition, although it often may do, especially in famine conditions. Overall sufficiency of diet is usually measured in calories but a qualitative lack of vitamins or protein can still occur, particularly in specific food cultures (Howe 1977). Kwashiorkor and marasmus relate, for example, to protein deficiency (and more generalized protein-energy malnutrition); pellagra (niacin deficiency) is associated with some sorghum-based diets; and beriberi (thiamine deficiency) is linked historically with rice cultures (Learmonth 1978, 1988; Trusswell 1985).

Failure of any food to be available leads to *epidemic undernutrition* (famine), which may occur seasonally in many Third World countries when crops fail or have been insufficiently planted. Tragically, famine can also occur on a larger and longer scale when environmental, economic or political conditions become changed or unstable. Whilst economic development in nations does not always correlate directly with levels of health, by and large it does correlate with undernutrition and malnutrition in that the richer the country, the better able it is to feed its citizens. However, even in middle-income countries, many of the poorest people living in urban margins or in poor rural areas suffer from malnutrition or even famine, and the diagnosis and management of malnutrition then has to become an important public health task (Trusswell 1985). A major health and welfare issue arising from malnutrition and undernutrition is not only the immediate excess mortality that the latter in particular causes, but the long-term misery both create. They open affected people to many infections and some degenerative illnesses; make their quality of life much less and, in a vicious circle, reduce their ability to work and feed themselves. The upper-income countries in the Third World rarely see indigenous undernutrition or true deficiency diseases. The problem characteristically, although not exclusively, pertains to the poorer countries.

Epidemiological transition and demographic transition

It has long been recognized that societies seem to pass through various changing patterns of morbidity and mortality during the development process, even if not all the stages and sequences are identical in every case. In general, health improves, morbidity and mortality rates fall and come from different causes, and life expectancy increases; this comprises the 'epidemiological transition' (Hellen 1986; Omran 1971, 1977). These changes generally come with modernization and appear to be part and parcel of the process. However, they seem to occur at a different pace in different countries. The causes and mechanisms of the health–illness–death process are very complex as they encompass numerous biological and socioeconomic factors. Whilst biological factors may technically be associated with ill health and mortality levels, they may often be brought into action, mitigated or worsened by lifestyles, levels of living and environmental exposures (Ruzicka 1986).

Demographic transition

It is generally accepted that it is not possible to identify precise correlations with many of the changes in mortality and morbidity within the epidemiological transition except in certain specific instances such as vaccination and the eradication of smallpox, although even in this case improved living standards were also important. However, the epidemiological transition is closely related to many changes in the growth of populations. Demographers and, to an extent, historical, population and medical geographers, have for a long time debated the evolution of fertility patterns, family size and longevity when societies modernize. In particular, the population-fertility literature has generally revolved around the investigation of 'determinants of fertility' (see, for example, Bulatao and Lee 1983). The search for a 'grand theory' has not met with total success, but it has nevertheless proved valuable in highlighting empirical trends and some generalizations concerning population change. The theory of demographic transition has focused primarily on the explanation for the decline in fertility; the onset of mortality decline and its causes were less conspicuous in the context of the theory (Caldwell 1982; Ruzicka 1986; Thomlinson 1965). There is not general consensus that mortality decline was the major determinant of fertility decline although interactions almost certainly took place. From the point of view of health care providers, both aspects of the demographic transition theory are important but in particular the stimuli of change and rates of future change are crucial.

The general trend suggested by demographic transition theory is that, from a period of low population growth when deaths and births roughly balance each other (infant mortality rates are high and life expectancy is low), some sorts of health and social improvements occur that allow more people to survive and, for a while, population growth can be quite rapid and family sizes large (Notestein 1945). The need for large numbers of children to replace those lost through high infant mortality gradually diminishes and, eventually, the social and economic benefits of having smaller families may be recognized as 'modernization' spreads. Fertility control replaces natural fertility. Family sizes tend to stabilize at a lower number and standards of living rise whilst societies as a whole become more affluent. Eventually, a stable population size may be achieved, and there may even be some slight reduction as deaths from natural causes in old age tend to outweigh the number of births.

This depicts a straightforward and perhaps simplistic and deterministic demographic transition. Whilst most societies today can undoubtedly be observed to be at various stages in the transition, it is subject to many checks and balances. Its rate of occurrence has varied tremendously both internationally and historically, and reverses may even occur in some unusual circumstances. The seemingly simple core of the demographic transition theory is that fertility declines appreciably, probably irreversibly, when traditional, non-industrial (usually agrarian) societies are transformed by modernization or development into bureaucratic, urban-oriented societies (Beaver 1975; Jones 1981). This statement assumes many things: for one, that a simple industrial–economic modernization will occur in societies and that it will be accompanied by changes in lifestyles, living conditions, aspirations and, of course, health levels. There are many reasons why such a simple progression may not be followed and, indeed, modernization theory and the orthodox development orientation it implies are not wholly accepted by many researchers (Kitching 1982).

Nevertheless, there is undoubtedly evidence that elements of the demographic transition concept can be identified in most societies (Findlay and Findlay 1987; Verhasselt 1985). In so far as the demographic transition relies on fertility and mortality decline, this has been a source of some debate. In reality, the causes and mechanisms of the health–illness– death process are very complex as they encompass both biological and socioeconomic factors (Correa and El Torky 1982; Ruzicka 1986; United Nations (UN) 1986a; Feachem *et al.* 1989) and their relationships to demographic structure and change are likewise complex. Undoubtedly, with the very considerable natural growth in populations (today almost exclusively in Third World countries), some contributions of both fertility and mortality change have to be considered. Explanations have evolved, however, since the 1930s and 1940s. Early-identified causes of population growth were often assumed to be reductions in mortality. The view that rapid population growth resulted from mortality decline in the presence of more or less stable fertility was initially generally accepted. However, by the 1960s, whilst reductions in mortality were still seen to be the prime causes of accelerated population growth, it became evident that the expected reduction in fertility to more stable population sizes was not occurring as rapidly as anticipated, and many writers maintained that rising birth rates were of greater significance to population growth than previously realized. Alarming trends were sometimes noted; for instance, some birth rates rising, rather than falling as the theory would suggest. Indeed, during the 1960s and early 1970s, it seems probable that only a few smaller developing countries actually experienced birth-rate declines. Social changes in others may have altered a previous balance so as actually to increase birth rates.

Nevertheless, by the 1980s, there seems to be consensus that pronounced fertility declines have occurred in many developing countries, especially in Latin America and East and South-East Asia. The most important countries that have not shown marked declines are probably Pakistan, Bangladesh and many of those in sub-Saharan Africa. India, Indonesia and especially China have shown particular decline, mainly through FP campaigns and changes in marriage patterns (Dyson and Murphy 1985). Indeed, China's fertility decline, of some 53 per cent in the decade of the 1970s, is the most rapid on record for a large nation, although the relative effects of socioeconomic development and government policies in precipitating the decline are not really well understood (Lavely 1984; Tien 1984) and there has been some popular reaction against the stringent family-size regulation of the one-child policy.

In general, the main questions in the debate revolve around the extent and timing of eventual fertility decline, in which there are also regional differences. Examining data for a number of Latin American and Central American countries, it seems that, with some exceptions, the early low fertility of the 1930s was followed by a peak in the 1950s and quite rapid decline by the post-1965 period. By contrast, there is a widespread view that fertility rises may well have occurred and are probably continuing in many areas of sub-Saharan Africa. Data are rather sparse and birth histories in the context difficult to interpret, but information from Kenya, for example, seems to indicate continued if limited upward trends in fertility (Dyson and Murphy 1985; Henin *et al.* 1982). Others suggest more definite increases: in spite of two decades of government-sponsored efforts to reduce population growth, Kenya's fertility level and rate of natural increase are at almost record levels. Natural increase is about 4 per cent per annum and total fertility close to eight births per woman. With such continuing high fertility, the outcome from the standpoint of population policy has been a 'highly conspicuous failure' (Frank and McNicoll 1987). In other countries, too, such as Malawi, recent surveys suggest that many women favour large families of eight children. Some suggest that, in the absence of broad-based socioeconomic changes, current efforts at fertility regulation may have few short-term or long-term effects (Sindiga 1986). This is very alarming for some poorer countries, and the policy implications of this type of research, indicating that pre-decline rises in fertility are common and may in fact continue, concern decisions to introduce, promote and maintain FP practices. The failure to achieve desired reductions may not be the result of poor programmes but may simply result from countervailing influences, especially poverty and lack of economic opportunities. It is increasingly acknowledged that cultural differences are crucially important in explaining the persistence of high fertility in, for example, parts of Africa and the rapid decline in other places, such as Thailand and other Asian countries (Caldwell and Caldwell 1987). It is important to recognize cultural and other factors and not to abandon programmes prematurely on the wrong bases. The Kenyan example is particularly worrying because the high fertility rate of about eight children per woman is quite recent and represents an increase from the six to seven children per woman similar to the rest of Africa in the 1950s and 1960s.

With such exceptions, the existence of varying types of demographic transition and its eventual effects are nevertheless widely recognized. The World Fertility Survey has done a great deal to document and account for fertility and reproductive changes in the Third World (see, for example, Cleland and Hobcraft 1985). However, of equal or greater interest to many epidemiologists, health planners, economists and medical geographers is that, with 'modernization', increasing affluence and life expectancy in most countries, a very different disease profile emerges from that of an underdeveloped or 'traditional' state. This has extremely important implications for the planning and allocation of health resources and manpower training to meet future needs (Colbourne 1976a,b; Joseph and Phillips 1984; Phillips 1981a).

Epidemiological transition: general aspects

The changing patterns of morbidity (illness) and mortality (causes of death) with modernization can also be placed in a perhaps deceptively simple but surprisingly consistent epidemiological transition model that parallels the demographic and technological transitions (Omran 1971, 1977). Epidemiological transition likewise assumes or implies a range of changes: in attitudes, education, diet, aspirations, urbanization, public health, and health care and its technology. Basically, it is proposed that societies during modernization will move from a period of high birth and death rates and low life expectancy (perhaps 40 years expectancy of life at birth or even lower) to a stable period when life expectancy will have increased to around 70 years or longer, and death rates and birth rates will have become much lower, often approximately balancing each other numerically.

During the early stages of epidemiological transition, infectious, parasitic and nutritional diseases will be the cause of the vast bulk of morbidity and mortality. By contrast, in the more advanced societies, such conditions will be responsible for only a trivial amount of ill health and mortality, although conditions such as measles, chickenpox and the like, which mainly affect children, will often persist. Generally, only pneumonia and influenza will be a real danger, and then mainly to the older age groups. On the other hand, in the early stages of modernization, the essentially chronic degenerative conditions associated mainly with older adulthood such as heart diseases and cancers will be relatively unimportant, although long-standing conditions related to parasitism and malnutrition may be important causes of morbidity. In more modern societies, chronic degenerative conditions rapidly seem to become responsible for the majority of morbidity and mortality. These are often regarded as 'Western' diseases but they are becoming increasingly visible in many Third World countries (Hansluwka *et al.* 1986; Hutt and Burkitt 1986; Lopez 1989; McGlashan 1982; Picheral 1989; Trowell and Burkitt 1981).

Trowell and Burkitt (1981) use the term 'Western' diseases in discussing what some have called the 'diseases of civilization'. Most are of uncertain aetiology but many undoubtedly do have environmental associations and, possibly, causes. Man is the only creature who profoundly alters his own environment and many Western diseases may be 'man-made' or man-induced, in that they essentially reflect the technological changes that have followed the Industrial Revolution. The environment in many Third World countries has been altered rapidly over the past 30 to 50 years and it has been argued that the pattern of environment-related diseases has likewise altered quickly.

Trowell and Burkitt (1981) recognize that future research may prove that their pioneering work contains errors but, provisionally, they list over twenty types of Western diseases that may be identified as increasing in the Third World. Some may be dietary as the reversion to traditional diets has been associated with regression; others may be more related to stress and social environment and more influenced by the adoption of Western, urbanized lifestyles in Third World countries. The list includes many common conditions such as obesity, coronary heart disease, essential hypertension, diverticular disease and many forms of cancer.

Deaths or illness due to injury, accidents and violence tend to make up a small if important proportion of mortality and morbidity, and certainly lead to considerable loss of work and reduced quality of life. Unfortunately, accidents often happen to children and young adults, and frequently occur at higher rates in the less developed world than in developed countries as workplace safety, housing and road conditions are poorer. Epidemiological transition, it appears, can sometimes be advanced by the concerted application of modern medical knowledge. However, most changes seem to be related to much wider developments in living standards and ways of life, of which active medical care, preventive medicine and public health are but a part. Arguably, the eradication of smallpox is the sole example of complete, medically based eradication of an infectious disease (Strassburg 1982). Indeed, as noted in Chapter 1, the correlation between increased health and more health care is not always direct (Howe and Phillips 1983).

Omran's Epidemiologic Transition Theory and its variants

Omran (1971) has suggested five propositions on the Epidemiologic Transition Theory:

1. that the theory begins with the major premise that mortality decline is a fundamental factor in population dynamics;
2. that during the transition, a long-term shift in mortality and disease patterns occurs, in which the chief causes of death become degenerative and man-made diseases, displacing pandemics of infection;
3. that during the transition, the most profound changes in health and disease patterns occur among children and young women;
4. shifts in health and disease patterns characterizing the transition are closely associated with demographic and socioeconomic transitions that are part and parcel of modernization;
5. distinctive variations in the pattern, pace, determinants and consequences of population change support three basic models of epidemiological transition.

The theory or model is obviously complex and subject to considerable spatial and temporal variation. Three main successive 'phases' can be identified in the transition, according to Omran: the age of pestilence and famine, the age of receding pandemics and the age of degenerative or man-made diseases. These may, of course, be vastly differentiated in their exact development and it seems that, today, some Third World countries are experiencing a combination of the second and third stages. This has major implications for their health care requirements and planning. In addition, at least three main categories of disease determinants influence the transition: ecobiological (disease agents, host resistance and environmental factors): socioeconomic, political and cultural (standards of living, health, hygiene and nutritional habits); and medical and public health determinants (emergence of preventive strategies and effective curative theories).

Interactions seem to occur among the epidemiological transition, demographic changes and socioeconomic changes. This is a complex area of research, and one in which it is very difficult to detect accurately cause and effect. The ways in which these interactions develop seem to produce at least three basic 'models' of the epidemiological transitions as suggested in Omran's (1971) fifth proposition. These are the classical or 'Western' model, the accelerated model and the delayed model. Examples of the Western model include most developed countries in Western Europe such as Britain, France and Germany. The accelerated model is to be seen in Japan and in many NICs such as Hong Kong and Singapore. The delayed model is perhaps the 'contemporary' model, relevant in many Third World countries today. These countries exhibit a slow, unsteady decline in mortality, often only evident in the last two decades, in which public health measures have been a major component, frequently involving internationally sponsored medical packages. It seems that these have often helped to reduce overall mortality but have left in some countries persistent high fertility and rendered many vulnerable to long- or short-term famine and sometimes to malnutrition. Sadly, there is evidence that mortality decline even from infectious diseases has begun to slow down and stabilize at higher national levels of mortality than anticipated. In parts of South and East Asia, Ruzicka and Hansluwka (1982) have noted that there should be scope for further reductions even under present technologies of disease prevention and treatment. Why this has not happened involves complex social differences, slowing of economic growth rates, changing population structures, the impact of health strategies, and the supply and distribution of food. No single factor can be isolated as the cause of persistent, apparently unexpected, high mortality in many Third World countries.

Important differences in the experience of epidemiological transition have become evident during the past few decades between the three main continents in which Third World countries are to be found: Africa, Asia and South America (see below). It seems that the differences are, if anything, even increasing. As early as 1971, Omran pointed to the utility of developing 'submodels' of the transition theory for different countries, particularly with respect to the varying responses of fertility and socioeconomic conditions to national development programmes. Today, the differential rates of emergence of 'Western' diseases and reduction of infectious conditions may also be added to submodels. In all, they make it difficult to generalize about Third World epidemiological transition today.

An equally clearly defined epidemiological transition to that in general health is also apparent in dental health, in which malignant and discrepant dental occlusal relations occur increasingly with urbanization and change in Western societies. In a cross-cultural survey, Corruccini (1984) noted that over three-quarters of people in groups classified as 'aboriginal' had a dental classification indicating ideal occlusion, whereas only some 42 per cent of industrialized peoples fell into this category. Put another way, it is suggested that only 3.5 per cent of persons in aboriginal populations would have severe malocclusion compared with 35 per cent of persons in industrialized populations. Corruccini suggests that this throws the weight of suspicion onto environmental rather than genetic aetiological factors. Evidence of the existence of this parallel dental epidemiological transition is, of course, of great significance in indicating the future need for dental health care facilities in modernizing Third World populations.

Two instances of epidemiological change

The difficulty of generalization about epidemiological transition is exacerbated by a lack of detailed case studies in Third World countries, in part a consequence of the paucity in quality and availability of data referred to earlier. It is possible to refer here to evidence for epidemiological transition in Hong Kong and Thailand. It may be noted that South-East and East Asian countries as a whole have generally experienced fast demographic transition, even overtaking European countries, where changes started much earlier (Leete 1987). It seems that they are likewise experiencing rapid and possibly more extensive epidemiological transitions, and comparative research on countries in East and South-East Asia will be important and may shed light on delayed transitions in the poorer developing regions (where, unfortunately, data are often less readily available).

Table 2.1 **Hong Kong: epidemiological change – percentage of all deaths from various causes (from Phillips 1988a, based on various official sources)**

Year	Percentage of all deaths					
	infectious and parasitic conditions (excluding pneumonias etc.)	Neoplasms	Heart disease	Cerebro-vascular diseases	Diseases of digestive system	Diseases of respiratory system
1951[a]	23.6	4.2	5.5		15.0	27.4
1961[a]	16.2	12.1	9.9	7.5	7.7	14.8
1970[a]	7.9	19.1	15.0	8.7	5.3	15.0
1975	4.0	24.2	15.6	11.0	4.6	15.8
1980	3.1	24.8	15.3	13.2	4.3	15.3
1985	3.1	29.4	16.5	11.8	4.2	16.4
1988	3.0	29.8	16.9	11.7	4.1	17.2

[a] Data regrouped according to different versions of International Classification of Diseases

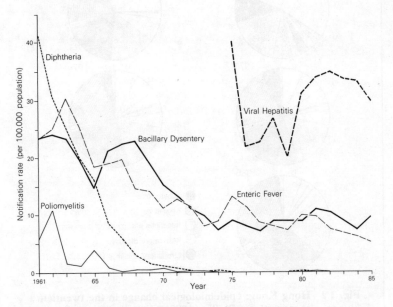

Fig. 2.1 **Hong Kong: notification rate of major infectious diseases, 1961 to 1985 (from Phillips 1988a)**

Hong Kong has, for practical purposes, experienced a very rapid epidemiological transition since the 1950s (Phillips 1987a, 1988a). In a period of less than 40 years, infectious diseases have moved from being responsible for almost one-quarter of mortality to barely 3 per cent, mortality from cancers has increased from 4 to 30 per cent, and deaths from heart and circulatory diseases now comprise a further 30 per cent, up from 5.5 per cent in 1951 (Table 2.1). Life expectancy has increased tremendously (for example, in the period 1971 to 1984 it increased from 68 to 73 years for males, and from 75 to 79 years for females). Virtually all infectious diseases

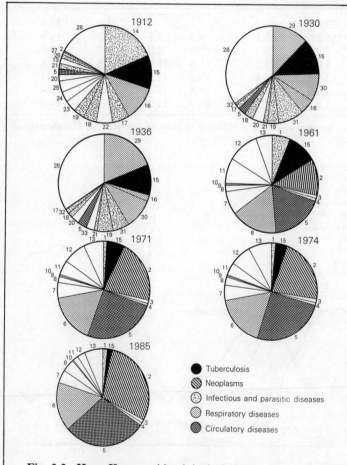

Fig. 2.2   Hong Kong: epidemiological change in the twentieth century (from Phillips 1988a)

have declined (Figs 2.1 and 2.2). Of infectious diseases typical of a Third World country, only tuberculosis might be said to remain and this is a threat only amongst older (mainly male) residents. Whilst it is difficult to draw general conclusions from a small, highly urbanized territory of fewer than six million persons, the Hong Kong evidence does show an impressive and very rapid epidemiological transition in only a few decades. Singapore, it seems, has followed a broadly similar pattern and speed.

Thailand, too, seems to be following a similar transition, although the effects are not so notable. Figure 2.3, whilst complex,

KEY
1 Infective and parasitic
2 Neoplasms
3 Endocrine, nutritional, metabolic, immunity disorders and blood
4 Nervous system, sense organs and mental disorders
5 Circulatory system
6 Respiratory system
7 Digestive system
8 Genito-urinary system
9 Complications of pregnancy, childbirth and puerperium
10 Skin, subcutaneous tissue, musculo-skeletal system and connective tissues
11 Congenital anomalies and certain conditions originating in the perinatal period
12 Symptoms, signs and ill-defined conditions
13 Injury and poisoning
14 Plague
15 Tuberculosis
16 Pneumonia
17 Smallpox
18 Malaria
19 Diarrhoea
20 Beri Beri
21 Dysentery
22 Paralysis and convulsions
23 Development diseases
24 Old age
25 Unknown
26 Syphilis
27 Typhoid
28 Other causes
29 Broncho-pneumonia
30 Bronchitis
31 Infantile diarrhoea
32 Enteric, Diphtheria, Cerebro-spinal fever
33 Nephritis

Note: Nos. 1–13 relate mainly to the period from 1961 onward
Nos. 14–33 relate mainly to the earlier period
No. 15 (tuberculosis) is common to both

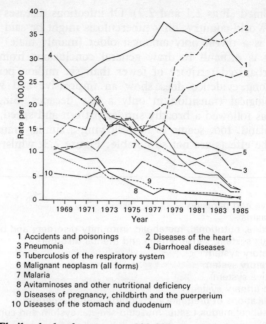

Fig. 2.3   Thailand: death rates per 100 000 population for major causes of death, 1968 to 1985 (from Institute for Population and Social Research 1988)

shows the decline in the crude death rate for most infectious diseases such as tuberculosis and diarrhoeal diseases, and a marked increase in mortality from heart disease and cancer (Institute for Population and Social Research 1988; Porapakkham and Prasartkul 1986). Of course, it might be argued that changing age structures underlie these changes, and this is in part true although, in both case studies, age-adjusted rates indicate the importance of mortality (and associated morbidity) from non-infectious Western diseases. However, whilst early gains were made in the battle against tuberculosis in Thailand between 1969 and the mid-1970s, subsequent declines have not been as great and neither has there been consistent success against malaria, indicating the difficulty of eradication in a large rural population (Fig. 2.4). This emphasizes the differences between a large Third World country and a small, rapidly developed territory such as Hong Kong. In Thailand, there has been a gradual linear increase for many apparently non-infectious diseases during the period 1970 to 1983, with circulatory and ischaemic heart disease showing a rapid rate of increase but from relatively low base levels (Fig. 2.5). It is, of course, important to note the initial level of any given disease in the community when comparing relative changes over time.

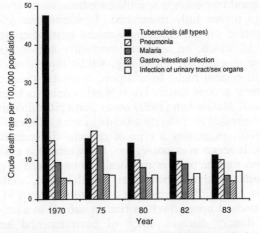

Fig. 2.4 **Thailand: crude death rates per 100 000 population from infectious diseases, 1970 to 1983 (based on data from Porapakkham and Prasartkul 1986)**

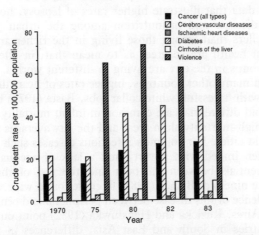

Fig. 2.5 **Thailand: crude death rates per 100 000 population from non-infectious diseases and violence, 1970 to 1983 (based on data from Porapakkham and Prasartkul 1986)**

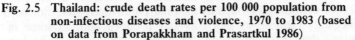

Different epidemiological experiences within countries?

In the previous chapter, reference was made to the fact that there are well-recognized urban–rural differences in health and access to health care within countries. This has important implications for epidemiological transition in specific countries, many of which have been by no means fully researched. It seems that many Third World countries are experiencing a mixed form of epidemioligical transition, in which, on average, morbidity and mortality from degenerative diseases are increasing, whilst those from infectious diseases still remain high. In addition, however, these conditions afflict different groups within Third World countries to greater and lesser extents. McGlashan (1982) notes that epidemiological transition had progressed to different extents in ten Caribbean islands by the late 1970s, suggesting a type of regional differentiation in its occurrence. It seems reasonable, too, to assume that epidemiological transition may be progressing locally at one speed in rural areas and at another within urban areas. Furthermore, well-to-do urbanites may be rapidly developing a Western pattern of mortality whilst the poorest urban dwellers remain subject to a host of infectious and dietary diseases. Lack of environmental health, bad nutrition, low wages and urban squalor mean that many infectious diseases are still a danger to the urban poor.

Evidence for intra-urban socioeconomic differentials in health and health care is abundant. Harpham *et al.* (1985), for example, summarize data that illustrate higher rates of leprosy, hookworm, diarrhoeal diseases and malnutrition among the urban poor and shanty dwellers than among those living in the richer areas. Differentials in health are so great as to mean that, in effect, these different groups in the city are living in different worlds. In Hong Kong, as in many other countries, higher rates of heart disease are associated with 'stressful' white-collar jobs. Basta (1977) illustrates that threefold differentials are common in infant mortality rates between the high-mortality slum areas and the city averages for many Third World cities. For common infectious diseases such as tuberculosis, often linked with poverty and a lack of adequate health care, differentials between the poor and the rest of the city of Manila were ninefold. Bianco (1983) likewise found wide variations in the incidence of this disease between peripheral and central areas of Buenos Aires. Ruzicka and Hansluwka (1982) point out that, in many countries in South and East Asia, differences in mortality levels of various subgroups in national populations have not been appreciably reduced as mortality has declined and, in some instances, they have increased. Disadvantaged groups have benefited far less than the more advantaged segments of population from any progress in disease and mortality control.

It has also usually been assumed that Third World urban health levels are better than the rural (Akin *et al.* 1985). Basic sanitation, health facilities, education and cash-employment opportunities are, it is felt, more likely to be available in most urban areas than in rural areas, where they may be totally unavailable.

However, when aggregate urban–rural data are considered, it may be that city health statistics appear better than rural ones only because either the urban poor do not feature in official statistics or, alternatively, their inclusion along with data for the much richer areas and inhabitants results in a very misleading average for the city's health. A disaggregated picture is likely to show that the urban poor are often in reality in a worse state in terms of nutrition and health than the rural poor. This may particularly be the case in socially less-organized urban areas, where the family support and food that might be available in many villages are non-existent. A considerable and often under-researched problem for poor city dwellers has become the provision of sufficient food for themselves and their children (Pryer and Crook 1988). Crowding, lack of basic sanitation and unclean water may also be the norm for many of the urban poor, particularly in many African and South Asian cities, which puts them at great risk from infections. Therefore, intra-urban differentials in health need to be accurately established for most Third World cities before data can be realistically compared with those for rural areas. At present, statistics illustrating urban–rural differences in health, as in the UN demographic yearbooks, for example, should be used with caution as urban figures in particular may represent a misleadingly optimistic 'city average'.

Epidemiological transition is therefore apparently a concept that needs to be applied with caution in many Third World countries. Only perhaps in the NICs, where health services are on the whole more uniformly available and data more reliable, can the concept be used with much confidence for present and future health care planning. This does not wholly invalidate it, however. The underlying trends of the transition must be recognized but, just because Western diseases are emerging, the infectious scourges cannot be ignored.

Epidemiological change: international patterns

In spite of such warnings, it is possible to outline the general transition over recent decades and to note varying speeds and types. Pyle (1979) provides one of the more succinct accounts of international changes in causes of mortality. Taking the four years 1947, 1956, 1965 and 1974, leading causes of death were extracted from UN demographic yearbooks covering four different revisions of the International Classification of Diseases. An increasing number of countries provided mortality data at each period although Indian data were not available until 1965 and data for China and the Soviet Union were missing from the reports. The data were subjected to factor analysis, a technique that shows up groupings of related diseases at each period in the data set. Given that there were more Western nations reporting at earlier periods and gradually increasing numbers of developing countries, and that no allowance is made for population size or density in the various countries, Pyle's analysis still provides a very interesting picture of disease pattern changes at the international scale.

Various groupings and spatial patternings of diseases appeared at each period. In 1947, clusters indicating a prevalence of chronic and degenerative diseases such as heart disease, cancer and stroke (which were statistically associated) were mainly to be seen in North Western Europe, North America, Australia and Argentina. By contrast, associated clusters of measles, malaria, bronchitis, diarrhoea, typhoid and avitaminosis tended to focus on the developing nations in Africa, Latin America and, at the time, Iberia. By 1956, the chronic–degenerative disease cluster had grown to include diabetes; rheumatic heart disease, influenza, whooping cough and smallpox formed a looser cluster affecting a range of nations. Again, the infectious and deficiency disease cluster was associated mainly with tropical and subtropical nations. Iberia had moved into an intermediate position, experiencing a mixture of chronic and degenerative and also infectious and parasitic conditions.

By 1965, the cancer, stroke, major heart diseases and diabetes cluster was joined by hypertensive diseases, nephritis, syphilis and cirrhosis. Pyle (1979) detects a strong link between levels of economic development and such disease distributions. However, by 1974, associations were less easily discernible. Some technical matters relating to deficient reporting and changing disease classifications may in part explain this, but there is also the possibility of the stronger emergence of Western diseases in many developing countries. It was clear that Third World countries still scored the highest for incidence of infectious and parasitic conditions, but the chronic and degenerative group showed some changes. Parts of Latin America, Southern Africa and South-East Asia had moved into the medium range on this factor; along with North America and Australia, certain areas of Eastern Central Europe and notably Iberia had moved into the highest category. Other high incidence of the degenerative group remained in North-West Europe; Japan and New Zealand were also above average. However, some countries of southern Latin America such as Chile and Uruguay were scoring relatively less highly than in 1965, although their scores on infectious and parasitic conditions still appeared among the highest groups. They seemed therefore to be developing a very mixed epidemiological distribution, which has probably continued to today.

Epidemiological transition therefore seems well illustrated at a world scale in Pyle's (1979) research. For more recent periods, it is interesting to compare the mortality patterns of different regions. It seems that there remain substantial regional variations in health status and epidemiological profiles. At the broadest level, East Asia and the Americas have about 20 more years of life expectancy than tropical Africa and 10 years more than Northern Africa and South Asia (Knowles 1980). Significant variations in the major causes of mortality have been emerging among regions of the Third World and, importantly, as noted earlier, areally within countries and between groups in them.

Using WHO mortality data for developed areas and an estimate for developing areas, mortality attributable to major causes of death around 1980 has been compared for the different regions of the world (Hakulinen *et al.* 1986). Interesting trends emerge from an examination of Fig. 2.6. Whilst infectious and parasitic diseases are pre-eminent in Africa and South Asia, this is less marked in Latin America and, indeed, diseases of the circulatory system are the most important single group cause of mortality in East Asia. Overall, infectious and parasitic diseases claim one-third of all deaths in the world, and four in ten of deaths in developing countries. Perhaps surprisingly, mortality due to injury and poisoning is almost

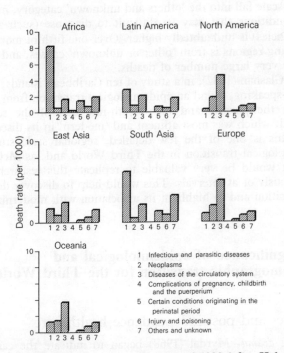

Fig. 2.6 **Mortality profiles by region, around 1980 (after Hakulinen *et al.* 1986)**

independent of the level of development of the region. More importantly, however, it seems that, although diseases of the circulatory system and neoplasms are the two most important causes of death in the developed countries, more than 50 per cent of all deaths due to these causes actually occur in developing countries. This indicates that 'Western' diseases are now well established in many non-Western countries. This fact is of the utmost importance in epidemiological terms and for health care planning and provision. Indeed, if variations in age structure are taken into account, it is possible that the relative incidence of many types of cancers is as high in developing countries as in the developed world (Howe 1986; Parkin 1986). With the increasing ageing and longevity of populations, this has profound implications for future needs for health care provision in many Third World countries.

In spite of the progress of epidemiological transition, infectious and parasitic conditions still comprise the most common group of causes of deaths in the world. However, about one-quarter of all deaths occur from diseases of the circulatory system. Neoplasms, certain conditions originating in the perinatal period, and injury and poisoning each account for an estimated 5 to 8 per cent of deaths in the world. However, since almost one-fifth of deaths at a world scale fall into the 'others and unknown' category, mortality from conditions that may be difficult to diagnose (such as some malignancies) is undoubtedly higher. Over one-fifth of mortality in developing regions is from 'other or unknown' causes, and this involves a very large number of deaths.

McGlashan (1982), in a study of ten Caribbean islands, all now English-speaking, found an epidemiological transition from St Vincent, at the poverty and high death-rate end of the scale, to Trinidad, which was most affluent and 'modern' in its disease pattern. This is one of the few detailed, regional scale studies of epidemiological transition in the Third World and, as McGlashan notes, it would be very valuable to replicate this research either continuously or at intervals. This would help to discover details of the transition and to highlight its association with modernization.

Significance of epidemiological and demographic transition for the Third World

Pre- and post-independence health care

In *Asian drama*, Myrdal (1968) began to indicate the early significance of epidemiological change in many of today's Third World countries and particularly to pre- and post-independence health. Early impacts of modern health care were often limited. For example, the first European doctors to work in South and South-East Asia and much of Africa were too few in number to cater for any but colonial and military personnel, other Europeans and a very limited number of native persons in the upper social strata. Some very rudimentary forms of 'Western' medicine of the times did filter down to workers and their families, in recognition of the relationship between work and efficiency and in the hope that the locals with whom Europeans might have daily contact would be relatively well. However, for most people, health remained as poor as it had been in pre-colonial days. Missionary medicine did touch a small proportion of local people in many African and Asian countries and, in them, colonial governments also often began to train native assistants in Western medicine. Some also went abroad to study, but numbers of doctors trained were few and standards often low and, on return, most remained in the main centres. Towards the end of the colonial era in Asia, only Malaya, Ceylon and the Philippines had any hospital network to speak of and auxiliary personnel were also very scarce. In much of Asia, the number of doctors and hospital facilities per capita was negligible (Myrdal 1968).

However, for the countries of Latin America, the majority of which have a 150-year history of independence, the foregoing discussion does not easily explain the current distribution of health resources, but it can, to an extent, help to point up the significance of the demographic and epidemiological transitions for these countries. It may be necessary to look to the dependency theorists or Marxist schools of thought for some explanation of how the health systems remained essentially insufficient even in these independent countries and how curative medicine rather than social improvements was as prevalent (and restricted) in them as in many colonized countries. Their poverty and exploitation during the nineteenth and early twentieth centuries arguably placed them in a position little better than the contemporaneously colonized lands to develop their own infrastructure and housing along 'modern' lines. For the majority of their citizens, modern care and facilities did not exist any more than they did for local residents in colonies.

Whether it is thought that access to 'modern' medicine in colonial countries was rationed and restricted as a means of social control of the masses (Banerji 1979; Sanders 1985; Turshen 1984), or expanded mainly as a means of legitimizing the colonial state and creating and maintaining the basis of reproduction of labour power in colonial economies (Leng 1982; Manderson 1987), it has generally been accepted that 'public health services' as understood today were relatively poorly developed in most such countries in the nineteenth and early twentieth centuries. 'Modern' medicine had begun to be developed along systematic and scientific lines in Europe from the eighteenth century, even if detailed understanding of (infectious) disease transmission was still some time away. However, the argument is generally that, initially, medical care in colonies was provided for the colonial élite, those in their direct employment and for labour involved in export industries.

In Europe and North America, as the nineteenth century progressed, Western medicine became increasingly concerned with preventing illness, and this is highly significant in the Western epidemiological and demographic transitions (McKeown 1965, 1976). However, indigenous medicine in the colonized lands, to which most local people had to have recourse, did not generally develop along the same lines. Many colonial regimes can also be criticized for their lack of investment in health infrastructure other than curative facilities, but it is evident that some regimes did have considerable interest in the health of their people. They were, of course, limited by the knowledge of the time, by the tiny numbers involved in technical and social aspects of disseminating health information and by miserable budgets. In Hong Kong, for example, many governors and prominent officials in the nineteenth and early twentieth centuries pressed for the upgrading of sanitation, housing and education as well as of health facilities, but financial support from London was minimal (Phillips 1988a). Most colonies therefore had to rely on meagre revenues gathered themselves. It seems that here and in many other cases there were genuine humanitarian as well as economic and other motivations. Some improvements may be noted with regard to infectious diseases such as smallpox, for which vaccinations were introduced early in the nineteenth century in many Asian countries, and also plague and cholera, against which some measures were taken in the nineteenth and early twentieth centuries, in a number of countries.

Towards the end of the colonial era (pre- and post-war), rudimentary maternal and child welfare campaigns had been initiated in many colonial countries but, on the whole, most efforts remained curative and, by force of circumstances, were reactive mainly to dangerous infectious diseases. The 50 years preceding the independence of many African and Asian countries saw the First World War, the Great Depression and the Second World War, and anti-colonial and internal struggles up to the last in many countries. Therefore, not only were funds for wider social and preventive improvements severely limited but arguably the conditions for much concerted effort over the timespan required were not auspicious. Rural areas tended to receive even less formal health care than urban areas. In addition, the beginnings of rapid urban growth were evident in many countries, with attendant problems in housing, facilities and employment.

However, the pre-independence distribution of health facilities has often been perpetuated after independence. For example, in Kano State, Nigeria, there was very little health care provision in colonial times except for Europeans and some urban-dwelling Africans. Stock (1985, 1986) reports that many spatial and class disparities that characterized colonial health care have remained: Kano has 10 per cent of the state population but 85 per cent of the medical doctors (see Chapter 4). The lack of rural medical services and distortions in health-sector spending favouring hospitals perpetuate the underdevelopment of rural health. High mortality and morbidity continue, especially in rural areas. In other countries, regional variations in the supply of hospital beds, physicians and other health care provisions are often as wide as or wider than inter-country differences (Akhtar and Learmonth 1986; Akhtar 1987; Diesfeld and Hecklau 1978; Myrdal 1968). Severe rural–urban differentials in provision and accessibility are often typical (Chapter 4).

Demographic transition really only became significant in the post-independence era in South Asian and many other Third World countries (Myrdal 1968). Technical and other interventions in health were to become of great significance in reducing mortality but the infrastructure has been insufficient to keep pace with population growth and epidemiological change. However, it is even more evident in the late 1980s than it was in 1968 that efforts to prevent and cure disease, and to improve quality of life, will increasingly require reforms in the fields of nutrition, sanitation, hygiene, housing and education as well as in the supply of physicians, paramedical staff and health care facilities. Medical technology without major inputs in these and other fields will provide isolated and, probably, faltering, attacks on ill health.

In the post-independence era (in the early days of Third World-hood), many countries started out with seriously inadequate or poor quality health facilities. Myrdal (1968) documents the poor situation in many South Asian countries in terms of measurable health provision in the early 1950s and mid-1960s; in terms of the often non-quantifiable aspects of sanitation, hygiene and housing, matters were probably even more serious. With an inadequate supply of health personnel and health facilities, and lacking many of the much wider social and physical environmental improvements applied in the West, the nascent Third World was set to face rapid demographic and epidemiological transitions relatively unprepared. Populations were about to increase very rapidly; survivorship and dependency rates were to grow both in youth and old age, and many different health care needs were to emerge. Curative health services were going to continue to be important, but preventive services were to gain new significance. The problems of young children and mothers were gradually to change and many Third World populations were to face an expanding, ageing population.

Almost entirely novel health concerns were, and are, yet to emerge, such as the needs of ageing Third World populations for geriatric care (UN 1986b). Whilst they may not be directly health care concerns, the changing demands of chronic ailments and ageing bodies will present enormous challenges to many countries in the provision of social care. They cannot be dealt with simply by institutional or personnel provision; they require societal involvement, care in the community and the involvement of families in social care that is, sadly, often being lost. Hellen (1981, 1983), for example, considers the long-term implications of epidemiological transition for public policy and developmental planning in Egypt and Nepal. He highlights data paucities and the need for increased recognition of the phenomenon by high government levels, as the populations of both countries are increasing by some 2.5 per cent annually and dependency rates are increasing with accompanying epidemiological changes. Because of the speed and scale of such changes, the challenge presented is almost entirely novel in most developing countries; the solution will prove to be very difficult and may be impossible.

How many worlds for health?

The Third World is often thought of as rather uniform in terms of health and health care. However, this is manifestly not so, as evidence presented so far emphasizes. In statistical terms, the morbidity and mortality in cities such as Hong Kong, Singapore and Seoul are at much lower levels and from different causes from those in, say, Calcutta, Lagos, Manila and Lima. Many countries of Latin America, East and South-East Asia (apart from the NICs) are in positions intermediate between the extremes of Third World countries. Qualitatively and quantitatively, health care provision is generally if not inevitably of a much higher standard in the NICs, and becomes of lower standard, the poorer the country. There is also as a general rule an increasing discrepancy between health care in urban and rural areas and between the élites and poorest, the poorer the country considered.

In terms of both demographic and epidemiological statistics, what is thought of as the Third World is manifestly comprised of many different 'worlds' – groups of similar countries, perhaps, or different people or regions within individual countries. Although just under one-third of the world's population lives in South Asia, almost 40 per cent of all deaths occur there, with relatively high crude annual death rates of about 15 per 1 000. By contrast, East Asia has almost half this crude rate (7.5 per 1 000) and Latin America 8.8 per 1 000, whilst Africa has a yet higher rate at 18 per 1 000 (rates in individual countries within these regions vary, of course). Indeed, in part because of the populations' age structures, East Asia and Latin America have crude death rates similar to, or even lower than, those of Europe, North America and Oceania. However, because of the population totals involved, only about 5 per cent of the world's deaths annually are from the more developed countries.

The diversity within the Third World is illustrated in Table 2.2. If the very roughest indicator is used, the difference between 'less developed' and 'least developed' countries on crude death rates, the former have death rates of some 12.1 per 1 000 compared with the latter's 17.1 per 1 000. Death rates in the 'least developed' countries are over 40 per cent higher than in the somewhat more developed Third World. Around 1980, total actual numbers of deaths per annum in the least developed countries alone were running at approximately three times the number of deaths in the 'developed' world.

When morbidity is considered (as opposed to mortality), data become even more difficult to obtain, particularly for many of the poorest countries. Inferences may be drawn regarding the incidence of, say, various cancers in different parts of the developing world from works such as those by Howe (1986) and Parkin (1986). Obviously, such statistics depend heavily on diagnostic and treatment efficiency. Howe (1977), McGlashan and Blunden (1983), Trowell and Burkitt (1981) and the UN (1986a, b) provide important information on global incidence and specific country incidence of many types of morbidity and mortality. However, paucity of reliable data on national morbidity is a major confounding feature of much research, and renders detailed cross-national comparisons of Third World countries almost impossible. At present, most researchers are reduced to making 'guesstimates' like those noted earlier for the global burden of conditions such as malaria and tuberculosis.

Demographically, the Third World displays even less homogeneity than it does epidemiologically. What is perhaps the most basic indicator, expectation of life at birth, varies in the examples chosen in Table 2.2 from around 45 years for Mali citizens to 76 years in Hong Kong. Many of the example countries (selected to show the range of 'worlds') still have expectations of life in the 45- to 59-year range. Relatively few countries have expectations in the high 60s except for the NICs and some such as Costa Rica and

Table 2.2 How many worlds in health? Health-related indicators in selected countries ranked by U5MR (from UNICEF 1989)

	Population growth rate (%)		Crude rates[a]		Total fertility rate[b]	Contraceptive prevalence (%)[c]	U5MR[d]		Infant mortality[e]		Life expectancy (yrs)[f]		% Adults literate[g] M/F	Polio Immunization (% 1-year-olds)
	1965–80	1980–86	Death 1960/87	Birth 1960/87	1987	1981–85	1960	1987	1960	1987	1960	1987	1985	1981/1986–87
Very high U5MR (>170)														
Mali	2.1	2.3	29/31	50/50	6.7	1	370	296	210	170	35	45	23/11	–/8
Malawi	2.9	3.2	28/20	53/53	7.0	1	364	267	206	151	38	48	52/31	68/50
Nepal	2.4	2.6	26/15	46/40	5.8	15	297	200	186	129	38	52	39/12	1/40
Bangladesh	2.7	2.6	22/16	47/42	5.4	25	262	191	156	120	40	52	43/22	1/8
Nigeria	2.5	3.3	24/16	52/50	6.9	5	318	177	190	106	40	51	54/31	24/21
High U5MR (95–170)														
India	2.3	2.2	21/11	42/32	4.2	34	282	152	165	100	44	59	57/29	7/50
Indonesia	2.3	2.2	23/11	44/28	3.1	40	235	120	139	85	41	57	83/65	–/70
Guatemala	2.8	2.9	20/9	49/41	5.6	25	230	103	125	60	46	63	63/47	42/18
Botswana	3.5	3.5	20/12	52/48	6.1	29	174	95	119	68	46	59	73/69	71/88
Middle U5MR (31–94)														
Brazil	2.4	2.2	13/8	43/29	3.3	65	160	87	116	64	55	65	79/76	90/99
Philippines	2.9	2.5	15/8	46/33	4.2	33	135	75	80	46	46	64	86/85	44/73
China	2.2	1.2	19/7	37/20	2.3	74	202	45	150	33	47	70	82/56	–/77
Low U5MR (<30)														
Jamaica	1.5	1.5	10/6	39/26	2.7	52	88	23	62	18	63	74	–/–	37/82
Costa Rica	2.6	2.4	10/4	47/28	3.2	68	121	23	84	18	62	75	94/93	85/89
United Kingdom	0.2	0.1	12/12	17/13	1.8	83	27	11	23	9	71	76	–/–	71/85
Hong Kong	2.1	1.2	7/6	35/16	1.7	73	65	10	44	8	65	76	95/81	94/86

Nations are listed in descending order of their 1987 U5MR. Data may not be given for precisely the same years in all countries

a Annual number of births or deaths per 1 000 population
b Number of children born to a woman in all her fertile years
c Percentage of married women aged 15 to 44 years using contraception
d Annual number of deaths of children under 5 per 1 000 live births
e Annual number of deaths of infants under 1 per 1 000 live births
f Years of expectation of life of newborn children
g Percentage of persons aged 15 and over who can read and write

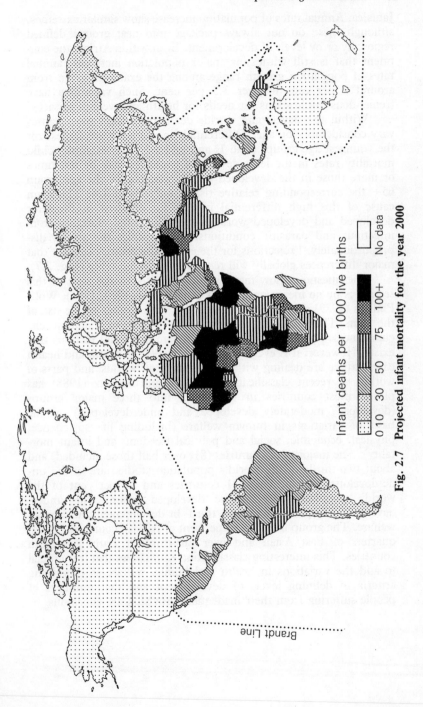

Fig. 2.7 Projected infant mortality for the year 2000

Infant deaths per 1000 live births

☐ No data

■ 100+

75

50

30

☐ 0 10

Jamaica. Annual rates of population increase show similar extremes, although these do not always package into neat groups defined regionally or by levels of development. Even within Africa, the continent that is still witnessing major population increases, annual rates of population growth range among the examples given from around 2 per cent to over 3.5 per cent. Such variations have tremendous implications for needs for health and welfare services.

Within the developing world, death rates from most causes vary considerably by age. Differentials in mortality are largest for the youngest age groups (0 to 1, and under 5). For example, child mortality rates in the least developed countries may be ten times or more those in the developed world, whereas for the age group 65+ the corresponding relative risk is only about 1.4. The main cause of this high differential in risk for children in the least developed and developed world is the differential mortality from infectious and parasitic conditions, which afflict the young disproportionately. Projections for the end of the century suggest that major differences globally will remain in child mortality (Fig. 2.7).

The question, 'how many worlds?', raised at the start of this section is by no means original. Worsley (1964, 1979, 1984), Wolf-Phillips (1979) and others have posed it with respect to the use of the term 'Third World', in view of the variety of economic circumstances, political alignments, non-alignments and factions that exists. However, it is even clearer with respect to health and health care that we are dealing with a wide range of 'worlds' and parts of worlds. A recent classification by Tata and Schultz (1988) has placed most countries in the world into three major groups (developed, moderately developed and underdeveloped) on the basis of variations in human welfare (including life sustenance; physical, economic, social and political freedom; and infant mortality). The majority of countries (81, over half those included) and about two-thirds of the world's population studied are in the underdeveloped group. Only 21 countries and 14 per cent of the world's population are in the developed group. The underdeveloped group clearly comes 'third' in development and human welfare. The group includes 93 per cent of African countries, three-quarters of East Asian and over one-third of Latin American countries. This interesting classification emphasizes that it is crucial to add the variations in health and human welfare as classifying criteria in defining levels of development and that numbers of people suffering from their inadequate provision are enormous.

Chapter 3

Traditional and modern health care in the Third World

In addition to the many differences in economic development, population, cultural, ethnic and other characteristics, the nature of Third World health care systems is also highly differentiated. Some countries are more reliant on private care or self-help; others have tried to adopt truly comprehensive public systems. This chapter discusses the nature of health care in the Third World (its sources; its traditional, modern and informal sectors; and the like). In Chapters 4 and 5, the organization, delivery and distributional systems are considered in more detail. In organization terms, as we shall see in Chapter 4, most countries in theory follow a broadly similar pattern. The government, through its Ministry of Health (MOH), usually provides a publicly funded network of institutions, in general based on a pyramidal hierarchy, for both administration and facilities (see Fig. 4.1). In this, there are usually a number of urban-based major hospitals, a tier of smaller regional or district hospitals, a layer of rural health centres providing a more or less full range of modern services and, finally, a subcentre network of health posts (variously termed), often manned by volunteers or peripatetic professionals and ancillary workers. However, in reality, the private sector is often left to provide much care in an uncoordinated manner.

The hierarchy described above tends to provide the official support or input for public health care and planning. Care and services may be via 'top-down', vertical programmes, or may involve greater focus on grass-roots, community-level activities, sometimes referred to as 'horizontal' programmes. However, whichever strategy or combination of strategies is adopted in organizational terms, often the full service and support system does not exist in practice or it is seriously short of resources, buildings, personnel, equipment or medicines. It is also crucial to recognize that the nature of health care resources is often varied and extends beyond formal, Western-type care. However, whilst generally short of resources, systems are rarely short of patients and potential patients, and in many cases the sheer weight of numbers threatens to overwhelm public provision. This is often particularly true in the poorest and intermediate countries. Public health care systems in many African, Latin American and South Asian countries are often so overburdened as to provide less than the minimum of realistic care. Table 3.1 shows the great variation in ratio of population to trained personnel, and in expenditure on health. Whilst simple correlations are misleading, it is evident that pressure on personnel and expenditure is highest in the countries with highest under-5 mortality rates. It must also be remembered that distributional inequalities can greatly exacerbate some of these pressures on services, particularly in certain districts.

Modern or Western-oriented health care systems may be supplemented by other important modern-sector sources of care (traditional sources are discussed below). One is the social security system based on facilities or institutions, usually hospitals, serving government or privately enrolled workers who are entitled to use them (this is generally a very small proportion of the population in most Third World countries). Akin *et al.* (1985) suggest that health care facilities ostensibly provided for the military and armed forces can also sometimes be a source of public health care. This may be of major importance in war zones, and in countries with military regimes where the high numbers in the military may have access to care for their relatives and dependants. Indeed, in some countries, military facilities may account for a large proportion of hospital beds and doctors; in Iran and Iraq, for example, such facilities had high priority through the 1980s. Likewise, in regimes such as Mozambique in the mid to late 1980s, the disruption of life caused by the poor security situation has meant that virtually the only health facilities with any supplies at all are related to the armed forces. In some countries, or at certain times, the use of military or military-provided health facilities may become quite widespread, especially in times of emergency.

There is also often a significant charitable, religious or international aid agency 'sector' of health facilities in many countries. Strictly speaking, these agencies may sometimes be supplementing with money, personnel or resources other existing facilities but, particularly in the case of religious organizations, they often provide their own facilities. These generally offer free care or care at nominal cost for needy groups. The problem is that they do not as a rule provide systematic coverage, although in certain countries or parts of countries or at times of crisis, such facilities – almost invariably externally funded – can provide significant proportions of care. It is not easy to identify the overall contribution of charitable-religious provision, especially in the health-related sector, but in some countries it may be very considerable. In Malawi, for ex-

Table 3.1 Resources for health and other indicators in selected countries ranked by U5MR (based on data from UNICEF 1989 and other sources)

	% Government expenditure on health[a] 1986	% of total household consumption on medical care[b] 1980s	Population per Physician 1965	Physician 1981	Nursing person 1965	Nursing person 1981	% Births attended by trained personnel 1983–1987	% Urban population 1965	% Urban population 1985
Very high U5MR (>170)									
Mali	1.7	1	55 510	26 030	3 360	2 280	27	13	20
Malawi	6.9	3	46 890	52 830	–	2 980	59	5	–
Nepal	5.0	–	46 180	28 780	–	33 390	10	4	7
Bangladesh	5.3	–	8 400	9 690	–	19 370	–	6	18
Nigeria	–	3	29 530	9 400	6 160	2 690	–	15	30
High U5MR (95–170)									
India	2.1	3	4 880	3 700	6 500	4 670	33	19	25
Indonesia	1.9	2	31 740	12 330	9 500	2 300	43	16	25
Guatemala	–	13	3 690	–	8 250	1 360	19	34	41
Botswana	5.0	4	27 460	7 400	17 720	700	52	4	20
Middle U5MR (31–94)									
Brazil	6.4	6	2 500	1 300	1 550	1 140	73	50	73
Philippines	6.0	4	–	6 850	1 130	2 640	–	32	39
China	–	–	3 790	1 730	3 050	1 670	–	18	22
Low U5MR (<30)									
Jamaica	6.7	3	1 990	2 830	340	550	89	38	53
Costa Rica	19.3	7	2 010	1 440	630	–	93	38	45
United Kingdom	12.6	8	870	680	200	120	98	87	92
Hong Kong	9.3	6	2 460	1 290	1 220	790	–	89	93

[a] Data are not strictly comparable because of variations in the importance of private-sector health care
[b] Expenditure on medical care, private and public, relative to household consumption

ample, the organization Médecins Sans Frontières provides care for refugees in formal camps, which would otherwise place a huge burden on the thin public PHC network, especially in the south of the country. In Zambia (when Northern Rhodesia), missionary societies were responsible for almost all rural care (Henkel 1984), and in Zaire, in the mid-1970s, estimates suggest that mission groups provided up to 75 per cent of the country's rural modern health services and employed 30 per cent of the nation's health manpower. Mission hospitals in Ghana were estimated to account for 30 per cent of all hospital beds (Akin *et al.* 1985).

An important feature of charitable expenditure is that it may be strongly focused on specific sectors (such as MCH or curative services) or in specific areas (such as rural localities), particularly in some ex-colonial countries. Former colonial powers and religious–charitable organizations from such ex-colonial powers may also be of significance in health and many aid or development projects. This is particularly noticeable, for example, in many French West African countries, and in former British colonies, where the Overseas Development Administration may assist health care projects with capital or personnel costs (the wider role of aid in health care is discussed in Chapter 8).

In many countries, charitable–religious or general voluntary-sector provision may be more or less formally integrated into the modern national health care system. In Ghana and Malawi, for example, this occurs with mission hospitals. In Hong Kong, the voluntary sector is subvented by the government for most of its running costs and also for some capital costs. It has become integral to the overall health and social welfare system and today provides, for example, 38 per cent of hospital beds. It also provides important welfare and residential facilities for groups such as elderly, handicapped or indigent persons.

In spite of the activities of public and charitable organizations, the practical impact and coverage of free or publicly provided medical care tend to be very small in many poorer Third World countries. In almost all except for some socialist regimes, extensive if fragmented private-care networks have developed at all levels of the health care hierarchy. Often these are the only sources of care in systems where the public sector is very busy and lacks even basic facilities and supplies. The private sector, for example in Uganda, has frequently been the only source of medicines for patients in public hospitals. However, the effective coverage of qualified, modern-sector private practitioners is generally small, catering for the élite and middle classes. In many countries, private practice is permitted or tolerated for poorly paid professionals 'moonlighting' from the public sector. This is common in the Philippines and Jamaica, for example, and the supplementary income from private practice enables the public sector to retain employees it might otherwise lose.

Nature of modern facilities

The nature of the health care hierarchy in the modern, Western sector in most countries is that it generally incorporates (in theory, at least) the full range of facilities familiar to the developed world. Hospitals – general or specialized – with inpatient and outpatient provision exist, as do networks of clinics and surgeries usually linked by a national referral system. There are in reality important distinctions, however, between many developed and developing countries in the functioning of facilities. In practice, the referral system in the developing country's hierarchy will often be ignored and may only exist in theory. The nearest hospital with any form of outpatient or accident and emergency department may well be used for general consultations and PHC, regardless of its specialization. In a manner of speaking, health care delivery can become much more generalized, and medical personnel at all levels have to expect much greater variety of casework than would be anticipated in a hospital-oriented system in a developed country.

This may be illustrated by the use of emergency rooms (accident and emergency, or casualty, departments). Strictly, these should be used as their name implies, for accident and emergency cases. However, in many Third World countries (and, of course, increasingly in Britain, Europe and North America), such venues have become the settings for almost any types of medical consultations. They are frequently looked upon as a convenient 24-hour alternative to public or private primary care facilities (especially for out-of-hours care). People tend to have faith that they will receive some attention, and believe that diagnostic equipment or medicines are more likely to be available in the emergency departments than elsewhere. Such utilization behaviour results in long queues and waiting times, hinders attention to real emergencies and turns casualty departments into general outpatient clinics. Such usage is officially discouraged but perforce tolerated in numerous countries.

Complexity and diversity

One of the major features of formal, modern health care provision (and of more traditionally based services, also) in many Third World countries is that of complexity. Within the modern sector, often very basic, minimal public services, frequently provided by many levels of authorities, coexist with a wide range of private services. Mexico, for example, has both federal and state-level public services and facilities, aimed at different categories of its population (manual workers, government employees and the remainder of the population). In addition, numerous types of private facility exist, mainly urban-based, but offering choice for those who can afford them. In Malawi, both the MOH and local government provide PHC centres, the former offering some supervised care free of charge, the latter offering care by unsupervised paramedical workers but charging a relatively expensive fee for medicines. Which facility is used will depend on chance of location and accessibility. A very small sector of private care exists, although it is far too expensive for the vast bulk of the population in this poor country. In the somewhat wealthier countries such as the Philippines and Jamaica, however, fairly extensive public sectors coexist with large private sectors, as is the case in many other countries in South-East Asia and Latin America.

The private sector generally concentrates on lucrative curative health care or relatively inessential services such as cosmetic surgery, but the public sector is generally struggling to provide preventive and promotive health care as well as curative services in an inadequate infrastructure and with insufficient funds. The contrast is often striking between high-cost private clinics, in which the allegedly most modern treatments and drugs are available, and public wards and emergency departments, denuded of decoration and even blankets and bedding, and frequently lacking medicines. This is particularly evident in many of the lower-middle-income Third World countries (not the poorest) such as Jamaica, Mexico, the Philippines, Thailand and Brazil. In the private sector in Bangkok and Manila, clinics for specialist cosmetic surgery, orthopaedic and radiological treatment, and treatment of sexually transmitted diseases do a good 'trade' with paying clients. In some such cities, state-owned hospitals frequently run out of essential drugs and equipment, and function with underpaid medical and nursing staff who have to 'moonlight' in private practice to make a living.

Whilst systems grow increasingly complex, and the range of often inappropriate or marginally required private clinics multiplies, the formal linkages between the public and private sectors often dwindle or are non-existent. In Manila, for example, the public sector nominally buys space in plush private hospitals in the business district of Makati, but such capacity is strictly limited and available only to a fortunate few public-sector patients. Perhaps one of the major drawbacks of these mixed systems, in which resources are very unevenly spread, is that those who can afford to pay can be exposed to far too many investigative procedures and expensive and sometimes unnecessary treatments. By contrast, the poorest citizens who cannot pay but who need modern medicine have to rely on a denuded and minimal public sector; alternatively, or in addition, a wide range of self-treatment and traditional sources may be used. In these circumstances, promotive, preventive and also curative medical care are very difficult to implement and, in any case, care is often attempted in isolation from social and physical environmental improvements that might be of greater underlying significance to health (see Chapter 5).

It has been recognized for some time, and is becoming increasingly apparent, that it is impossible to separate the nature of health care systems from the societies that they seek to serve (Hours 1986). They are created within specific social, cultural and economic structures, and, even if the health care is 'imposed' externally, it has to adapt to local expectations, beliefs and norms if it is to have any popular relevance. It is increasingly acknowledged that certain modern scientific medical treatments may not only be economically and physically inaccessible to the bulk of Third World populations but, moreover, frequently be considered unnecessary or inappropriate by them.

Nevertheless, when choice between therapies is presented, there is still evidence to show that the decision to use, say, Western medicine is inhibited not so much by unscientific attitudes but rather by the political and economic factors that limit its effectiveness and by the availability of alternatives. This is a crucial recognition: Lasker (1981), for example, illustrates that, in the Ivory Coast, the choice of therapy depends more on accessibility (particularly in terms of time) than on the characteristics of the individual patient. This is of relevance when unequal access to various types of modern care is discussed in Chapter 4 and utilization of care examined in Chapter 6. The physical provision of modern care (in particular), often economically or politically influenced, will be a crucial determinant of utilization.

Resources for health in Third World systems

Pluralistic health care systems, discussed in more detail below, are common in many Third World countries, although they are by no means confined to the developing world. The resources for care and sources tapped are often very wide, which contrasts with the legal and cultural tendency this century in the developed world for health care to be sought largely from formalized, biomedical outlets. The resources may be conceptualized as an *ethnomedical system*, which encompasses the total medical resources that are available to, and might be utilized by, a community and society, including its biomedical and traditional forms of therapy (although many definitions of ethnomedicine itself focus only on the latter type).

The acquired knowledge, resources (formal and informal), organization, behaviour and strategies (traditional and scientific; indigenous and imported) that a community or society utilizes for individual or collective well-being comprise an ethnomedical system in its broadest sense. Good (1978a), following Kleinman (1980), regards an ethnomedical system as incorporating the full complement of health care strategies acceptable to some or all members of a community, including biomedicine, traditional medicine and self-help. Good explains that an ethnomedical system evolves from a people's view of the world and life; it incorporates theories and accepted explanations of the nature and causes of illness and the appropriate and expected remedies. It is therefore very much influenced by social and cultural factors, and interpersonal relations.

An ethnomedical system may be summarized as comprising three main spheres, although the relative weight of each will vary from culture to culture and also over time (Fig. 3.1). The *popular* sphere of health care is generally the first to be encountered in all cultures; it comprises a range of more or less knowledgeable sources, including the 'lay referral system', in which individuals, family or others believed to be authoritative are approached before more formal sources (Freidson 1970). Kleinman (1980) has suggested that as many as 70 to 90 per cent of all illness episodes even in the United States are managed within the popular sector; the

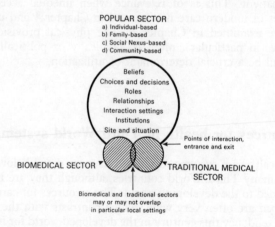

Fig. 3.1   **An ethnomedical system (after Good 1987a)**

figure is certainly as great or greater in most Third World countries, although in some circumstances the division between the popular sphere and traditional sphere as sources of help may be somewhat blurred. The other two spheres, the *biomedical* sector and the *traditional* medical sector, may be more or less discrete entities, with greater or lesser contact, overlap, interdependence or even congruence (as in the case of China, discussed later). For example, Simpson (1983) considers that, in Costa Rica, popular, traditional medicine is basically separate from scientific medicine but there are overlaps in certain specific areas involving some practitioners and illnesses (Fig. 3.2). In general, it seems that licensed practitioners of orthodox scientific medicine do not participate in the traditional system but that certain peripheral, ancillary workers such as nursing aides or pharmacists may do so. This example illustrates that there may be variations in cooperation between the two sectors depending upon the professional levels under consideration.

Good (1987a) summarizes an ethnomedical system as encompassing folk knowledge and beliefs; traditions, symbols and values related to health, illness and disease; a society's causal theories and taxonomies of sickness; supportive social institutions (groups,

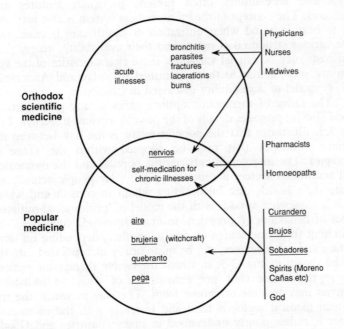

Fig. 3.2 Overlaps between orthodox scientific and popular medicine (from Simpson 1983)

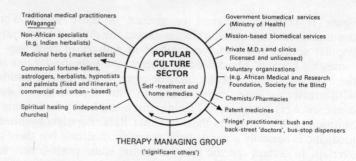

Fig. 3.3   The range of therapeutic options in many Third World countries (from Good 1987a)

families, dispensaries, hospitals); recognized specialists (traditional and modern; professional and paramedical); and the spatial arrangement and interaction between the various physical settings in which various phases and elements of illness and therapy are diagnosed, evaluated and administered. This provides a usefully broad conceptualization of the components of a health care system. The spatial arrangements and interactions, in particular, appear to be important in Third World settings because transport, information flows and accessibility often present particular features and problems. The concept of the ethnomedical system is also very useful to bear in mind when utilization of health care is examined. The various structural elements and their availability, accessibility and costs may be crucial variables; these characteristics of the system are very similar to those identified by Aday and Andersen's (1974) model of accessibility discussed in Chapter 6.

The range of therapeutic options varies in any given setting; Good (1987a) provides details of the possible options in Kenya. Figure 3.3. illustrates that the popular sector is the link between the various strategies that may be adopted within the range of therapies. The interaction between the popular and the biomedical and traditional sectors is crucial; typically, lay people actually activate their health care by deciding whom to consult and when. This is somewhat at odds with the model of 'professional-initiated' types of behaviour so prevalent in most developed countries. The switching from one source of care to another, depending on satisfaction and other factors, can be quite neatly incorporated into the model shown in Fig. 3.3, in which the twelve therapeutic options are representative (but not exhaustive) of what an individual Kenyan may be able to choose from. The way in which the traditional medical sector is used and interacts with the biomedical sector is rather poorly understood in many countries and Good's research provides important conceptual and empirical insights into this complex issue.

Good's (1987a) study suggests that traditional medicine is a significant resource of health care throughout Kenya and this is apparently so in most other Third World countries. In spite of the fact that many people questioned may underplay or deny any association with traditional medicine (having to an extent been conditioned to believe in Western medicine or to conceal use of traditional medicine), about one-quarter of respondents in a survey of users of modern facilities in Nairobi claimed to have consulted a traditional healer at some time (the real figure is probably higher). About one-third reported the personal use of herbal remedies. Two-thirds knew of traditional practitioners working in their home area. The attitudes to traditional practitioners of even the users of modern facilities were positive and only 28 per cent said they should not be licensed (Good 1987a).

Traditional medicine

The maldistribution of health care personnel and resources between areas of many Third World countries, and particularly between urban and rural parts, is well documented and is discussed in Chapter 4, although it has generally been studied almost exclusively in terms of modern or Western-type facilities and personnel (for which some official data usually exist). However, this sector may be of limited relevance in terms of availability, costs or cultural acceptability to many residents, particularly but not exclusively those in rural areas. The paucity of Western-style medical personnel, exacerbated by their maldistribution and frequently unaffordable charges, especially in the poorer Third World, is counterbalanced to some degree by the existence of traditional medical practitioners. It is estimated that these are the basic providers of health care in various guises for as many as 80 to 90 per cent of the rural population in countries in South Asia and Africa, and some writers suggest that pre-scientific medicine covers 80 per cent or more of all African populations (Koumaré 1983) and that pre-scientific medicines of various sorts involve directly or indirectly 80 per cent of the world's population (Scarpa 1981). Therefore, this chapter now focuses on these important sources of care.

Cultural, social and psychological acceptance of health systems other than the modern scientific has been long established and recognized in the majority of Third World countries. In many countries, particularly in Africa and Asia, prior to European settlement or contact, traditional medicine, intertwined with magic and religion, was important in influencing the conduct of public and private affairs. It also acted curatively (Ulin 1980; Ulin and Segall 1980). Today, such 'social control' elements and influences of traditional medicine persist, but the practical medical aspects of traditional medicine (of various sorts) are increasingly being acknowledged. Now that there are growing numbers of indigenously raised and trained doctors of Western medicine, the European (and particularly missionary) misunderstanding, scepticism, and even fear, of many aspects of traditional medical practices are fading. The time is ripe in many nations for fuller collaboration of modern with traditional medical sectors, although there are often considerable obstacles to overcome.

Traditional medicine exists in various forms and under a range of names; the term 'indigenous medicine' has often been applied as an alternative to scientific, cosmopolitan medicine (biomedicine), and the wider term 'alternative medicine' is increasingly in use (Cai 1987; Patel 1987). Other terms include ethnomedicine, folk medicine, fringe, pre-scientific and culture-bound systems. There is some confusion, for the terms do not necessarily mean identical things, and neither are they exclusively to be applied in the Third World. Aspects of their utility are increasingly being recognized internationally but we should also remember that, historically, various forms of alternative medicine were (and are) in general use in countries of today's developed world (Bhardwaj 1980).

Virtually every human community has responded to the challenge of restoration and maintenance of health (broadly speaking) by developing a 'medical system': this may be thought of as 'the pattern of social institutions and cultural traditions that evolves from deliberate behaviour to enhance health' (Dunn 1976: 135). Research has revealed much about the nature and form of such medical systems, which have ranged considerably in formality and coverage. The study of these systems has emerged in the discipline of 'ethnomedicine', which involves the study of beliefs and practices stemming from indigenous cultural development, rather than being explicitly derived from modern medicine (Yoder 1982).

Ethnomedical systems, as discussed earlier, may nevertheless be more broadly defined to encompass the total medical resources available to, and utilized by, a community or society. Fabrega (1977) sees ethnomedicine as being the study of medical institutions and the ways in which human groups handle disease and illness in the light of their cultural perspectives. Some writers expand the term 'ethnomedicine' to include contemporary allopathic medicine (Foster 1983). This can lead to some confusion but, nevertheless, certain key features of any system, such as its extent, legal basis and incorporation into formal health provision, may be analysed. In this context, it is useful to bear in mind the biomedical distinction between 'disease', which relates to bodily dysfunction, and 'illness', the individual experience of disease. Modern biomedicine tends to focus principally on disease, whilst ethnomedicine is often felt to be broader, to a greater or lesser extent focusing on the illness in its social, cultural and familial settings, sometimes seeking explanations and cures far beyond the immediate 'disease' itself (Neumann and Lauro 1982); it may be said to be more 'holistic'. However, as discussed below, this image may not be wholly accurate, particularly in large settlements where traditional medicine may be as impersonal as modern medicine!

Medical pluralism

The existence and use of a wide range of sources of medical care, traditional and modern, static and evolving, are generally known as 'medical pluralism'. This may take the form of pluralism in the coexistence of multiple systems of medicine (traditional, modern and 'folk'), giving multiple choices to individuals, or it may mean pluralism within a particular system, allowing access to various levels and types of care (Minocha 1980). The significance of medical pluralism for many Third World countries, especially the poorer ones, is that, whilst virtually all governments wish to bring modern health care to their populations, the means and resources for this often do not exist. The recurrent and capital costs of expanding modern health care are enormous and exploding; many African countries, for example, face economic and political disruptions that severely curtail their attempts to expand modern health care. By contrast, the influence of traditional medicine is extensive in virtually every African country (Good 1987a), and in other continents. After self-treatment, traditional medicine is generally the main provider of health care, especially to the rural poor.

In Swaziland, for example, over 5 000 traditional medical practitioners (TMPs) provide a TMP to population ratio of 1:120, and at least 85 per cent of the population is thought to utilize their services. In Malawi, in the late 1980s, there were fewer than 150 qualified doctors for the population of almost eight million, a ratio of well over 50 000 persons per doctor, compared with some 5 000 TMPs (a ratio of about 1:1 600). Therefore, 'medical pluralism' inevitably exists, although it varies regionally. Traditional medicine and TMPs may intuitively be felt to cater mainly for rural dwellers, but they also have considerable, sometimes overlooked, influence on the lives of town dwellers, as indicated by Good (1987a), Maclean (1971) and others. Traditional medicine may be particularly important to the urban poor (Ramesh and Hyma 1981) and those living peripherally, many of whom are new arrivals, the semi-urban peasant class as they have been called in Mexico. However, many socioeconomic groups, and not only the poor, may make use of traditional health providers, often concurrently or in association with modern services. Traditional and modern facilities therefore coexist, often complementarily but sometimes in conflict.

An example of medical pluralism with multiple health systems has been recognized in Sri Lanka for over a century but to some extent it was made legally explicit only in the 1980s. The health care system is highly diversified and pluralistic (Nordstrom 1988). The most basic analysis points to at least three main sources. Cosmopolitan medicine is provided free by government-run hospitals and dispensaries, and for payment by private practitioners. There are several forms of indigenous medicine, divided into the professionalized (university-trained), and traditional non-professionalized, a distinction corresponding roughly with Ayurveda and Sinhala medicine. Ayurvedic medicine has in Sri Lanka come to imply the dispensing of herbal and allopathic medicines (although strictly the latter may be used only by modern physicians). Sinhala medicine provides the majority of traditional medicine on the island, usually dispensing only herbal remedies. There are also other treatments such as acupuncture and homoeopathy growing in use but mainly in urban areas. In addition, a number of ritual and religious healing traditions supplement health care services – exorcistic specialists, Buddhist priests, lay priests, astrologers and fortune-tellers. These divisions are to some extent stereotypes of the Sri Lankan system but they are readily recognized by the general population and those analysing the system. The patient population, however, realizes that there are actually a number of different forms of medical practice *within* each of the major healing traditions; moreover, many practitioners, regardless of training, offer a combination of treatments and the lines of classification among them are blurred (Nordstrom 1988).

Medical pluralism clearly exists in many developing countries and it is increasingly recognized in the developed world, especially in North America, where alternative medicine is often supplementary or complementary to, or actually a substitute for, modern clinical medicine. Leslie's (1976) book *Asian medical systems* showed the existence of multiple interacting traditions and that therapies based on the classic humoral texts are still widely practised. It seems that such revitalized learned traditions can coexist with cosmopolitan medicine, homoeopathy, folk traditions, possession cults and so on (Pfleiderer 1988). Equally importantly, however, the acknowledgement of medical pluralism by researchers, governments and providers may mean that modern Western medicine need not automatically or uncritically be regarded as the norm and local beliefs need not be seen as an impediment to improved health care.

There is nevertheless a continued difficulty in many countries in obtaining information on traditional medicine, as data are scarce and not systematically recorded. This is often compounded by an official negativism, sometimes the result of attitudes inherited from colonial times and imbued in Western-trained doctors. As Turshen (1984) discusses, traditional medicine was historically frequently suppressed at the instigation of Christian missionaries, sometimes on the basis of misunderstanding or fear, and, in countries such as Tanganyika and others, this deprived a growing number of Africans converted to Christianity of a store of traditional medical knowledge and a source of self-reliance. Today, some governments continue to regard traditional medicine as backward, non-modern, and as not fitting in with competitive, especially capitalistic, societies. Such values continue to emphasize the expansion of costly, hospital-based, doctor-dependent, almost inevitably urban-biased health care systems, beyond the economic and physical reach of many Third World people, rural or urban. Good (1987a) adequately illustrates this in the case of Kenya.

Types of traditional medicine

The blurred nature of the boundaries between modern and traditional medicine and within each of these groupings themselves has already been noted, but some general categorizations of indigenous practitioners have nevertheless been derived. Neumann and Lauro (1982) identify four main types:

1. Spiritual or magico-religious healers;
2. herbalists;
3. technical specialists such as bone-setters;
4. traditional birth attendants (TBAs).

The first group, *spiritual or magico-religious healers*, is the most wide-ranging and includes the most respected healers and witch doctors but also many fringe or charlatan practitioners. This group has received considerable anthropological, sociological and medical attention. The inseparability of traditional medicine from religious and moral cultures, noted by Good (1987a) and others, was clearly identified in the classic writings of anthropologists such as Evans-Pritchard (1937) based on extensive fieldwork in the Sudan, and, later, by the work of physicians based on years of observation and research whilst working in colonial countries such as Rhodesia and Nyasaland (see, for example, Gelfand 1964). More recently, the connections between 'primitive religion' and healing have been documented in detailed fieldwork in Bahia, Brazil, by Williams (1979). In this study, the emergence of the local religion and the Indian, African and European influences on it and on subsequent healing practices and rituals are explained. In certain circumstances, for example in Thailand, traditional beliefs and practices may sometimes be fused with the most serviceable and appropriate features of Western medicine as in the 'doctor monk' (*Maw Phra*) schemes using Buddhist priests with a basic medical training (Gosling 1985).

Herbalists, as the name implies, focus on the use of medicinal plants and formulations; knowledge is sometimes passed from healer to apprentice, whilst, at other times, it is more formalized, being set down in herbal formularies. Much recent interest has focused on the evaluation of the chemotherapeutic efficiency of herbs and, as noted in Chapter 7, considerable research is being conducted in many countries into the nature and potency of herbally-derived medicines. *Bone-setters*, similarly, have a technical, albeit limited, focus to their work. In some societies, they bear resemblance to practitioners of physical medicine or chiropractic; some bone-setters historically have derived their skills from religious training or following physical exercise or involvement in the martial arts. Certainly, skilled bone-setters may be well known locally as sources of help after accidental injuries.

Traditional birth attendants who are predominantly female, assist mothers at childbirth. A TBA will generally have acquired her skills by delivering babies herself or by working with other TBAs. They are almost ubiquitous in Third World countries and many early hopes of involving traditional practitioners with modern health care revolved around them (Pillsbury 1982). Today, training programmes for 'upgrading' TBAs, teaching literacy, aseptic technique and recording of basic demographic and vital information are frequently the major manifestations of community participation in PHC. Traditional birth attendants have many different names nationally and locally, for example, *hilot* (Philippines); *dai* (India); *dukun bayi* (Indonesia); and *partera* or *comadrona* (various Latin American countries) (Cosminsky 1983). Virtually every society provides some system for dealing with the practical and emotional issues of childbirth and this usually includes patterned sets of beliefs and practices concerning pregnancy, delivery and the puerperium.

Over two-thirds of births in the world are delivered by local or traditional midwives or birth attendants who are not trained in formal, Western medicine. Often they are locally recognized as possessing important skills and knowledge relating to childbirth and children. Sometimes, however, they may merely be older female family members or friends who assist in the delivery and who are not generally recognized in the community as 'birth attendants'. In some settings, particularly rural, they may be responsible for 90 per cent of all deliveries (see Chapter 7). The term 'traditional birth attendant' suggests a rather narrow range of functions related only to the delivery itself but many TBAs (who are predominantly females) provide a wide variety of care and advice relating to the period before and after the birth. The preferred term is therefore sometimes 'traditional midwife', although this can provide a spurious air of reliability and knowledge.

Traditional midwives are typically middle-aged or elderly women, who practise as a part-time occupation. Their own experience of childbirth and their skills are usually locally recognized and respected. Western-trained midwives, by contrast, are often younger, sometimes with a nursing background, often single and childless and not local. Their supervisory role over TBAs can, of course, be a natural source of conflict and needs careful diplomatic handling. The TBAs will often be held in high esteem locally (although this varies), be well known and speak the local language or dialect. However, they may be accorded relatively low status by hospital personnel and those formally trained in Western medicine. Such attitudes have therefore to be carefully managed; they have created obstacles in some experimental cooperative programmes (Cosminsky 1983).

There have probably been more Third World health projects and programmes that have incorporated TBAs (indigenous midwives) than have involved other types of traditional healers – perhaps as many as twenty times more, although this has not been accurately quantified. Many have been relatively localized and small-scale projects, but Pillsbury (1982) has noted some 44 countries in which traditional midwives had been given formal training by the early 1980s and utilized as service providers in modern-sector projects. The WHO and other organizations have clearly identified TBAs as major resources in the attempt to extend PHC as a whole (and MCH in particular) to populations, especially in rural and poorer areas. As a result, numerous training programmes have been started to 'upgrade' the skills of traditional midwives, and introduce them to safe and sterile delivery practices, vaccination requirements and vital data recording. Their roles have therefore often been more widely interpreted than purely midwifery, and have incorporated family health, FP and preventive medicine.

Traditional midwives are therefore often regarded as a means of speedily introducing some family health care to large numbers of people, relatively cheaply. Success may be measured in the reduction of infant and maternal mortality and this has certainly been achieved in many countries. In the Philippines, traditional midwives have been involved in health care for about 30 years. More recently, they have been working directly with modern nurses and midwives in the locally based, *barangay* PHC programme (Phillips 1986a).

However, some programmes have been less successful than they might have been because of a lack of knowledge of the actual skills and beliefs of the traditional midwives. The illiteracy of many TBAs has also sometimes been a problem in training and data collection. A useful study of TBA training and utilization in seven countries shows how programmes have been established in six countries and planned in the seventh (Mangay-Maglacas and Pizurki 1981). The Philippines, for example, is the first country to have carried out a national survey of TBAs as a resource. In the 1970s, it appeared that there were some 31 000, a ratio of one TBA to every 200 women in the reproductive age group 15 to 44 years. In sheer numerical terms, TBAs therefore provide a major source of potential personnel for family health care.

It should also be noted that mothers themselves can become resources for community health development. They can help, for example, in the identification and treatment of common health problems such as diarrhoeal illnesses among children, and show that these ailments can be prevented or effectively treated. Bender and Cantlay (1983) cite a Bolivian example in which programmes for training one or two mothers locally in each community in basic curative, preventive and helping skills have been grafted on to existing mothers' clubs. The *colaboradoras* can subsequently help to transfer their knowledge to other mothers in the community. Similarly, 'model mothers' have been used in some Thai villages to encourage adoption of FP methods. 'Model mothers' are themselves selected and trained on the basis of being of child-bearing age, intelligent and locally respected, but having only two children. They may be able to encourage other women in their locality to use contraceptive methods to limit family size (Sirikulchayanonta 1989). Recent findings indicate that 'model mothers' may significantly increase the uptake and continuance of FP methods (see also Chapter 7).

Social attitudes to traditional medicine

Traditional views of causes of illness: influence on health care acceptability

To an extent, the differences among the four main categories of TMPs arise out of varying representations of 'causes' of illness, and Foster (1983) suggests at least seven within ethnomedical research.

These include angry deities who punish wrongdoers; sorcerers and witches working for hire or personal reasons; spirit possession or the intrusion of an object into the body; and the 'evil eye'. These are sometimes referred to as magical or supernatural causes, although Foster prefers the term 'personalistic', as the aggression or punishment is directed against a single person as a consequence of the will and power of a human or supernatural agent.

By contrast, explanations of illnesses may be in terms of natural causes – naturalistic. For example, the intrusion of heat or cold into the body may be believed to upset its basic equilibrium: the balance of humours (the *yin* and *yang* of Chinese medicine). This must be restored if the patient is to recover. To an extent, Foster (1983) considers that personalistic explanations are predominant in the traditional systems of Africa, pre-conquest America, Oceania and indigenous Siberia, although not to the exclusion of naturalistic explanations, which are predominant in humoral pathology, Ayurveda, Unani, traditional Chinese medicine, homoeopathy and naturopathy. The explanations of illness adhered to locally are of significance to health care delivery and utilization, in that they may well determine the mix of traditional medicine available and the propensity to use modern-sector services (if available) for specific conditions.

Stereotypes concerning traditional medicine

It is useful to be able to categorize traditional medicine, but it is also important to note that several stereotypes contrasting traditional and scientific medicine have emerged. These may actually hinder the incorporation of useful aspects of traditional medicine into modern health care systems because, whilst the stereotypes are not all negative, some are rather overoptimistic as to the reality of traditional medicine. Like most stereotypes, many have elements of accuracy but they tend to lack flexibility and depth of appreciation.

Stereotypes suggest first, for example, that traditional medicine is holistic, whilst modern medicine sees only the disease. This might be true in relatively isolated, small-scale societies, but in large Asian and African villages and towns, there is probably almost as much impersonal treatment by traditional healers as there is by practitioners of modern medicine. The holistic appeal of traditional medicine – that it considers the patient as a whole person, in his or her domestic and social setting – may in fact be perpetuating a false image.

Secondly, traditional healers may be stereotyped as old, highly respectable people, who may become valuable allies in PHC because of their status. Whilst this may again have an element of truth, research in Mexico suggests that health training for young, literate people is a more effective approach to providing practical care than working through established shamans. There may also be amoral elements to many traditional therapists (particularly those involved in personalistic explanation of disease), as they may actually cause illness through sorcery; they take no oath attributing primacy to the patient, or to use their powers for good.

A third stereotype suggests that traditional people dichotomize illness into two categories: 'folk' and physician-curable. This 'adversarial' model is used to explain or predict the choice that traditional people will make in seeking help. However, whilst it may have some validity in the years immediately following the introduction of modern medicine to traditional people, it appears soon to lose its easy predictive accuracy. Health care utilization is affected by a great many variables including costs, accessibility, preferences, confidence and the affective behaviour of the provider (see Chapter 6). No single simple model can really accurately predict behaviour, particularly in a crisis.

Finally, Foster (1983) identifies a stereotype that implies that modern physicians practising in traditional settings are frequently ignorant of traditional medicine, fail to understand it and have difficulties communicating with patients. He feels this is based again on the antagonistic mode of analysis and that, in reality, many modern physicians do understand and appreciate the aetiologies to which their patients subscribe. Indeed, with the advent of more locally trained health professionals, many may be personally familiar with indigenous beliefs. The doctor–patient communication problem is perhaps more apparent than real, although it does undoubtedly exist in modern as well as traditional settings. Much research shows that physicians find it hard to communicate with modern patients, so there should be little surprise if similar barriers occur occasionally between them and more traditionally oriented patients.

These stereotypes indicate that many assumptions regarding the potential role of traditional medicine in modern systems, and indeed assumed barriers to its incorporation, should be critically tested. Some optimistic overassessments of the real potential and value of traditional practitioners in modern systems may have been made but, likewise, unwarranted objections may also have been raised. Nevertheless, it must not be forgotten that some herbalists do not possess real skills or even local respect, and Learmonth (1988) is correct to note that traditional medicine, like Western medicine, has its iatrogenic casualties. Cases of blindness resulting from traditional remedies have been noted (McGlashan 1969; Queguiner 1981) and many unborn and newly born children have

suffered at the hands of unskilled or quack TBAs. It would be helpful if these facts were publicized locally so that people would be
specifically warned, to avoid the discrediting of all traditional medical practices by association and rumour. In this context, it is now
appropriate to outline briefly the various legal attitudes to traditional medicine and to discuss the government policy options
that have recently been identified.

Official attitudes to traditional medicine

Some legal aspects

Academic research findings and the encouragement of bodies such
as the WHO have been prompting the biomedical establishment
over the past decade to adopt a somewhat more open mind about
the contribution and potential efficacy of certain elements of
traditional-based systems in many countries. The attitude on the
part of the international medical establishment has in the past
tended toward the sceptical and, as Vuori (1982) suggests, many
health professionals and authorities believe, and would wish traditional medicine to be, 'dead as the dodo'. Nevertheless, far from
being extinct, traditional medicine seems to be alive and thriving.
Estimates suggest that it may be the principal if not the only source
of medical care for two-thirds of the world's population, and pre-
scientific medicines of various sorts are immensely widespread and
their use may involve about 80 per cent of the world's population.
Ramesh and Hyma (1981) suggest a similar percentage for the
coverage of traditional indigenous practitioners in Tamil Nadu,
India. In Nigeria, Chiwuzie *et al.* (1987) declare that TMPs are
'here to stay' and are the choice of the majority of the people for
reasons of culture, cost and availability. In spite of controversy
about treatments, over 70 per cent of Nigerians still consult
traditional healers.

Therefore, numerous examples support the contention that
traditional medicine is not only alive but thriving, although many
official health services have been reluctant to recognize this and
evaluate its contribution. The 'inescapable reality' that Western
medicine has little or no chance of becoming available in the
foreseeable future to many people, particularly in the poorer Third
World, is now forcing authorities to re-evaluate their own stances
on traditional medicine. This was encouraged after the mid-1970s,
when the WHO began to develop policy guidelines to assist Third
World countries wishing to conduct research, initiate pilot

programmes and subsequently implement training and treatment strategies in traditional medicine. Various technical booklets have been produced, including a handbook for administrators and planners that gives specific information about various traditional systems such as Ayurveda and Unani (WHO 1978b), and also an overview of traditional practices in WHO regions (Bannerman *et al.* 1983).

The concept of cooperation between modern and Western systems is attractive in general terms (Maclean and Bannerman 1982) and numerous limited experiments have been conducted, frequently with TBAs but often resisting the incorporation of other traditional healers into national health care systems (Pillsbury 1982). In addition, Chiwuzie *et al.* (1987) show that doctors, medical students and traditional healers all tend to favour cooperation and/or integration under certain conditions or for certain purposes (see Tables 3.2 and 3.3). However, few countries have actually taken formal, positive steps to reorganize their legal and organizational bases of health care delivery to incorporate traditional medicine completely. Nevertheless, Good (1987a, b), based on his analysis of the situation in Kenya and elsewhere in Africa, suggests that a formal policy

Table 3.2   Attitudes of doctors and medical students to integration of Western and traditional medicine, in Benin, Nigeria (after Chiwuzie *et al.* 1987)

Opinion	Doctors (%)	Medical students (%)
Integration favoured	20.7	27.3
Integration conditionally favoured	50.0	30.7
Integration not favoured	29.3	42.0

Table 3.3   Traditional healers' views on cooperation with Western-trained doctors in Benin, Nigeria (from Chiwuzie *et al.* 1987)

Types of cooperation favoured	Number of practitioners
In the same institutions	81
In separate institutions	31
In special institutions	26
In some fields, e.g. orthopaedics and psychiatry	23
None	14
Total	175

decision to pursue specific areas of collaboration could yield health benefits for both urban and rural populations. In some countries such as Nepal, traditional practitioners have been trained as tuberculosis and leprosy referral agents and have produced significant upgrading of health standards in the face of general lack of success in PHC. They have apparently helped improve attendance at rural health facilities because of their effective communication with rural dwellers, although improving attendance was felt likely to be their chief contribution to raising health standards (Oswald 1983). They were therefore, in this instance, bringing more people into contact with formal health services and increasing confidence in PHC rather than acting curatively themselves.

Categories of legal regulation of health care

Four broad categories of legal regulation of health care are recognizable (Stepan 1983: 292), which produce varying systems with respect to traditional medicine:

1. *Exclusive (monopolistic) systems*, where only the practice of modern, scientific medicine is recognized as lawful. Other forms of healing are excluded and sanctions taken, although enforcement varies from one country to another.
2. *Tolerant systems*, in which, whilst only activities based on scientific medicine are recognized, the practice of various forms of traditional medicine is legally tolerated, at least to some extent.
3. *Inclusive systems*, in which systems other than scientific medicine are regarded as legal, and their practitioners may practise their form of healing, in conformity with certain standards.
4. *Integrated systems*, in which there is official promotion of the integration of two or more systems within a single, recognized service. Integrated training of health practitioners is official policy.

Certain countries, notably but not only in the West, have developed monopolistic, *exclusive systems*. Often this is ostensibly to protect the public from unqualified practitioners but deeper analysis may suggest that the scientific medical hierarchy is powerful in lobbying to maintain its monopoly. These regulations were often reproduced in colonies of Western powers; for example, in the Belgian and French territories, regulations were generally based on a monopoly of modern scientific medicine practised by licensed professionals. In virtually all African countries, the state has control over medicine and divides its practice into authorized, legal, official, and unauthorized, illegal, unofficially tolerated or repressed (Fassin and Fassin 1988). However, the theory and practice of such legislation often do not coincide. Sometimes health laws expressly prohibit certain forms of healing (such as by supernatural powers), and may be broad, operating in the case of Honduras against naturopathy, homoeopathy, empiricism and certain other practices deemed to be 'harmful or useless'. However, in countries or regions in which expensive, modern medicine is inadequate and unable to satisfy even the most basic health needs, and where the people are imbued with a belief in traditional forms of healing, such prohibitions on traditional medicine are unrealistic. 'The dead letter of the law does not interfere with the daily practice of all sorts of traditional healers' (Stepan 1983: 295). Nevertheless, although perhaps unmolested, healers have no legal standing or official recognition. Such situations, however unsatisfactory, are widely accepted by governments in numerous Third World countries and the *de facto* toleration of many forms of indigenous healing is the case in many countries in the Middle East, Africa, Central and South America.

By contrast, *tolerant systems* also exist in some developed countries such as Germany and Britain, which do not prevent non-physicians from providing non-orthodox care, although the practice of modern medicine is of course strictly regulated and attempts to deceive the public into falsely thinking qualified medical care is being provided are unlawful. Similar tolerant systems are to be found elsewhere in developed countries and have been growing in the developing world. In the former, this is in line with extending individual freedom to choose therapies, and in the latter it is a practical recognition of the need to extend sources of care. Certain Latin American countries have a pattern of rather tolerant legislation and policies to some practitioners of traditional medicine, notably herbalists and TBAs. However, some African countries previously under French influence have been more cautious in movement towards liberalization of traditional medicine, although certain forms have been legalized in, for instance, Mali and Upper Volta (Burkina Faso).

In many former British colonies, where indirect rule via native hierarchies and minimal interference with local customs had been preferred, there has generally been a tolerant, liberal attitude to indigenous practitioners. Many are exempt from the general limitations on medical practice by non-professionals, although they were usually subject to certain restrictions on nomenclature and types of procedures permitted. In Hong Kong, for example, whilst still a formal colony, Chinese-style practitioners are tolerated but are prohibited from calling themselves 'doctor' and from undertaking certain types of operations, such as on the eye (Phillips 1984); they are also regarded as professionally unequal to Western-trained practitioners (Lee 1975). In Malaysia, the 1971 Medical Act allows a similar tolerance of traditional medicine to that found in Hong

Kong. Uganda has allowed the practice of any system of therapeutics, provided the person is trained and recognized by his community. Sierra Leone and Ghana have similar legislation dating from the 1960s and 1970s. Other countries such as Lesotho and Swaziland attempt to limit the practice of traditional medicine either to certain registered practitioners, or by placing restrictions on the performance of certain procedures. However, it should be noted that even 'tolerant' systems often have legislation prohibiting acts such as witchcraft in general or harmful witchcraft in particular (for example, Malawi, Tanzania and Uganda).

Inclusive systems attempt to regulate legally two or more health care systems that coexist. This is widespread in South Asia, where indigenous medical systems not only are tolerated but are actually part of the State-regulated structure of health care. Inclusive systems have generally evolved where the traditional systems have a long and popular history (indeed, much longer than that of scientific medicine), and they have formal medical traditions, literature, training and research. In the Ayurvedic system, for example, the organizers emphasize the necessity to combat charlatans. Since independence in India, considerable sums have been allocated to the development and teaching of traditional medicine, and a Central Council of Indian Medicine is responsible for the regulation and teaching of Ayurveda, Siddha and Unani (Stepan 1983). Although indigenous and cosmopolitan medicine are not formally integrated in India as they are in China, there is much *de facto* integration between the different sections of the Indian medical system (Leslie 1975). The situation is similar in Pakistan. Sri Lanka established a Department of Ayurveda within its Ministry of Health in 1961, and the importance attached by the Sri Lankan government to traditional medicine, particularly Ayurveda, is evident by the creation of a Ministry of Indigenous Medicine in 1980.

Integrated systems go a step beyond the 'inclusive' category, in which the modern and traditional are still formally, if not wholly functionally, separate. The policy of the WHO is generally to encourage some type of integration to optimize health care coverage, but Stepan (1983) suggests only China and Nepal have integrated their systems in any realistic sense. The earlier comments about the activities of traditional practitioners in Nepal imply they may have a relatively modest role at times, although Dhungel and Dias (1988) note both official encouragement for integration and fairly frequent co-use of modern and traditional facilities. It seems, too, that the Democratic People's Republic of Korea has, since 1980, enacted legislation to combine traditional therapeutic methods with modern diagnosis, including research and training in traditional medicine. Overall, however, integration is unlikely to be easily achieved (Bibeau 1985).

In general, it appears that increased involvement of traditional medicine in formal health provision creates new pressures for legitimation. As Fassin and Fassin (1988) note from Senegal, the healers who are the most inclined to search for official recognition tend to be those who have the weakest traditional legitimacy, and new sources of legitimation may be necessary. The interplay of power bases is complex and newer health-related groups often feel the need for official recognition under new sets of rules; secure traditional healers may not feel this need so acutely. Therefore, legislators seeking integration must ensure that effective elements and sectors of traditional medicine are included, but that uncertain or even dangerous practitioners are excluded.

Policy options

Only a few countries such as India and Sri Lanka seem to have taken serious steps to promote traditional medicine nationally on a large scale. China, of course, has progressed considerably towards integration. However, some countries are lagging in their promotion of traditional medicine and it seems that many still associate it with a stigma of backwardness or underdevelopment, rather than regarding aspects of indigenous medicine as a resource. Relatively little has been done in the majority either to review legislation or to create the legal framework for indigenous medicine to flourish. It is possible to relate the legislative typology above to the range of policy options open to planners, and four main options present themselves (Joseph and Phillips 1984; Kikhela *et al.* 1981).

1. *Making traditional medicine illegal* is an option pursued by some Third World countries within monopolistic (exclusive) systems. Algeria in 1976, Honduras and certain other countries have adopted this approach, although it may be regarded as a state of self-deception since people still customarily have recourse to traditional sources.

2. *Informal recognition*, the *laissez-faire* approach, may allow traditional medicine to exist, with regulation only intervening to prevent abuses or certain types of practices. Healers therefore have no formal protection or licensing, and the public has little real knowledge of their officially recognized skills. Tolerant systems such as those in Hong Kong, Singapore, Sierra Leone, Ghana, Lesotho and Malaysia adopt this attitude.

3. *Simple legislation* may be introduced to govern the practice of traditional medicine. Licensing announces who the healers are but,

as most people probably know this already, it does little to afford them any guarantee unless there are serious attempts to introduce some forms of qualifications and control of unlicensed practitioners. Much of South Asia does adopt this type of approach, with formal qualifications and recognition of many forms of traditional medicine. In practical terms elsewhere, however, neither qualifications nor controls are generally enforced. As with inclusive systems, this approach may be suitable for those types of traditional medicine that have established and formalized development and skills.

4. *Gradual cooperation with healers* is the option favoured by the WHO, which itself has a Unit of Traditional Medicine. It implies that research and evaluation will be undertaken and that thorough revision of laws will allow the proper incorporation of healers. This should enable healers to become professionalized but hopefully without losing any popular appeal. It does, however, demand attitudes of open-mindedness on the part of both modern and traditional practitioners, who must be prepared to cooperate and recognize each others' skills, albeit if in specialist areas. The integration needs to be in rural and urban areas, wherever systems coexist, so that traditional medicine is not relegated to rural locales and to peasant status. A useful principle is for healers with specialized skills to be encouraged to act as specialists. For instance, healers and TBAs have been found to be important in psychiatry in Senegal (Sène 1983), Mali (Coppo 1983) and elsewhere in Africa (Koumaré 1983). Nevertheless, it is generally recognized that most traditional practitioners will tend to be primary care, front-line health agents (Kikhela *et al.* 1981).

A model for integrating traditional and modern health care

Good (1987a) illustrates a type of integration that might be suitable for agrarian communities in countries such as Kenya (Fig. 3.4). His model suggests the need to emphasize community-based preventive and curative care within the social boundary of the community. It envisages that TMPs (probably well-regarded herbalists and midwives) will have been identified and selected in their communities, and be receiving training to assume a VHW role. When necessary, referrals may be made within a hierarchy via a health centre or dispensary (level C) to a district or mission hospital (level D). The A- and B-level villages and communities would be visited on a regular basis by a peripatetic health centre team, who would review, evaluate and reinforce the biomedical skills of the TMPs, consult

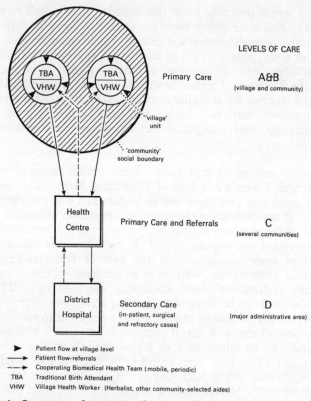

LEVELS OF CARE

Primary Care — A&B (village and community)

'village' unit

'community' social boundary

Health Centre — Primary Care and Referrals — C (several communities)

District Hospital — Secondary Care (in-patient, surgical and refractory cases) — D (major administrative area)

▶ Patient flow at village level
→ Patient flow-referrals
- - → Cooperating Biomedical Health Team (mobile, periodic)
TBA   Traditional Birth Attendant
VHW   Village Health Worker (Herbalist, other community-selected aides)

Fig. 3.4   Structure of a proposed cooperative health care system (from Good 1987a)

jointly with them on new and continuing local cases, and replenish their supplies of common drugs and medicines.

Locally adapted versions (Good's (1987a) emphasis) of this scheme should in certain circumstances help to expand access to a better quality of care, facilitate simple treatment and provide a continuous care even when the health centre team cannot be present. They would also make effective use of respected TMPs and TBAs, reduce costs and unnecessary travel to health centres, encourage communities to take greater initiatives in determining solutions to their own health needs and, hopefully, combine the best elements and eliminate the least desirable aspects of local traditional medicine. The avoidance of unnecessary visits to health centres is a valuable contribution of the local screening and referral aspect of the model, because dispensaries can be clogged by as many as 30 to 40 per cent of attendances involving community-preventable problems (Good 1987a).

Case studies of traditional and modern medicine

Malaysia

Malaysia's population of some seventeen million people is characterized by ethnic diversity: about half are Malays, one-third Chinese and 10 per cent Indians, and smaller percentages comprise Ibans, Kadazans, native aborigines (Orang Asli) and others. This is accompanied by a diversity in types of traditional medicine, each type reflecting the cultural characteristics of one of the ethnic groups. Heggenhougen (1980) and Chen (1981) identify at least three distinct groups of traditional medicine in addition to modern medicine, which has made considerable advances in Malaysia. These are, first, traditional 'native' medical systems, secondly, traditional Chinese medical systems and, thirdly, traditional Indian medical systems. It is instructive to consider each briefly as an illustration of the considerable medical pluralism within the alternative, traditional sector itself (which it is sometimes tempting to view as uniform). In addition, the movement of patients from one traditional system to another and to the modern sectors, and the overall incorporation of TBAs into health care, is interesting.

Traditional 'native' medicine in Malaysia is particularly diverse and no two systems are identical although they do share common features, such as the concept of illness as being both physical and supernatural. The Malay, Iban and Kadazan systems are identified by Chen (1981). In the Malay system, people's actions or avoidance of certain actions may be held responsible for many types of illness. The *bomoh* (traditional Malay medicine men) and *bidan kampung* (TBAs) have a number of therapies varying from minor and major rituals to use of drugs, mainly herbs, by the *bomoh*, and to traditional birth-delivery practices, and bone-setting. Traditional Iban medicine has similarities to the Malay medicine but, as the Iban are largely animists whilst the Malays are Muslims, there are differences. In particular, according to the Iban philosophy, ill health is not clearly distinguished from other forms of misfortune and all are quite often seen as the workings of *hantu* (evil spirits), who are to be found everywhere. As with other 'native' systems in Malaysia, there is a strong belief in *semangat* (soul-substance), which, on leaving the body, may be influenced by *hantu* or other evil powers.

The Iban approach to illness can be to drive away *hantu*, retrieve lost *semangat* and tend to the *ayu* (a secondary soul-substance). Whilst most will know how to deal with minor matters by offerings, the Iban make reference to a minor medicine man (the *dukun*) as a next step and, if this fails, a *manang* (shaman) will be called to perform effective rites. Sacrifices and offerings may be necessary.

The Kadazans of Sabah have a traditional medicine system similar to the others but with some unique features. Good and bad spirits are recognized, and various charms may be necessary to protect, for example, newly born babies from *rogon* (evil spirits that cause illness by stealing or abusing souls or by putting certain things such as worms into the body). The Kadazan have a belief in seven souls rather than one, located in various parts of the body. They also have a female traditional healer, a *bobolian*. In addition to rituals and sacrifices, the Kadazan use up to eighty plants as medicines.

Chinese medicine, like Ayurveda, is based on the understanding of balance of elements, with imbalance causing disease. Whilst there are specific approaches or schools of thought within Chinese medicine, it is felt that the two elemental forces *yin* and *yang* should be in harmonious balance. Traditional Chinese medicine in Malaysia follows the classic concepts and therapeutic practices, which can include use of herbal remedies, acupuncture and moxibustion, and its formulary monitors and may incorporate modern drugs. Many Malaysian Chinese are economically and educationally of higher socioeconomic background than the native Malays, and they view traditional Chinese medicine as complementary rather than antagonistic to modern medicine and move freely from one system to another. In this, attitudes are similar to those of many Singaporean and Hong Kong Chinese (Ho *et al.* 1984; Ho 1988; Lee 1980; Phillips 1984; Quah 1981).

In Malaysia, 4-year training courses are available in four schools of traditional Chinese medicine. Numerous herbs are used, some studies identifying over 400 in common use; medicinal teas are also very popular. Traditional medicines are dispensed by a variety of people, from roadside medicinal tea vendors to fully trained Chinese physicians who have completed the 4-year course. Some of these practise from Western-style offices, individually or in groups, or from traditional herbalists' shops. Many keep abreast of developments in acupuncture therapy in China and also dispense packaged standardized herbal remedies imported from China (see Chapter 7 on the use of traditional medicines). Traditional Chinese medicine in Malaysia has a long history of coexistence with modern medicine, and a hospital in Kuala Lumpur has both modern and traditionally trained doctors on its staff, although in different sections of the hospital. In addition, as in some other cities in the region, certain Malaysian physicians trained in modern medicine have included acupuncture in their range of skills, which is indicative of a generally broad-minded professional approach to pluralism (Chen 1981).

The third major group of traditional medical types in Malaysia incorporates a variety of systems originating in the Indian subcontinent. Although Chen (1981) notes that relatively little systematic research has been carried out locally on this sector, the Indian community certainly makes extensive use of various systems: Ayurveda, Siddha, Unani and homoeopathy (for definitions, see Bannerman *et al.* 1983; Ramesh and Hyma 1981). It seems that Ayurveda is perhaps the most common and, like the Chinese systems noted earlier, this postulates that a balance of elements maintains health, whilst imbalance causes disease.

Indian traditional medicines are imported into Malaysia from numerous manufacturing pharmacies in India and a wide range of Ayurvedic drugs is used (some may only be applied by certain healers). By contrast with the native traditional practitioners in Malaysia, the Ayurvedic practitioners and most other Indian practitioners have had formal, sometimes lengthy, training in colleges in India, in one of the over 100 institutions (many of which are affiliated to universities) awarding degrees in traditional medicine. Postgraduate training is also available, principally in Ayurvedic medicine. There is considerable scope for research into the use of traditional Indian medicine in Malaysia, for example, among Tamil workers on some rubber plantations who appear to be placing considerable reliance on traditional Indian medicine even though free modern medical services are provided (Chen 1981). This implies a strong cultural and psychological attachment to traditional medicine even though it has to be paid for.

Malaysia therefore presents a very interesting case study of medical pluralism in an ethnically diverse and rapidly modernizing society. It embraces two of the three great systems of traditional medicine (Arabic, Hindu (Ayurvedic) and Chinese), as well as an extensive network of varied types of 'native' medical systems (Kuang 1983). Indeed, as many as 20 000 *bomohs* minister to the health of Malaysians compared with fewer than 2 500 physicians (Vuori 1982), so many traditional practitioners are readily accessible. Nevertheless, modern-sector health care is also generally of an improving standard, with considerable attention being paid to the extension of PHC networks, especially in rural areas and rural service-centre settlements (Lee 1987).

In Malaysia, possibly four sets of forces influence the development, acceptance and integration of medical systems (Chen 1981): first, cultural and historical forces; secondly, political forces; thirdly, economic forces; and, fourthly, the influence of other systems. Here, we shall focus briefly on the first and third of these. Sick individuals appear to move easily from one system to another, and Chinese medicine, in particular, has been gaining strength. There are undoubtedly regional and urban–rural differences in both the nature of traditional medicine and the extent of modern medicine's availability but there has also been a certain amount of official support for traditional practices.

Cultural and historical factors are important in this multicultural land. Members of each cultural group may tend to adhere to their own systems of beliefs, but they still may have reference to other systems as well. However, the main cultural groups have some differing explanations of illness and ill health, so they generally seek cures in line with these explanations. In addition, the traditional medicine man may be very personally supportive and have time to devote locally to the patient by contrast with practitioners of modern medicine. Traditional medicine also provides the philosophical and ritual bases that, in the cultural perspective of each group, modern medicine lacks.

Economic forces, including the cost and accessibility of care, are particularly crucial in developing countries. Although government health services in Malaysia are relatively well developed, there remain transport difficulties and, in many rural areas, traditional medicine is still the only form of care easily accessible. This is an important factor in a large and relatively sparsely populated country (in Asian terms). Rural people may well be unwilling to risk their daily incomes to travel to distant modern facilities for perhaps minor illnesses, so they may perforce choose locally available traditional sources of care. This may, of course, be problematic in terms of preventive and promotive health care but, until the PHC network is ubiquitously spread, questions of economic and physical access costs will continue to favour traditional medicine, particularly in rural settings.

China

The Malaysian example illustrates a system in which, whilst many different groups use a variety of traditional medical types, modern medicine dominates officially and in practice. China has gone a stage further and is one of only two or three countries in which official policy is to give integrated equivalent status to both types of medicine. However, evidence suggests that, whilst an interesting blend of modern with traditional practice has been evolved (for example, the use of acupuncture and herbal drugs in some modern operations), traditional medicine has been rather selectively adopted.

Traditional Chinese medicine nevertheless is based on rich clinical experience and an ancient theoretical system with an extensive literature (Crozier 1968; Unschuld 1985; Wang 1983). Its use spread widely outside the Chinese heartlands because of the Chinese traders and settlements throughout South-East Asia. It has appeared extensively since the mid-nineteenth century in Chinese enclaves in North America and Europe, especially among earlier generations of migrants. It survives strongly, and thrives, among Chinese populations throughout East and South-East Asia, including Hong Kong, Taiwan, Singapore, Malaysia, Indonesia and further west (see, for example, Kleinman *et al.* 1975; Lee 1975; Phillips 1984; Quah 1981). During the 1970s and 1980s, training courses in traditional medicine were run for domestic and numerous overseas health carers, and the WHO set up a number of cooperation centres in China in traditional medicine (Hou 1986). However, in terms of its recent developments and incorporation into a modern health care system in a huge (in parts rapidly modernizing) Third World country, it is the domestic application of Chinese medicine and the accessibility of the system that have fascinated researchers (Cai 1988; Hillier and Jewell 1983; Leslie, 1975; Morley *et al.* 1983; Rosenthal 1987).

In the years preceding, and during, the Cultural Revolution of the mid-1960s, Mao Ze Dong sought very actively to promote Chinese medicine and to incorporate it in a modern way into China's health care system. It became a basic principle that practitioners of Chinese medicine must be 'united' with practitioners of Western medicine and that health work must be integrated with mass movements and serve the people.

Today, China has over 500 000 personnel involved in traditional Chinese medical services, of whom some 350 000 are traditional Chinese doctors: about one-quarter of the country's total doctors (Table 3.4). There are about 1 800 hospitals of Chinese medicine with over 160 000 beds and, in addition, there are many thousands more practitioners of traditional medicine in the ethnic minority areas of China. Most Western-style hospitals also have departments and pharmacies of traditional Chinese medicine. By the late 1980s, the country had twenty-eight colleges, thirty-seven medium-sized schools and fifty-seven academies or research institutes of Chinese medicine (Wang 1988). Chinese medicine therefore enjoys equal status with Western medicine and it is playing an increasingly important role. However, this has not always been so and it is only since the 1949 revolution that it has come to the fore officially.

Early post-Liberation attempts to modernize China largely fol-

Table 3.4 Professional medical workers in China (from *Beijing Review*, 1983)

	1949	1957	1965	1975	1980	1982
Total	541 240	1 254 372	1 872 838	2 593 517	3 534 707	3 957 804
of which:						
Technical workers	505 040	1 039 208	1 535 595	2 057 068	2 798 241	3 957 804
Doctors of traditional Chinese medicine (including those with secondary medical school education)	276 000	337 022	321 430	228 635	262 185	302 791
Pharmacists of traditional Chinese medicine		53 505	71 848	86 201	106 963	140 231
Senior technical workers (doctors and pharmacists of Western medicine, and senior nurses)	38 875	78 875	203 402	318 488	502 022	699 380
Middle-rank technical workers (practitioners and pharmacists of Western medicine with secondary medical school education, nurses and midwives)	103 277	341 637	619 870	938 353	1 174 435	1 223 238
Junior technical workers	86 888	228 169	315 045	485 391	752 636	777 303
Total number of doctors and practitioners of both traditional Chinese and Western medicine	363 400	546 296	762 804	877 716	1 153 234	1 307 205

Source: *Beijing Review*, Vol. 26, No. 46, November 1983

lowed the Soviet model but, even with considerable advances in the 1950s in health facility and manpower development, health services remained very inadequate through the 1950s and to the mid-1960s. This was exacerbated by regional maldistribution of resources and the concentration of much medical manpower in cities, and this urban bias has persisted in the 1980s. Data on medical manpower vary but, in the mid-1960s, it appears that there were some 320 000 doctors of Chinese medicine and some 72 000 traditional pharmacists. By the 1980s, the number of pharmacists had increased considerably but the number of doctors had decreased slightly. By contrast, in 1965, there were only 203 000 senior workers in Western medicine but this number increased to almost 700 000 by 1982 (Table 3.4). Until the 1970s, it appears that the number of practitioners of Chinese traditional medicine outweighed those of Western-style medicine.

The Cultural Revolution saw great but disruptive attempts to reorientate workers to the countryside and denigrate formal education (particularly Western) and to encourage mass participation in health, among other things (Sidel and Sidel 1979). Traditional medicine, still the poor relation in the mid-1960s, was to be more actively pursued and differentials between its practitioners and others were to be reduced. Medical training was drastically altered away from a formal, university-based, Western-style training to favour practical work in the countryside, which included the accelerated training of medical auxiliaries, in particular worker doctors and 'barefoot doctors', of whom there were in the late 1970s some 1.6 million helping China's rural population. However, their numbers have since been in decline and some estimates suggest that 40 per cent of them are no longer practising (Rosenthal 1987); the term 'barefoot doctor' was dropped after 1984 (see p. 171). Mao's attempts to upgrade and incorporate traditional Chinese medicine have been widely studied and regarded either as a laudable attempt to retain an ancient, appropriate form of care or as an unwise, desperate attempt for political and other ends to preserve a useless, fossilized system.

Rosenthal (1987) considers that Mao's motivation involved a complex of pragmatic factors that underlay the economic system evolved in the 1960s and 1970s and still influence the health system in the modernizing China of the 1980s and early 1990s. First, there was a desperate need for medical personnel, which could be met in part by using traditional medical resources. Secondly, there was a concomitant lack of capital for building facilities and for providing Western pharmaceuticals. Thirdly, the large, mainly rural population had faith in, and respected, traditional medicine. It was therefore arguably wrong to discard it completely. As a result, there are now over 550 hospitals of traditional medicine above the county level, and many more exist or are conjoined in general hospitals below this level. Nevertheless, observers during and since the Cultural Revolution have noted that the adoption and use of Chinese medicines and techniques have been selective. Acupuncture, for example, is widely used in modern and traditional facilities, and a limited range of herbal medicines is in common use, but generally under the supervision of a Western-style doctor. Nevertheless, departments and pharmacies of traditional medicine have been established in hospitals of Western medicine, leaving doctors and (presumably) patients a degree of choice. In medical training today, however, Western-style doctors tend to be in charge and all use extensively modern diagnostic techniques. Since the Cultural Revolution, over 280 000 doctors of traditional medicine have joined work in state and collective hospitals, medical schools and research institutes.

Traditional herbalists continue to evolve the remedies, but today these are tested and researched by modern pharmacists. Herbal medicines are being industrially produced in modern factories (as noted in Chapter 7), of which over 800 produce some 2 000 or more varieties of medicinal herbs (Wang 1983). Rosenthal (1987) discusses one such factory in Shanghai, which, for example, produces 230 standardized, packaged, over-the-counter traditional medicines with some quality control, and with national and overseas distribution. However, this industrial approach to production is very different from the small-scale ancient use of traditional medicine, in which a herbalist would monitor the patient and vary the prescription and strength from time to time, according to the patient's changing condition. The modern factory approach eliminates much flexibility and standardizes the process, but it does produce a recognized group of patent medicines that are used locally and internationally. Research is also widely conducted into traditional techniques such as moxibustion and acupuncture, and modern methods of development and evaluation are nowadays applied (Rosenthal 1987). Aspects of traditional practices and therapies may be included in various branches of medicine, such as psychiatry, in addition to Western techniques or where they have been less than effective (Tully 1985).

The underlying policy of incorporating traditional Chinese medicine into a modernizing health care process might be said to have been relatively successful over the past 40 years or so. However, this did require the direction and initiative of a powerful leader as well as popular acceptance; under other circumstances, major efforts to modernize medicine might well have been along hierarchical Western (or Soviet) lines. The large numbers of traditional practitioners were adopted as a health care resource rather than being regarded as a hindrance. They were given important official, professional and legal recognition, whereas before the Communist revolution, although widely used, traditional Chinese medicine was regarded as illegal and was discriminated against professionally (Wang 1983). Economically, as Rosenthal (1987) suggests, traditional medicine has enabled the extension of medicinal treatment to rural areas that have few funds for modern pharmaceuticals and equipment. There is evidence that traditional practices and medicines are still most widely used in the remoter areas of China and, today, the nearly 700 000 rural medical practitioners often use both Western and traditional therapies (Wang 1988). In political terms, traditional practitioners have helped to link the peasants to the modernization process, and the selection of local (politically acceptable) individuals for medical training as barefoot doctors also helped earlier in this process. Overall, it could be said that the efficacy of Chinese rural health care lies in prevention rather than therapy (Huang 1988).

Recent directives from the Central Secretariat of the Chinese Communist Party appear to reaffirm that Chinese and Western medicine are held to be equally important (Cai 1988). The use of traditional medicine should not be abandoned, it is stated, but Chinese medicine must make full use of advanced science and technology and modern measures so that further development can be ensured. It seems that the policy of integration of Chinese and Western medicine is to continue and they should cooperate with one another. This is facilitated because there are today three types of doctor in China: traditional, Western-trained, and Western-trained with qualifications in traditional medicine (Wang 1988). These categories give the real appearance of professionals working together, and goals of complementarity and integration appear to some extent to be being achieved. However, this has been largely because of considerable political and economic support of the better, tried-and-tested aspects of traditional medicine, which moreover has a long history and a huge national following, particularly among a predominantly rural population. Therefore, it is doubtful that the Chinese experience will provide a realistic model for an integrated health care system for certain other Third World countries where traditional practices are less predictable and less effective. Care must be taken in the uncritical extrapolation of the Chinese example to all Third World settings.

Urban and rural differences in traditional medicine

Earlier in the chapter it was suggested that traditional medicine tends to be stronger or relied on more extensively in rural than in urban areas. It has nevertheless survived and, indeed, flourished in many urban and peri-urban settings (in virtually all Third World countries). There is, however, evidence to suggest that urban traditional medicine may take on a somewhat different character from that of the remoter rural areas of any given country. This is perhaps because practitioners become exposed to more varied forms of medical competition from the pluralistic systems that develop in most cities. Patients may also be more accustomed to shopping around among the wide range of accessible health-care options that tend to exist in urban settings. Urban residents are, for instance, far more likely than their rural counterparts to have ready access to free public health care services, to modern pharmacies and to a range of alternative sources (Durkin-Longley 1984; Lee 1973, 1975). They not only may become more conscious of the competing therapeutic options but also may become more price conscious. In addition, urban residents are more likely to be involved in cash payment for health care (particularly traditional sources), whereas payment in kind may be more prevalent in rural locations.

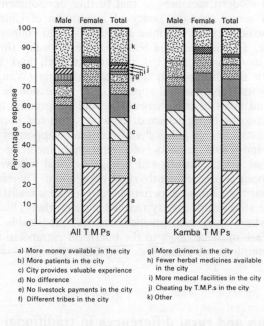

a) More money available in the city
b) More patients in the city
c) City provides valuable experience
d) No difference
e) No livestock payments in the city
f) Different tribes in the city
g) More diviners in the city
h) Fewer herbal medicines available in the city
i) More medical facilities in the city
j) Cheating by T.M.P.s in the city
k) Other

Fig. 3.5   **Perceived differences between practice of traditional medicine in urban and rural areas of Kenya (based on data from Good 1987a)**

From the provider's perspective, there appear to be quite important differences in the practice of traditional medicine in urban and rural areas. Although there are relatively few studies that specifically investigate urban and rural differences in the practice as opposed to the general availability and use of traditional medicine, Good's (1987a) Kenyan study included questions to some forty-five TMPs in the Mathare sub-areas of Nairobi, Kenya. Figure 3.5 summarizes his findings; the monetary rewards and numbers of patients available in the city are obviously higher than in rural practice. This featured in 43 per cent of responses from all TMPs and 51 per cent of responses from the TMPs who were Kamba people (from Kitui district, near Nairobi). However, there were also subtler differences, relating to the availability of herbal medicines, other medical facilities, and breadth of experience in the city. Nevertheless, a reasonable proportion (14.7 per cent of all TMPs and 12.5 per cent of Kamba TMPs) suggested there was little or no difference between urban and rural practice of traditional medicine, so the issue is not clear-cut. Along with urban–rural differences in availability of traditional medicine, and the differences in utilization discussed in Chapter 6, the attitudes of practitioners to urban and rural practice obviously form an interesting area of future research in health care provision. The continued success of traditional medicine in urban areas may well depend on how it is perceived by practitioners as well as patients.

Conclusions

This chapter has emphasized the diversity and pluralism that prevail in Third World health care provision. They have many implications for utilization, which will be subsequently discussed. There is nevertheless a tendency for specific types of medical system components to prevail in certain areas, although often separate systems and subsystems exist. To date, an urban-modern versus rural-traditional health care dichotomy has been implied, although many rural areas do seem to have a reasonable spread of modern facilities. In addition, the density of available health services varies considerably locally and nationally and provides greatly varying access to all forms of health care.

It is important to note that the frontiers and interfaces among and between the components of the broadly defined ethnomedical systems are not as clear-cut as some figures in this chapter might suggest. Much has been written about the relationships between medical systems, and the 'relative strength' of subsystems and, indeed, their internal integrity and consistency will vary geographically. Medical systems do not prevail to the same degree in all places and the concept of geographical areas of concentration as the 'core areas' of any medical system and the remaining areas as their 'periphery' has been suggested (Streefland 1985). The frontier of a medical system may be considered that part of the periphery in which the system is increasing, with the 'interface' the borderline between medical systems (see also Good *et al.* 1979). The position of this frontier, and its width, form and persistence, may be determined by many social, cultural, economic and legal factors. A case study of Nepal suggests that there the development of modern Western medicine is characterized by centralization, growth and a commercial–capitalist nature which influences the place of the frontier but the shape of the frontier is influenced by factors such as tourism, labour migration, foreign aid and physical geographical conditions (Streefland 1985). Such factors will aid or hinder the spread of modern health care in any given situation.

If it is accepted that there is great overlap among medical systems (in some cases involving considerable integration), it is reasonable to conclude that great diversity will characterize the frontier and interface among systems and the health systems that develop there. The circumstances at any frontier and the medical system's manifestation there are rarely static or uniform. Ideas and beliefs vary; influences on the modern and traditional systems change and those who come into contact with a medical system, particularly at its frontier, tend to experience only one facet of it. For example, it makes a considerable difference whether one experiences modern medicine through a modern urban hospital, or via the activities of a newly introduced VHW, or by information from fellow villagers who may have worked as porters in a mountaineering expedition or as soldiers abroad (Streefland 1985). It may, in fact, appear to the person that there are many different types or variants on the same medical system. If differences are very big (as, for instance, between a modern urban hospital and a VHW's outpost), then the systems themselves may almost appear to be different although they are, in fact, based on the same broad principles. It seems reasonable to suppose that similar conclusions may be reached when outsiders come into contact with indigenous systems. This recognition is important for a fuller understanding of, and empathy with, the great variety in the nature of health care in the Third World. We all tend to have images based on only partial information about health care systems. Rarely is it possible to derive unambiguous conclusions about the nature of health care since it is neither a homogeneous service nor uniformly available across any country.

Chapter 4

Health care in Third World countries: aspects of distribution and accessibility

In the majority of developing countries, health care implies much more than access to medical facilities. It should also consider availability of safe water, advice and education, and adequate nutrition. However, much health planning in the Third World has focused on the physical provision of health care facilities (which equate with illness responding, and less often with preventive and promotive services), for the very good reason that there has been a marked, absolute deficit of facilities overall or locally in many countries. This chapter focuses on access to health care at a general level within nations (aggregate provision and service distribution). Access to various specialized services and for specific groups of the population is considered in subsequent chapters. Health services are discussed in spite of the acknowledgement that 'health' levels in communities are rarely clearly correlated with the objective physical provision of health care facilities. Rather, they are influenced by a parcel of services (often included in the basic needs and PHC approaches) and overall improvements in living standards. The limitations of a sectorally discrete analysis of health care facilities should therefore be borne in mind.

Some issues related to access to health care

A discussion of access to services arguably should begin with a number of distinctions:

1. between physical (potential) accessibility and revealed accessibility (utilization);
2. between equity and equality of provision;
3. between quantity and quality of services.

Many of these concepts have received considerable philosophical and practical consideration in the medical and social sciences. In the first place, the definition of 'accessibility' is rarely clear-cut. Accessibility may be considered a slippery notion, meaning, in general terms, that something is 'get-at-able' (Moseley 1979). It is useful to distinguish between *locational accessibility* (a measure of proximity) and *effective accessibility*, dependent on having the ability, mobility and time to reach a service. In health care terms, the provision of a facility of a given type within a specified distance of an intended user population is frequently considered to give more or less equal access to all 'potential' users – hence the derivation of the concept of 'potential' accessibility (viz. because a facility *exists*, it *may* be used). However, research over a number of years has emphasized that many variables other than physical availability may intervene to prevent or distort utilization. Prominent among these is the existence of recognized need to use a facility, closely followed by the financial ability to use it (charges, transport costs and the like), the physical ability to attend and the sociopsychological readiness to utilize it. The clarification of the influence of such variables has formed a major research focus in the developed world and research in the Third World has been of growing importance. Utilization and variables influencing it form the focus of Chapter 6, and detailed discussion will be deferred until then.

Other constraints that influence utilization (or effective accessibility) include time–space variables: facility opening times or the days of provision have to coincide with the times at which individuals can reach a service point and must therefore take into account their other commitments and transport availability. In jargon terms, these may be 'coupling constraints', which effective planning should aim to minimize (Carlstein *et al.* 1978). These constraints may be particularly crucial in influencing 'effective accessibility' (utilization) of health care services, especially those of a more 'voluntary' or elective nature, such as preventive and promotive services (including screening, immunization and FP). In many rural Third World countries, one of the greatest challenges to health care planning is the extension of effective accessibility.

The distinction between *equity* and *equality* of provision is complex but important. Equality of provision implies the arithmetic division of available facility resources equally among the population, possibly by a formula adjusted for demographic criteria such as local age structure. Equity, by contrast, implies 'justice' in distribution, in which those who for some reason require more of a service will be provided with more than their equal share (Smith 1979). These persons or groups might then become targets for special provision because of their relatively high requirements. This involves the problem of how to define and measure *needs*, the solution to which has, for practical purpose, eluded medical and social scientists to date. Indeed, at least four types of need may be recognized in the health care delivery field (Bradshaw 1972) and the planning of provision based on need will be affected by which is selected. 'Normative need' is professionally defined or determined, often by allegedly objective tests or criteria; 'felt need' is perceived by an individual and may or may not be amenable to 'objective' identification; 'expressed need' is felt need turned into action by seeking or demanding a service; finally, 'comparative need' involves comparison of the relative requirements or needs of groups within the population (possibly by localities, or social, economic or ethnic subgrouping). Groups who do not receive services that they apparently require and others obtain might be in 'comparative need'.

The identification and, indeed, the value of knowing levels of need in the population to be served, seem subject to medical and political question. It is self-evident that much greater levels of 'need' exist in virtually all Third World countries for virtually every type of medical service than can absolutely be met. In many cases, it would be politically most undesirable for official providers to identify vast amounts of need for any given service, which then could not possibly be met. Therefore, vague and often unsatisfactory rankings of need are often all that is achieved. However, occasionally, it might be politically and practically expedient to highlight certain types of need (for MCH services, vaccination, essential drugs or the like) in order to stimulate donations by target-oriented relief agencies.

The distinction between *quantity* and *quality* of service is also particularly acute in many Third World countries. For example, in the developed world, the inclusion on the list of medical practitioners of old and infirm doctors, or the use of outmoded inefficient buildings, is well known and may make real quality of care less than it appears. However, in the Third World, just because facilities are identified on paper, there is sometimes little reason to believe they exist at all or in fully fledged form in practice. Many countries, for example, have planned and even built networks of primary medical units that are in theory staffed by doctors and nurses, provided with medicines, beds and vehicles, and embedded in a referral hierarchy. In reality, however, many a facility might be staffed by relatively lowly trained field workers, who have no professional support, medicines, equipment or vehicles, and no opportunities to refer to more appropriate services their more difficult cases or those beyond their skills. The 'quality' of service available therefore often does not equate with that which allegedly or quantitatively exists.

A qualitative issue in care that is underlaid by quantitative deficiencies is the absence of medicines from hospitals and clinics in many of the poorest Third World countries such as Uganda. This is a major issue influencing qualitative access. Deficiencies in supplies are also to be seen in some facilities in relatively better-off countries, such as Jamaica and the Philippines. In addition, the manning of health units (especially in rural districts) by part-time, poorly trained, underqualified or unqualified staff, and certainly by too few professionals (as in the Philippines and many other countries), is also widely recognized. This leads to vast differences in the 'objective' quality of services available. Variations in provision can, in addition, occur according to time and day. At certain times in certain facilities, especially at the primary level, only stand-in staff or community workers may be on duty. The nurse, midwife or doctor may be away from the post on visits to the community or absent for other reasons, sometimes 'moonlighting' in private practice. Another quite common feature is the peripatetic visiting of some sites by mobile teams, or circuit doctors or nurses. Therefore, only on certain days (possibly widely spaced) will a trained professional worker be available at the facility in question. All these features need to be recognized when the issues of quantitative and qualitative access to health care are considered. They are often very sensitive local issues.

The health care hierarchy

Conventionally, health care planners in the developed world have tended to conceptualize the provision of services in a hierarchical form. Ubiquitously available primary and family care services form the base, and more specialized services form the upper tiers, until virtually uniquely specialized institutions are reached. These higher levels are often found only in larger settlements and usually in the capital or largest city in a country, according to generalized rules of urban size ranking. However, even in the developed world, there exists no single, uniform hierarchy with a fixed division of functions and referral paths between strata. The great variety of health care delivery systems (arising under different professional, political and socioeconomic arrangements) means that there are numerous international differences in hierarchies and access to their various levels.

The concept of a health care hierarchy is basically founded on central place system notions, in which certain threshold populations within a given travel distance are provided with a specified level of care. As greater levels of specialization above first aid and simple primary services are required, the hierarchy enables patients to be referred upwards to higher levels, generally in larger settlements

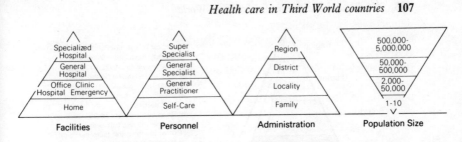

Facilities	Personnel	Administration	Population Size
Specialized Hospital	Super Specialist	Region	500,000-5,000,000
General Hospital	General Specialist	District	50,000-500,000
Office Clinic Hospital Emergency	General Practitioner	Locality	2,000-50,000
Home	Self-Care	Family	1-10

Fig. 4.1 **The health care hierarchy: levels and services in a 'theoretical' system (from Joseph and Phillips 1984; after Fry 1979)**

(although a hierarchy also exists *within* large settlements). The hierarchy may be adjusted temporarily by mobile services bringing higher-level services (doctors, dentists, nurses, opticians) to the lowest levels. At times, mobile operating teams (generalists or specialist) may visit local areas and thereby bring secondary and tertiary level facilities to remoter localities.

In the Third World, the 'rigid' triangular hierarchy is not necessarily the norm or the desired model. The hierarchy in Fig. 4.1 may be substantially modified and may follow a much looser referral system, with mobile teams modifying the services available at various times in different localities (Fendall 1981; Fry 1979). In addition, whilst the incremental increase in specialization is inherent in the developed-world type of hierarchy, this is not necessarily so in developing countries. The hierarchy may be 'climbed' by the world-be patient merely to obtain any formal service, not necessarily one of a significantly higher level of specialization. For doctors and health care workers, too, increasing training opportunities and career development may be provided by climbing the hierarchy. Increasingly, however, in the Third World, a focus on higher-level training is being felt inappropriate for community needs, and training is desired and sometimes being provided more at 'grass-roots' level by teams or individuals travelling to, or living in, localities. This may form the essence of sound 'grass-roots' systems and community participation.

Hierarchies in developing countries

In spite of the difficulties and costs of providing specialist facilities and their dubious suitability, many developing countries have implicitly or explicitly adopted a hierarchical system of health care delivery. Sometimes, this is difficult to identify precisely, given the coexistence of public, private and charitable providers in formal

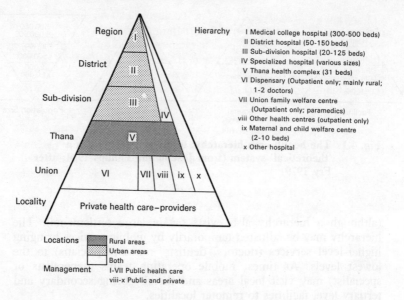

Region — Hierarchy
District
Sub-division
Thana
Union
Locality

Hierarchy I Medical college hospital (300-500 beds)
II District hospital (50-150 beds)
III Sub-division hospital (20-125 beds)
IV Specialized hospital (various sizes)
V Thana health complex (31 beds)
VI Dispensary (Outpatient only; mainly rural; 1-2 doctors)
VII Union family welfare centre (Outpatient only; paramedics)
viii Other health centres (outpatient only)
ix Maternal and child welfare centre (2-10 beds)
x Other hospital

Private health care–providers

Locations   Rural areas
              Urban areas
              Both
Management   I-VII Public health care
              viii-x Public and private

Fig. 4.2   The health care hierarchy in Bangladesh (after Paul 1983)

health care, as well as numerous types of traditional practitioners. The extreme urban–rural discrepancies discussed below can also make the identification of strict hierarchical levels difficult, and often what is available locally (especially rurally) can depend on fortuitous factors. However, Paul (1983) provides an example of the hierarchy of health facilities in Bangladesh. In this, hierarchical levels of specialization are related to location and management type (Fig. 4.2). Whilst noting the quantitative and qualitative inadequacy of facilities, their maldistribution and the fact that most people rely on private medical practitioners for health, this example provides a useful analysis of a hierarchy in which health care provision is related to the administrative levels of the country. The higher-specialization facilities are clearly located at the more important administrative levels. The lowest level of reasonably comprehensive care is the Thana Health Complex (a standard provision of thirty-one beds and one to five doctors). Below this, at the union level, are maternal and child welfare centres.

The hierarchical conceptualization enables the identification of urban or rural facilities and public or private provision. In analytical terms, the hierarchy may also be used to identify population to facility ratios at various levels, as can be seen in Bangladesh (Paul 1983), Thailand (Joseph and Phillips 1984), Kenya (Diesfeld and Hecklau 1978) and Nigeria (Okafor 1987). The services available to populations at each level may be calculated and measures of normative provision be compared for planning purposes.

For most developing countries, however, a planning system that is highly facility-oriented and that aims to provide a formal hierarchy and fixed referral system can result in administrative attention being paid to less immediately important aspects of service delivery. It can, for example, result in doctors and nurses spending a great deal of time on administrative matters related to referrals or being drawn into the bureaucratic machinery. It can also allow political rivalries between settlements, as those of certain sizes attempt to exert political pressure for a health service to be provided. In addition, for the populace, proximity to a facility of a given level does not guarantee accessibility if rigid referral systems are enforced. To achieve effective utilization, the system must be entered in the first place and the major task often becomes how to make the most effective 'first contact' with it. Therefore, access to any type of care can become the crucial element, whether this be the CHW, nurse, midwife, doctor or hospital.

The relative balance between public and private care is also often crucial, especially at the local level. The public system is frequently under such strain and so short of supplies, especially but not exclusively in the poorer developing countries, that it is regarded as a bad second-best choice by many. The private sector, it is assumed, at least provides some basic advice and access to medicines but it does not, by and large, undertake preventive measures and public health activities. In addition, private practitioners are frequently to be found only in bigger centres, where higher fees can be earned. They rarely participate in mobile extension services or in comprehensive PHC services other than curative procedures. These activities are left to the public sector (often to charitable or aid-funded providers), which further stretches its scarce resources.

Primacy in modern health care facilities

The distribution of settlement sizes has developed a marked 'primacy' in many (but not all) Third World countries. This means that the largest city (usually but not always the capital) grows to many times the size of the next largest and often dwarfs the urban hierarchy economically and in terms of services. The distribution of modern health care facilities, especially publicly provided hospitals and higher-order care, tends to mirror this but to favour disproportionately the largest centres. It is possible to regard the upper echelons of the hierarchy as parasitic in the health care system in that they cater for relatively fewer people than their budgetary allocations would warrant. For example, Manila's population is some eight million, about one-sixth to one-seventh of the Philippines total, and several times that of the next largest city (Cebu, which has a population of about half a million). Moveover, the Metro-Manila region, its urban sprawl and environs, contains some 25 per cent of the country's population yet has 43 per cent of total hospital beds (45 per cent of government beds and 41.5 per cent of private hospital beds) (Phillips 1986a).

This example is by no means unusual. Akhtar and Izhar (1986a,b), for example, cite the examples of India and Zambia, in which some 80 per cent of the total population are in villages but only have access to a very small proportion of the formal health care provision. In terms of higher-level hospital specialisms, such as open-heart surgery, the Indian case shows gross imbalances. Seven out of the eighteen hospitals offering this specialism are in Maharashtra state (five in Bombay alone); the small state of Kerala, with under 4 per cent of the total population, has two such hospitals, whilst none exist in Bihar, where almost 10 per cent of the country's population live. Uttar Pradesh, with 16 per cent of the total population, has only one such hospital. Doctors and dentists are likewise very much concentrated in the main centres, and Bombay, Calcutta and New Delhi may have as few as 500 persons per doctor. Elsewhere, there may be as many as 7 000 to 8 000 persons per doctor or, in some rural locations, even more. The distribution of persons per dentist is even more skewed; this ranged in the late 1970s from one dentist per 9 000 persons (approximately) in Chandigarh, to 1:626 990 in Bihar and 1:414 000 in Orissa. 'Primacy' seems to operate here at a state level; the 'higher-order' states with major cities are best favoured in terms of distribution of modern medical personnel and facilities.

Access to traditional practitioners, whilst not so widely documented or researched, shows similar distinct regional variations, but primacy is generally not so marked. The distribution of homoeopaths in India, for example, varies from 5 per 100 000 population in the north-eastern region to 28 per 100 000 in the eastern region of India. The ratio of traditional hospitals per million persons likewise varies, being highest in the southern region and lowest in the north-western region. However, the distribution of many forms of traditional medicine tends to be more even than is the case for much Western medicine and availability is generally higher (Good 1987a). This is, of course, one of the recognized strengths of traditional medicine, although regional variations and specialisms within it may still render traditional medicine differentially available both regionally and locally.

Kenya, like many developing countries, has a considerable degree of urban primacy, which has, historically, also been reflected in the distribution of specialist and general facilities. Until attempts to spread resources spatially more evenly in the mid-1980s, Nairobi's Kenyatta Memorial Hospital was really the only national specialist hospital. In 1974, over half of government-employed specialists and 50 per cent of post-internship medical officers worked there (Diesfeld and Hecklau 1978). Historically, 50 per cent of medical services were in Nairobi, provincial and district centres, reflecting the distribution of colonial administrative foci. Good (1987a) reports that 80 per cent of the national health budget even until recently has been taken up by residents of Nairobi, Mombasa and Kisumu, the three largest towns. It could be argued that, as half of Kenya's urban population live in Nairobi alone (the only city of more than half a million in the nation), the provision of hospital services does in fact mirror urban population and the capital's primacy. However, nine-tenths of the nation's total population live in rural areas, so such an argument may be persuasive to planners but hardly favours that rural majority! For them, utilization normally entails movement to urban areas or to the nearest provincial hospital. In urban areas, the doctor-to-population ratio is around one doctor per 5 000 persons but, nationally, this rises to 1:10 000, implying that some rural areas must be very poorly served.

Since the mid-1980s, therefore, Kenya has attempted to reduce the primacy of Nairobi in public and private health provision and has made districts the main unit for resource allocation. Each district is to manage its own resources, and it is intended that the development of district hospitals will reduce the rate of referrals to the capital. This will, however, be unlikely to affect the primacy of Nairobi in private health care, and some of the most expensive private care in Africa is located there. This is, of course, essentially inaccessible to the majority of Nairobi's population, who are poor, and the private hospitals will continue to serve an élite national and even international market.

Historical aspects of the health care hierarchy

The evolution of a top-down approach to health care in many Third World countries may be explained in most if not all cases by the imposition of modern, 'alien' medical systems onto people under colonial control (direct or indirect). The contemporary structure of modern medical systems reinforces the colonial influences, which favoured curative, rather than preventive, medicine, and this can be seen particularly in a number of African countries such as Kenya, Nigeria and Ghana (Fosu 1986; Muganzi 1989; Twumasi

1981; Yoder 1982); it is perhaps less visible in certain other regions. As noted in Chapter 1, it was often the case that access to preventive medicine was narrow and aimed only at improving the environments in which expatriate administrators lived. There were, of course, many altruistic attempts to extend this form of care but, arguably, the majority of efforts aimed mainly to serve the basic economic interests of the colonists. The bias of the bulk of health services was therefore usually towards curative medicine and urban areas (Leng 1982). Colonial rule and health programmes often even suppressed those rudimentary elements of indigenous public health that had existed in pre-colonial times (Waite 1987). Therefore, because much medical care in many Third World countries was only curative, many people cured of infections or parasitic ailments would return from hospital or clinic to unhealthy, reinfecting environments (Muganzi 1989). The provision of (curative) health care via a hierarchy also arguably made for easier control of access to the formal system of care, which enabled the rationing of modern health care as a means of sociopolitical control (Banerji 1979).

The emphasis on curative medicine reinforced the 'facility orientation' of health care, and this has often fostered the growth of 'top-down' hierarchical systems. In these, patients are referred to higher levels, which in theory possess greater skills and technical resources and which are the most highly regarded elements of the system. In historical terms, this vastly favoured the largest, often primate, cities in provision of health care, not only as the seats of governments and hence centres of investment but also as the apexes of established and growing hierarchies. In addition, when systems were initially introduced, the major facilities were most readily set up in the main towns or capitals; subsequently, regional capitals would receive investment but this meant that, with the few resources devoted to health provision in colonial days, areas outside the immediate sphere of such key settlements tended to receive very little in the way of formal investment in health care. Frequently, what health care was available in the rural areas would be provided by missionary bodies and the like. Henkel (1984) provides the example of the evolution of health care provision in Zambia, in which the pioneering role of various missionaries is highlighted. Many spread Western medicine as well as the word of God.

Historically in Kenya, as in many other colonial countries, vast urban–rural differences were found in the distribution of health care facilities according to the formal administrative hierarchy. This concentrated specialist and many other forms of care in Nairobi, with the seven other provinces having provincial hospitals as foci of 'quality' care. The hierarchical system, established early, did not encourage outreach services and these were relatively poorly financed until the financial and administrative reforms of the mid-

1980s attempted to disperse some levels and resources from the capital.

In Ghana, likewise, the organization of health services in a formal hierarchy reflecting the administration again led to neglect of many village areas and a concentration in urban sites. By the 1970s, the system focused on one teaching hospital, eight regional hospitals and thirty-two district hospitals. Over two-thirds of doctors but only 18 per cent of the population were concentrated in towns of over 20 000 persons (Fosu 1986). Even more striking is an analysis of expenditure, population to be served and hierarchical levels (Fig. 4.3). This suggests two hierarchies, one of expenditure and one of population to be served, but inversely related to one another. For the mid-1970s, expenditure on tertiary hospital care (specialized services), benefiting only 1 per cent of the population, amounted to some 40 per cent of health budget; expenditure on secondary hospital-care, serving only 9 per cent of the population, amounted to 45 per cent of the budget. By contrast, expenditure on PHC (especially promotive and preventive medicine), serving some 90 per cent of the population, was a mere 15 per cent of total health spending. It may be concluded that the evolution of the formal health care hierarchy in Ghana has led to the distribution of funds and personnel for PHC compared to hospital-based care in inverse proportion to the number of people that need to be reached by each.

Current inequalities in the distribution of Western-style health care thus often stem from the economic and political structures developed in colonial days. In India, for example, activities focused on port towns and strategic sites, raising the status of Western medicine in them beyond even the need of the colonial and local élite, and neglecting almost totally the hinterlands and the bulk of

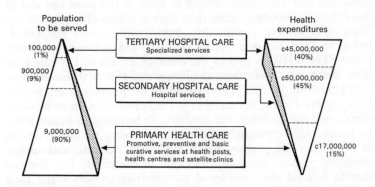

Fig. 4.3 Health care hierarchy and the inversion of expenditure to population served in Ghana (after Fosu 1986)

the indigenous population (Akhtar and Izhar 1986b). Disease and epidemics were not to affect trade and security. Local populations were cut off from modern medicine (Banerji 1979), but, ironically, indigenous systems were often discouraged and certainly neglected. The foundations for modern imbalances in the distribution of health care were therefore established early on.

Alternative perspectives on the hierarchy: the doctor on tap?

The provision of much health care and related services has in the past usually emphasized the prominent and paramount role of professionally trained workers, in particular doctors and specialists. Many people still tend to think of the primary health worker as a temporary and second-best substitute for the doctor and that, if financially feasible, people would be better off with more doctors and fewer primary health workers. However, the circumstances and needs of most developing countries, especially in rural sectors, lead Werner (1978) and others to a vigorous denial of this attitude. After many years of working with VHWs and primary health workers (Werner shies away from calling them 'auxiliaries'), Werner concludes that the role of the VHW is not only distinct from that of the doctor but, in terms of health and well-being, far more important. 'Health care' becomes a part of improved living conditions and is, as a result, considerably 'deprofessionalized'.

This discussion is continued in Chapter 5, but the reasoning behind Werner's (1978) conclusions has important implications for the notion of a 'hierarchy' in health care for Third World countries. Community or village health workers are often numerically the major resource for health, willing to work in the front-line and to share their knowledge, rather than store it within élite professions. Their jobs involve community improvement across the board, trying to stop sickness before it starts and actively promoting health. The VHW is part of the community; his or her role is to serve and not to profit from the illness and misery of his fellows.

Therefore, Werner (1978) argues for the primary health worker to be regarded as the *key* member of the health team (in its broadest sense), and the doctor as the auxiliary, to be called in as and when necessary. As a curative 'technician', the doctor would be on call as needed by the primary health worker for referrals and advice, attending perhaps the 2 to 3 per cent of commonly met illnesses that lie beyond the capacity of the informed populace and their health worker. The doctor might, in addition, be involved in the training of the primary health workers in the narrow area of health care called 'medicine'. Werner therefore proposes a rational exten-

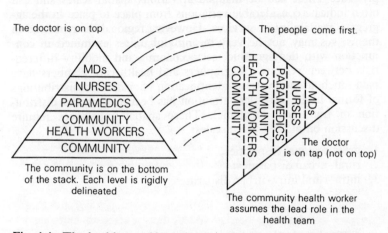

The typical pyramid

The pyramid as it should be

The doctor is on top

The people come first.

MDs
NURSES
PARAMEDICS
COMMUNITY HEALTH WORKERS
COMMUNITY

The community is on the bottom of the stack. Each level is rigidly delineated

COMMUNITY
COMMUNITY HEALTH WORKERS
PARAMEDICS
NURSES
MDs

The doctor is on tap (not on top)

The community health worker assumes the lead role in the health team

Fig. 4.4 The health care hierarchy to serve the people: the doctor 'on tap' (from Werner 1978)

sion of this philosophy: health care will only become equitable (socially just) when the skill pyramid of the conventional health care hierarchy is tipped on its side. The primary health worker will then be taking the lead, with the doctor on *tap* and not on *top* (Fig. 4.4).

This proposal has many interesting implications for accessibility. In terms of settlement hierarchies, it removes the 'theoretical' expectation that 'better' or higher-level facilities should automatically be located only in larger centres. It also reduces the visibility of barriers to upward referral in a system as, instead, the system is viewed as horizontal, with referrals between equal levels rather than to higher levels. Finally, and perhaps even more importantly, the psychological equality of community with health workers and professionals of all levels is more readily achieved when a rigid vertical hierarchy is removed and the equivalence of different functions stressed. As a result of fundamental attitudinal and organizational changes, both physical accessibility and revealed accessibility (utilization) might be considerably enhanced.

Geographical variations in the distribution of health facilities within countries

If physical accessibility is equated with availability of facilities or 'formal' health care, then differential ratios of persons per facility must provide some indication of relative spatial balance in the supply side. These can be mapped at various spatial scales and can often indicate considerable variations from place to place in the aggregate availability of services. However, regional distributions in themselves may not be very meaningful unless examined in conjunction with demographic, socioeconomic and mobility differentials between regions. Geographers and health care planners have paid much attention to the identification of spatial maldistributions of formal health care (less attention has been paid to the distribution of traditional medicine). These spatial imbalances require discussion on at least three scales:

1. gross regional disparities;
2. rural–urban disparities;
3. intra–rural/intra–urban disparities.

Regional disparities

The identification of disparities between different parts of countries has been a major source of research. Disparities are often very marked and there are often some areas that obviously have relatively far fewer, or far more, than their 'per capita' fair share of health service provision, to a much greater degree than could be justified by, say, demographic differences (or other variables potentially influencing need and demand). The scale of investigation is frequently limited by the nature of administrative units for which data are available, and the administrative subdivisions of a country may be very gross and reflect relatively little of the social geography of a country. However, such data are frequently all that are available and at least they provide some indices of different distributions.

Problems with the designation of regional availability measures are quite numerous and include data availability and accuracy, and scale of units. For example, data on specific types of health care facilities of personnel might be unavailable at a regional level or may be virtually completely fictitious. The question of scale is also important: an administrative subdivision in one country may, in terms of area and distances involved, be larger than another entire country, so care must be taken when looking simply at ratios of personnel or facilities to population, because physical distance plays its own important part. Distance may be incorporated in certain gravity-type measures (designed to estimate the relative accessibility weighted for population, facilities and distance between subregions), whereas other distributional measures such as the location quotient merely indicate quantitatively the share of a resource (such as facilities or personnel) that each region has, relative to the average for the whole (see Joseph and Phillips 1984).

There are numerous studies showing that Third World countries often suffer from severe regional imbalances in the distribution of formal health care provision. Akhtar and Izhar (1986a,b) illustrate the considerable overall regional and state variations in India during the 1970s in expenditure on health and family welfare. They also indicate the variations in hospital facilities and beds per capita at a district level. Their data highlight occasionally more than tenfold differences between the worst- and best-provided states in terms of hospitals and hospital beds per capita. Even if allowances are made for qualitative and other factors, such regional variations are indeed severe. In Africa, at a gross level, Stevenson (1987) illustrates the considerable differences between the four provinces of Sierra Leone, in which the more rural northern and eastern provinces are far more poorly provided in terms of facilities and health personnel per capita than are the capital and southern provinces. Elsewhere in Africa, Henkel (1984) and Mundende (1984) have shown that health services are very unevenly distributed in Zambia, on the basis of several indices, including ratios of hospital beds, nurses and doctors to population. Table 4.1 illustrates the extreme differences that persist between various provinces of the country, in spite of attempts between 1978 and 1981 to redress the balance. Some provinces, such as the northern and eastern, have well over double the number of persons per facility found in the better-provided provinces. This pattern has persisted from the past, and certain provinces appear to have been favoured over time in the provision of facilities (Fig. 4.5). The northern province, for example, seems to have experienced relatively low rates of change in all three periods mapped, whilst the copper belt saw high growth between 1965 and 1968.

Within Nigeria, Okafor (1987) illustrates inter-state levels of inequality for varying types of modern health facilities by means of a Gini coefficient (a measure in which a larger value indicates greater inequality of distribution). The coefficient indicates the extent to which health facilities are concentrated areally compared with another measure (need for health care, equated in this case with population distribution among the states). Figure 4.6 illustrates that there are considerable regional inequalities in the distribution of facilities relative to the population, and that levels of inequality are about the same for hospitals, health centres and maternity centres, but are lesser for dispensaries and hospital beds. The Lorenz curve (Fig. 4.7) shows that only about 32 per cent of the population as a whole have use of 50 per cent of dispensary facilities and about 60 per cent of health centres. Inter-state ratios of 'advantage' can be calculated, which in the Nigerian case show groups of more advantaged states (such as Bendel, Lagos, Imo and Anambra) and disadvantaged states (such as Sokoto and Kano), with ratios mostly below 1.0 on all health care provision indicators.

However, such measures only show how an *existing* amount of a service is distributed among the population. The measures do not take account of relative needs among population subgroups (although this refinement can be introduced), nor do they suggest that the existing level of aggregate provision is correct or even adequate. The comparison of values at different points in time can be useful to show how regions have converged or diverged. It does not, however, indicate whether quality or quantity locally has necessarily improved. Nor does this measure take account of the desirability of redistribution of some types of facility, which may only be providable in localized centres. It is, however, an extremely useful example of a measure of spatial equality of distribution, which may be applied regionally and also at a local level (to show intra-urban variations, for example). Okafor (1987) argues the case for using such regional inequality measures in a developing country for the statistical identification of problem areas in which provision falls well below standard. Often these are intuitively well recognized, but such measures might be used to prompt disadvantaged states to try to achieve a better expenditure on health.

Elsewhere in Africa, Diesfeld and Hecklau (1978), studying a similar time period, uncover similarly extreme regional variations in provision of formal health care in Kenya. The population per facility for health centres and dispensaries fluctuated considerably among the seven provinces, from some 43 000:1 to 84 000:1. Perhaps, however, the accessibility in terms of distance may be more crucial and this is naturally influenced not only by the availability of facilities but also by population density and transport availability.

Table 4.1   **Zambia: regional variations in the availability of hospital beds and health personnel; population per unit (from Akhtar and Izhar 1986b)**

	Doctors	Beds	Nurses	Medical assistants
Central	8 702	384	1 375	4 296
Copperbelt	4 311	296	695	5 475
Eastern	21 661	282	1 963	5 415
Luapula	14 505	301	2 052	3 968
Lusaka	2 998	325	847	6 527
Northern	17 730	286	2 376	4 579
North-Western	12 357	183	1 065	3 432
Southern	12 191	253	1 049	4 311
Western	15 993	257	2 350	4 427
Zambia	7 139	276	1 142	4 797

Plotting the catchment area of each hospital in Zambia also indicates that accessibility varied greatly among regions (Fig. 4.8). In
the Copperbelt, some 91 per cent of the population were within
30 km of an existing hospital; elsewhere, this ranged between 31
and 70 per cent, with the exception of the northern province, where
fewer than 30 per cent of the population were within this distance
of a hospital.

The influence of distance and physical access on utilization will
be discussed in Chapter 6 but, for now, evidence from Costa Rica
illustrates that, even in a system with almost universal coverage in
health care under social insurance legislation, there remain considerable provincial disparities in health care facility distribution
and utilization (Table 4.2). Discounting the case of San José, the
capital, there are still provinces that appear to be three times better
provided than others in terms of physicians or hospital beds per
capita. At the extremes, San José had in 1979 about 6.5 times more
physicians (per 10 000 inhabitants) and 5.2 times more hospital
beds (per 1 000 inhabitants) than did the province of Guanacaste.
A positive correlation was found between development indicators
(income, urbanization, employment in secondary or tertiary activities) and quality of health care coverage. As a general rule, the
rural areas lost in terms of provision of, and accessibility to, health
care (Mesa-Lago 1985).

The identification of regional imbalances in facility distribution
makes an interesting academic exercise, but in itself it will be of
little direct relevance to improving health care delivery in the Third
World unless translated into policy and action. Many of the

Table 4.2 **Provincial disparities in Costa Rican social security
public health care facilities (after Mesa-Lego 1985)**

Provinces	Physicians per 10 000 inhabitants	Hospital beds per 1 000 inhabitants	Medical visits per capita[a]	Composite index ranking
Alajuela	3.3	1.2	2.2	4
Cartago	3.6	3.6	1.8	3
Guanacaste	1.9	1.1	1.8	7
Heredia	2.7	0.5	1.9	6
Limón	6.0	1.7	2.6	2
Puntarenas	2.0	0.9	2.2	5
San José	12.4	5.7	3.0	1
Costa Rica	6.5	3.0	2.4	

[a] General and specialized medicine: excludes emergencies and dental
visits

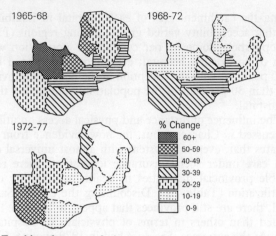

Fig. 4.5 **Zambia: the rate of change in provision of health facilities has not been even over time (after Mundende 1984)**

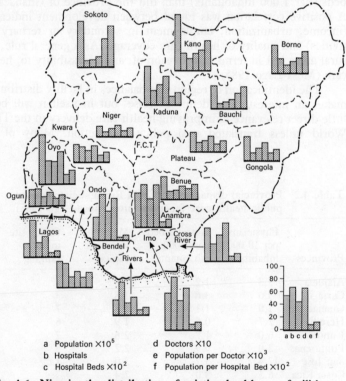

a Population ×10⁵   d Doctors ×10
b Hospitals   e Population per Doctor ×10³
c Hospital Beds ×10²   f Population per Hospital Bed ×10²

Fig. 4.6 **Nigeria: the distribution of existing health care facilities relative to population in the different states (based on data from Okafor 1987)**

programmes identified in this book have been aimed at broadly improving accessibility. Nevertheless, the overt aim of reducing *regional* disparities in health care may itself become an important policy objective, in part sometimes for reasons of increasing regional balance at an aggregate level, but also to avoid the political repercussions of continuing regional deficiencies. Regional disparities might be reduced by greater investment in underprovided regions or by encouraging the movement of resources and personnel from relatively well-off to poorer regions. This, of course, is often very difficult to achieve without firm direction, as few regions or cities wish to lose services, and health facilities may be relatively immobile. Planning policies may direct increasing proportions of future (public) investment to more disadvantaged regions. Tanzania took such a positive step in the 1970s and Maro (1987) points to the resultant reduction of regional inequalities in health provision and proximity to services, although the overall level of provision is still relatively poor. In addition, extra coverage of non-capital-intensive PHC might be directed to the less well provided regions to achieve greater provision at less cost in these underprivileged locations.

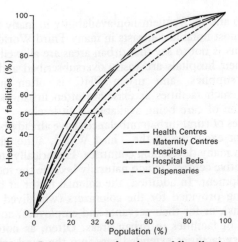

Fig. 4.7 Nigeria: Lorenz curve showing maldistributions for various types of facility relative to population (from Okafor 1987)

Rural–urban disparities

The apparent relatively good physical availability and shorter distances to health care in most urban areas (but particularly in

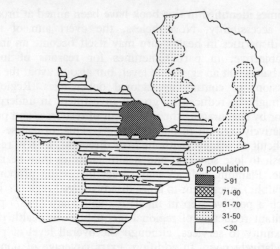

% population

- >91
- 71-90
- 51-70
- 31-50
- <30

Fig. 4.8 Percentage of population in each province in Zambia within 30 km of existing hospitals (after Akhtar and Izhar 1986b)

primate cities) and its frequent non-availability in many rural areas is one of the most notable contrasts in many Third World countries (Fig. 4.9). This is not to say that urban areas are all well provided; frequently, their hospitals are vastly oversubscribed and lack personnel and supplies, and urban PHC is often inadequate. Nevertheless, such facilities as exist are often urban-located, and give the illusion of care being available, if little else.

The causes of rural–urban imbalances have already been hinted at and are not exclusive to the Third World, although they are exaggerated in many developing countries. Historically, towns were the administrative centres, which naturally became the foci of major facility development. In addition, the colonial factor of health care primarily being provided for the colonizers (who lived mostly in the main towns), or for their servants and employees, added to the concentration of facilities in urban areas. Often, as noted earlier, only missionary facilities extended care into the rural areas, where otherwise very heavy reliance on traditional provision existed and persists.

Biomedicine (as opposed to traditional medicine) in particular often displays a distinct urban bias. It is 'aggressively technology dependent and resource consuming' (Good 1987a: 30), and this mutually reinforces its urban bias and the inadequacy and unmet need of rural areas. The differences in provision between rural and urban areas are often so great as to make national averages of

Percentage of total population with access to health services, 1980 - 86

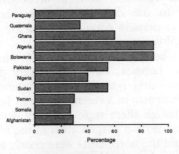

Percentage of urban population with access to health services, 1980 - 86

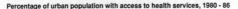
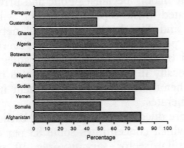

Percentage of rural population with access to health services, 1980 - 86

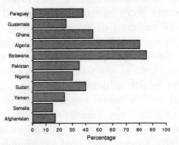

Fig. 4.9 Percentages of urban, rural and total populations with access to health services, 1980 to 1986

population to facilities almost meaningless. In Kenya, for example, it has been estimated that only 10 per cent of the country's doctors serve rural areas and that some 70 per cent of all doctors are in urban private practice. Doctor-to-population ratios range from 1:990 in the cities to 1:70 000 in rural areas (Good 1987a). Indian examples also illustrate the varying proportions of population having a nearby medical facility. These range from 84 per cent of urban residents having a medical facility within 2 km to under half this percentage for residents in rural areas (Akhtar and Izhar 1986b). Similarly to the Zambian example above, many rural respondents even in densely populated India are over 5 to 10 km from a medical facility.

By contrast, however, some of the smaller developing countries, such as Jamaica, have a relatively densely provided health care network (although still spatially uneven). The average distance to a health centre in a recent survey in Jamaica was found to be 2 miles, although there were still considerable rural–urban variations noted and certain rugged areas of the island (such as the Cockpit country and the north-east) were poorly served. However, there are significant urban–rural differences in availability of hospital services and the major specialist public and private hospitals are strongly concentrated in the capital, Kingston, with some capacity in Montego Bay and Mandeville. The rural network of smaller hospitals or PHC posts is supplemented by government clinics or facilities provided by large aluminium companies. The quality of care availability locally in rural Jamaica has also been strongly influenced by whether there has been investment in health care by industrial conglomerates.

The health care dilemma in Ghana noted earlier – the financial maldistribution, which concentrates some 85 per cent of expenditure on the hospital sector serving only 10 per cent of the population – is also mirrored by rural–urban imbalances stemming from this favouring of hospital care. Fosu (1986) found that some 67 per cent of doctors were in towns of over 20 000, which contained only about 18 per cent of the population; 86 per cent of all pharmacists were living and working in these larger towns. In the mid-1970s, Accra dominated health care, with the only teaching hospital, some 37 per cent of physicians, 46 per cent of pharmacists and 100 per cent of health educators. Communities of fewer than 20 000 persons (in which were found over 80 per cent of the population) had roughly only one-third of the national total of private- and public-sector physicians, midwives and nurses. Only in assistants, auxiliary nurses and nurse-midwives did these rural areas have over half the national total.

The uneven urban–rural distribution of modern health care facilities has already been noted in the Philippines. Elsewhere in East Asia, Soh (1980) reports that some 35 per cent of licensed physicians in Korea were working in the capital, Seoul, which has only about 20 per cent of the population. Even though the overall number of medical personnel was not really insufficient, spatial imbalance and a focus on the main towns (Seoul and Pusan) meant that as many as 15 per cent of the population (mainly rural or in small towns) were without any medical practitioners, modern or herbalist. A 5-year plan to establish comprehensive care has existed since the mid-1970s, and this aims ultimately to cover the country with health centres and hospitals (general and specialized). The unequal distribution of health personnel is regarded as one of the main underlying factors affecting health in Korea.

Urban bias in distribution of health facilities and personnel is also found in Pakistan and some interesting possible explanations for the evolution have been proposed. Zaidi (1985) presents data showing that extreme spatial maldistribution of health resources and personnel had arisen by the early 1980s and the distribution of health facilities in no way reflects the urban–rural split of the population. A total of 78 per cent of hospitals and 90 per cent of hospital beds were in urban districts, which also had 95 per cent of tuberculosis centres and 100 per cent of tuberculosis beds, and 66 per cent of MCH centres and 85 per cent of MCH beds. However, only some 28.3 per cent of the 1981 population of Pakistan lived in urban areas, whilst 71.7 per cent were in areas termed 'rural'. Although the overall provision of health facilities in Pakistan may be relatively favourable compared to that in many other poor Third World countries, the distribution within the country is heavily biased against rural areas. When the major city, Karachi, is removed from consideration, the picture is yet gloomier, so the 'natural' (primate) bias of the capital is not as pervasive as in some other countries. In particular, the physical access for nearly all urban people, not just residents in the capital, is better than that for ruralites. In most parts of the country, all urban dwellers have a public or semi-public institution within 2 miles; for rural dwellers, the proportion rarely exceeds one-third (Table 4.3). 'Urban bias' is also evident in the distribution of other facilities, and the maldistribution of water supply and sewerage facilities, which heavily favours urban areas, is of direct relevance to health. By 1983, some 77 per cent of urban dwellers had access to potable water supplies and 48 per cent had access to sewerage and drainage,

Table 4.3 Percentage of population within a 2- and 5-mile radius of public and semi-public health institutions in Pakistan (from Zaidi 1985)

| | 2 miles | | 5 miles | |
	Urban	Rural	Urban	Rural
Punjab	99.58	32.40	99.73	82.41
Sind	100.00	24.20	100.00	69.50
North-West Frontier Province	100.00	41.20	100.00	88.40
Baluchistan	100.00	28.70	100.00	28.70
Total	99.78	32.10	99.89	78.61

compared with only 22 per cent and 4 per cent of rural dwellers respectively.

Intra-rural disparities

There has been a tendency to regard the major problem of health services distribution in many Third World countries as being the maldistribution between urban and rural areas. However, a further complication is maldistribution within and between specific rural areas and between specific urban areas. In particular, there are often areas of rural deprivation and relative rural well-being within the same country in terms of physical provision of health services. In rural Bendel State, Nigeria, for example, free health care has been provided and access to general hospitals is therefore of considerable importance to the population. If there is no local access to public hospitals, the rural resident either has to make long trips to distant hospitals or has to patronize fee-charging hospitals or clinics. Therefore, clear intra-rural differentials in well-being might arise.

Such differences between rural parts of the same country are illustrated by a study of access to general hospitals in Bendel State, in which Okafor (1984) found very distinct variations in spatial provision between essentially rural local government areas (LGAs). An index was derived based on a population to hospital measure, transport availability, income spent on health care and the percentage of households travelling more than 8 km to the nearest general hospital. A multivariate analysis of these variables enabled the identification of the LGAs most deprived of the free medical attention offered by the state's general hospitals. Figure 4.10 illustrates that considerable spatial variations existed, and the additional complication arises that it was the LGAs that scored low on other indices of socioeconomic development that were most seriously affected by inaccessibility to general hospitals. Okafor stresses that this illustrates intra-rural variations in levels of deprivation, of which difficult access to services such as hospitals is but one aspect. In addition, the discrepancies between government social plans, which assume that all rural populations in the state have equal or reasonable access to health services, and the reality of the situation, are highlighted. One reason for the growth of such maldistributions is probably inappropriate expenditure of LGA health budgets on single hospitals relying on expensive, imported high technology. The use of simpler local materials to provide more widely dispersed cottage hospitals might be more in line with local needs and could help to reduce intra-rural disparities in access.

Further evidence of differences in provision between rural

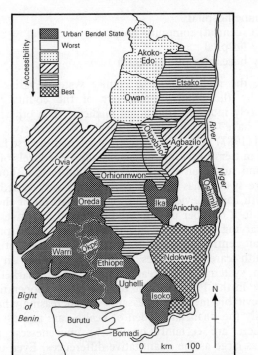

Fig. 4.10 Patterns of spatial inaccessibility to general hospital facilities by LGAs within rural Bendel State, Nigeria (after Okafor 1984)

areas is to be seen in yet larger countries. China has extreme variation in population densities and physical conditions. It is hardly surprising that even today's health care system has significant disparities among rural areas. The Chinese system is, to some extent, often regarded as a model of community-based PHC, focusing on the development needs of the most deprived populations, namely those in rural areas, and the combination of curative with preventive, promotive and developmental activities has been discussed in the previous chapter. Nevertheless, case-study evidence shows continuing imbalances in provision of facilities and in the extent of reliance on successful combination of traditional and modern practices in this large country.

The rural health care system in China in the early 1980s relied basically on five tiers:

1. production brigade health station (barefoot doctor, health aides, midwife)

2. commune hospital
3. district (central) commune hospital
4. county hospital
5. county bureau of public health

However, the reality of these county systems varies and is influenced by the relative prosperity of the county. Some, for example, rely more on traditional medicine than others; some, by contrast, have an almost exclusively Western-style approach. Rosenthal (1987) notes that there are particular diverse facilities and functions in tiers providing ostensibly the same levels of care (both in rural and suburban areas), reflecting contrasts in how the rural health care system has actually emerged. A very varied pattern of rural health care is evident from her comparison of the provision identified in a number of case studies. Local initiatives, historical factors, varying patterns of agricultural success and proximity to large urban centres all seem to influence the exact nature of local rural health care. Resources thus vary even in an ostensibly egalitarian system. The greater emphasis on market forces in agriculture in the 1980s and the decline of the cooperative medical system inevitably mean that peasants will increasingly have to bear individually the financial burden of health care and illness. In addition, there are certainly qualitative unevenessess in supply, probably as large as the quantitative differences. Even on the relatively crude indices of ratios of hospital and medical workers to population, Rosenthal found considerable variation between the four rural communes studied, and between them and China's urban areas, in which most modern medical technology is being concentrated.

Disparities undoubtedly exist within Third World rural districts, especially relatively large ones. In a study of health risks in the Kibwezi division of Kenya, half-way between Nairobi and the south-east coast, Ferguson et al. (1986) highlight important differences in access to health care within a single rural district. Internal communications in the area are difficult, yet it lies only 2 hours by road from Nairobi and 3 hours from Mombasa. Health care facilities, traditional and modern, were relatively few and, until the inception of a rural health scheme, the modern facilities were almost exclusively located on the axial road and rail routes connecting Nairobi and Mombasa. Therefore, inhabitants near to the main communication routes were likely to have had greater access to the existing health facilities and also to have been within striking distance of the main towns should higher-order services have been required. By contrast, the populations dwelling in the hill areas were far from the health facilities and travel to the urban areas would also have been much more difficult for them. This emphasizes the differences in accessibility to formal facilities within

Table 4.4 Access to modern health services in rural Guatemala: distance and time (from Annis 1981)

Province	Nearest MOH health post/centre	Hospital	Pharmacy	Private clinic	Private doctor
Sololá	3.9 km	22.2 km	6.0 km	7.3 km	13.0 km
	34 min	1 h 31 min	47 min	49 min	1 h 16 min
Totonicapán	8.0 km	24.5 km	7.7 km	16.9 km	19.4 km
	56 min	1 h 39 min	57 min	1 h 25 min	1 h 28 min
San Marcos	5.0 km	30.7 km	5.9 km	19.0 km	20.4 km
	54 min	2 h 19 min	59 min	1 h 46 min	1 h 49 min
Overall average	5.3 km	27.1 km	6.3 km	15.5 km	18.3 km
	49 min	1 h 57 min	56 min	26 min	1 h 35 min
Median distance	4.0 km	22.0 km	4.0 km	11.0 km	12.5 km

rural areas and the need for health extension to many rural dwellers. Since the early 1980s, the situation in the Kibwezi area of Kenya has been improved through the provision of both a centrally located health centre and a community-based health care programme involving CHWs and TBAs.

It may, however, be misleading to think of all Third World countries, and rural localities in particular, as suffering from poor access to formal health services. Annis (1981) provides the example of three large departments in Western Guatemala, in which, whilst there are differences in average distances to modern health facilities, the distances themselves are not great. The average distance of communities from an MOH health centre was only 5.3 km, although individual distances varied from less than 3.9 km in one department to 8 km in another. Therefore, even allowing for poor roads, overall physical accessibility was quite good (Table 4.4); however, utilization of MOH facilities was low because of poor perceived quality of care. This issue of the effects of distance and other variables such as quality of utilization is discussed further in Chapter 6. Nevertheless, whilst local differences in these departments are small, some other districts are served less well. In particular, peripheral Indian areas in the highlands are poorly served, yet in great need. The health system has also been disrupted by political instability and by natural disasters such as an earthquake in 1976 (Behrhorst 1984).

Intra-urban disparities

That most curative facilities are concentrated in urban areas in the majority of Third World countries – and indeed in others – is beyond dispute. However, the concentration of provision and health expenditure in urban hospitals and on urban health personnel is often a dubious benefit for the cities themselves, as it may divert resources from the preventive and outreach services so crucial for the health of the urban poor. Therefore, it pays to reconsider what aggregate urban–rural differentials might actually mean. Cities are very heterogeneous and almost certainly display more variation socially and environmentally than most rural areas, and the practical reality of intra-urban access to health care probably varies as greatly as does access between rural areas. If reliable disaggregated data concerning different urban sub-areas are available, then the conditions of the urban poor and the rural poor will almost certainly be found to be more similar than averages make them appear.

For example, the nutritional status of the urban poor may often be worse than that of their rural counterparts. The axiom of 'urban being better' may only apply to aggregate physical distance to specialist health facilities that are either so crowded or so expensive as to be in effect unavailable. It is also well recognized that physical propinquity does not equate with revealed accessibility or utilization (Joseph and Phillips 1984). Recent research for the WHO suggests that in many cases the apparently better-off health care position of poor urban areas may in fact be counterbalanced by poorer health status of urban than rural populations. Harpham *et al.* (1988), for example, cite many studies that show more malnourished children among the low-income urban than rural populations.

In Thailand, for example, infant mortality rates are thought to be higher in Bangkok than elsewhere in the country. In Haiti, Port-au-Prince's infant mortality rates in poor areas are almost three times those of rural areas, whilst the rich in the same city show rates comparable to those of the urban USA. In terms of disease incidence, in the Ivory Coast, tuberculosis rates, with an annual incidence of infection of 1.5 per cent, range from 0.5 per cent in rural areas to 2.5 per cent in Abidjan and 3 per cent in the more deprived urban areas, where the disease also strikes at younger ages. Again in the Ivory Coast, socioeconomic differences in food availability showed worse nutrition for certain urban groups than for equivalents in rural areas. Similarly, in San José, San Salvador and Guatemala City, the prevalence of second- and third-degree protein-calorie malnutrition was similar to, or even above, that in rural areas.

Oni (1988) illustrates that wide intra-urban variations in child mortality exist in Ilorin, Nigeria, in which mortality was much higher in low socioeconomic areas than in medium- and high-status areas. Data from this study are instructive and show the range of intra-urban differentials in facilities and education, and their relationships to child mortality. Many variables, including housing and environmental conditions, spacing of births, use of breast-milk substitutes and the like, vary considerably from one sub-area to another. The city is shown to be anything but uniform in its dangers and life chances.

It is probable that the differences in socioeconomic and environment conditions between sub-areas of cities render city-wide statistics virtually meaningless. It also seems that, despite the evidence to show urban concentrations of high-order health care facilities and numbers of physicians, the relative standards of health care for slum and shanty dwellers may often be well below the reasonable minimum. Higher costs of living in cities may also outweigh the higher urban wages; food quantity may be reasonable but good fresh food may be less readily available. Women may have more opportunities to work in towns, but may leave their infants in the care of inexperienced young children. Feeding of the young may suffer and the children's exposure to the greater risks in the urban than the rural environment may easily counterbalance the city's advantages of access to health care. Hart's (1971) 'inverse care law', according to which those in greatest need of care have the worst access to it, seems to operate as much in the Third World, especially in cities, as it does elsewhere. Many health care researchers are currently noting that less attention is paid to the increasingly quantitatively and qualitatively serious health problems of the urban poor than is generally paid to the health service problems of those in the rural areas. This is particularly true of urban PHC, which is often inadequate.

An important feature of access to modern health care facilities in urban areas is their uneven availability in peripheral, peri-urban sites. Peripheral areas, whether of high or low status, have often grown rapidly in Third World cities and some such locations have been very poorly served with formal health care, either because their growth has occurred in a haphazard, unplanned way, outstripping the official provision of facilities, or because of an absolute lack of capacity. As it is often the poorest who live on the shanty peripheries and who have the least ability to travel to health care sites, they are doubly disadvantaged. In Banjul, the Gambia, the peri-urban area was identified as the least-served location, contrasting with the concentration of services in the city. Similar problems are seen in many other Third World cities, including Nairobi (Harpham *et al.* 1988), Ibadan (Iyun 1983) and Kingston (Bailey and Phillips, 1990). In Kingston, Jamaica, the poorer inhabitants of the peripheral sites have little choice of facilities and many travel to the university hospital casualty department.

Figures 4.11 and 4.12 illustrate the concentration of many health facilities in the relatively better-off areas of Kingston. However, peripheral residents both rich and poor seem to have considerable distances to travel for health care, although the burden of travel is much less for the richer residents. The poor within urban areas may have access to certain cash-earning employment but they often have no access to any formal social services or social security system. Often, their housing conditions and wider family support, especially for newcomers, are less satisfactory than they might be rurally. Equity in terms of health care, or even minimal effective accessibility, may be in reality denied to many of the urban poor.

Even the most fully developed, institutional social security systems in developing countries channel resources to only a small and privileged section of the community. Usually this will consist of a proportion of those in formal wage employment, waged employees themselves often comprising only a small proportion of the popula-

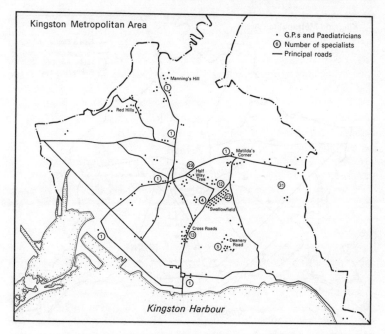

Fig. 4.11 **Kingston, Jamaica: intra-urban distribution of doctors (from Bailey and Phillips, 1990)**

tion. In India, for example, only some five million out of a population of more than 650 million are covered by social security schemes through their formal employment (MacPherson 1987). As only the rich and élite are usually covered by social security systems, these do not provide the opportunity they can do elsewhere to extend help (in the form of welfare or health benefits) to the bulk of the population, urban or rural.

What is the answer to improving potential and revealed (effective) access to health services (and social services) in poor Third World cities? Primary health care concepts, it is argued, are as relevant to urban health care systems as they are to national systems or rural subsystems. The discrepancy between the allocation of resources and health needs is just as marked within cities as it is between town and country. Gaps are widening between the urban rich and poor, between need and provision, and between 'haves' and 'have-nots' in health care. Possibly, the relatively good endowment of hospital facilities in certain Third World cities should be coupled with PHC policies and community health programmes; this perhaps could be achieved by urban hospitals serving well-defined catchment areas and interactively stimulating PHC within them (see

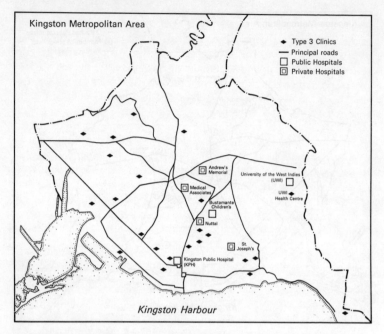

Fig. 4.12   Kingston, Jamaica: intra-urban distribution of hospitals (from Bailey and Phillips, 1990)

Chapter 8). Sadly, the reality in many countries is that neither public nor private health services are reaching the urban poor. On the contrary, private services are increasingly abandoning the poorer and declining areas, and under-resourced public-sector services are unable to meet the welling demands of the urban poor.

Some difficulties involved in extending access to health care

In most countries, attempts are being made to extend access to health care but there are, of course, numerous practical and theoretical problems in doing this, both regionally and locally. Financial and manpower shortages and bottlenecks are but two of the most obvious. Logistical problems involving availability of transport and supply of drugs and dressings, and systematic problems of responsibility, referral and the like, can all tend to combine to frustrate many worthy health extension projects. In addition, the political will to extend realistic health services beyond urban élites often may not exist.

An underlying difficulty in extending any service including health care to the poorer areas of Third World cities in particular is that of their scale and rapid growth. Only a few atypical city states, such as well-to-do Singapore and Hong Kong, and certain NICs mainly in East and South-East Asia, have managed to improve significantly their urban planning and service provision for poorer populations. This has often been in conjunction with public housing schemes and new towns development (Phillips and Yeh 1987). By contrast, the rapid expansion of cities in virtually all poorer Third World countries has outstripped the expectations and planning capabilities of their governments.

An example of this rapid expansion is to be seen in Pikine, a poor settlement on the northern edge of Dakar, Senegal, which has grown from virtually nothing in the early 1950s to over 600 000 by the mid-1980s. It is essentially a relocated city to control the growth of Dakar. However, the health care needs of this rapidly growing settlement were largely neglected until after the mid-1970s, when the conjunction of government and foreign aid allowed the development of a system of PHC posts (one PHC post to 10 000 people). This system was planned on a spatial catchment basis, and each post was intended to serve a radius of 500 m, but actually serves 23 000 people or over double the envisaged norm (Figs 4.13 and 4.14) (Guindo *et al.* 1986; Laloe *et al.* 1986). However, not only are services still well below what is desirable, but Salem (1989) suggests that the acquisition of community facilities is more a measure of the organizational capacity and pressure applied in local politics than of the real needs of specific locales. Health committees may be manipulated by politicians whose representativeness may well be open to question. This involvement of local politics, particularly in a rapidly growing urban environment, is another problem or facet of improving health care provision, and reflects a type of corruption endemic in many systems. Other studies have identified problems involved, for example, in extending PHC strategies within national systems such as that of the Philippines, where new approaches to intersectoral and interhierarchical cooperation are needed (Phillips 1986a).

An example of the problems involved in taking health services to the people is to be seen in Caracas, Venezuela (Rakowski and Kastner 1985). A major objective was to improve the use of central public and maternity hospitals by providing patients with a full range of local, peripheral services on which they could rely. There was a wish to shift the emphasis from curative to preventive services, and to promote client participation in health-related programmes. The experiences of one health service module (with the pseudonym *El Libertador*), located in a *barrio* of some 2 200 people and with a zone of influence extending to some 21 000 to

Health facilities

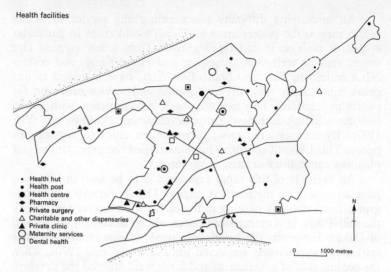

* Health hut
• Health post
● Health centre
◆ Pharmacy
▲ Private surgery
△ Charitable and other dispensaries
▲ Private clinic
○ Maternity services
□ Dental health

0   1000 metres

N

Fig. 4.13　Pikine, Dakar (Senegal): intra-urban distribution of health care facilities (after Laloe *et al.* 1986)

24 000 persons, are of interest.

The establishment of the health centres in the *barrios* was supposed to provide local access for clients to many of the same general health care services available in hospitals. Obligatory health programmes included in such centres concern FP, pre- and post-natal care, emergency and inpatient care, and vaccinations. 'Rural penetration' schemes were also initiated from the centres to extend services to the more destitute or difficult-to-reach parts of the neighbourhood (peri-urban places, in reality). Centres' optional programmes include those which, in theory, respond to local community needs, such as MCH and oral rehydration programmes. *El Libertador* centre was inaugurated in 1981 with one physician, but had gradually grown to involve sixteen regular staff, including a coordinator, two rural physicians, four nurse aides, a dentist and three social services staff. The experiences of the centre illustrate a number of general and specific problems that impeded the attainment of the Ministry of Health and Social Welfare's goal of extending coverage to a greater proportion of needy people.

First, there were administrative and organizational structural difficulties. The initial autonomy of centre staff was usurped in reorganization, and this led to dissatisfaction. Channels both for referral of patients and for administrative matters were unclear; problems of information flow were apparent, and were associated with serious logistical difficulties. Physicians were expected to as-

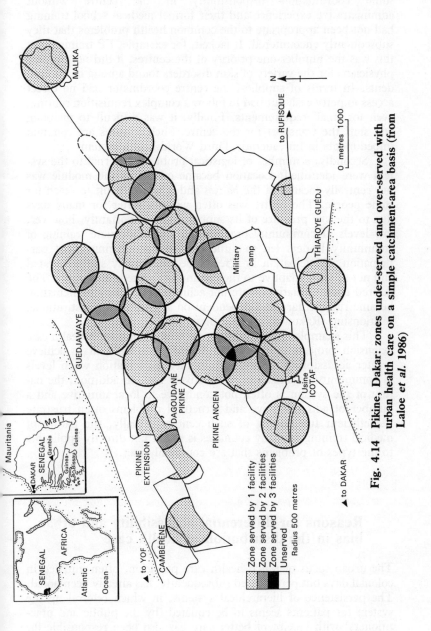

Fig. 4.14 Pikine, Dakar: zones under-served and over-served with urban health care on a simple catchment-area basis (from Laloe *et al.* 1986)

sume coordination responsibility in the centre without administrative experience and their formal medical school training had not been appropriate to the common health problems that they subsequently encountered. It lacked, for example, FP training, yet this was the number-one priority of the centres; it did not prepare physicians for the variety of skin disorders found among *barrio* residents. In terms of supplies, the centre coordinator had no direct access to petty cash but had to follow a complex requisition routing, even for small requirements. Finally, it was difficult to maintain and staff the transport for the centre. Such features are common impediments in bureaucratic Third World health systems.

Secondly, a number of logistical problems external to the system were identified. Location became crucial as the module was not centrally located in the *barrios* and it was difficult to reach for some people. The centre was often without water for many days due to the low pressure of its supply. Most importantly, however, low levels of community organization and inadequate training of community leaders led to difficulties in encouraging client participation. Participation as a result became largely staff-generated and not as such adaptive to the community's needs and wants. The desired client initiatives were not achieved and client participation became rudimentary and dependent on a paternalistic institutional relationship (Rakowski and Kastner 1985).

This example illustrates many problems common in health care extension projects in the Third World. It is difficult to achieve greater accessibility through community participation when levels of community organization are relatively low. In addition, the nature of the system is often not conducive to local initiative and a number of administrative and structural problems often frustrate the efficient functioning of such centres. Finally, the nature of medical training in many countries is as yet not directly applicable to the types of problems that are commonly met.

Reasons for differential accessibility and urban bias in the distribution of health care

The urban focus of much health care provision, often initiated in colonial days but perpetuated subsequently, has already been noted. The persistence of hierarchical systems, in which referral up the system for patients seems to be equated (by the public and practitioners) with receipt of better care has also been responsible for an image of 'bigger is better', and the view that 'better' is usually found in the city. Promotion structures for staff have also tended to be linked, whether deliberately or not, with movement 'up' the hierarchy. Therefore, characteristically many systems have tended to focus both higher levels of care and more investment into the main urban areas. In many ways, this is purely a reflection of urban primacy discussed earlier and, whilst primacy does provide some advantages of agglomeration for national economic development, it is also a hindrance to the development of more widely accessible and egalitarian, decentralized health care systems.

Differentials in levels of provision among different regions and subregions of countries have often developed and been perpetuated by resource allocation systems that are not sufficiently sensitive to the requirements of demographically varied populations. Levels of provision have also been historically derived and based on out-of-date population and needs criteria. It is also the case that, in certain countries, regions with greater political strength (sometimes resulting from ethnic group allegiances) have been able to attract and retain more than their fair or equitable share of health resources. In addition, the budgetary allocations in most ministries tend to follow established lines and to support existing facilities and projects. This means that in very tight financial circumstances little money is available for new allocations to undeserved areas. Nevertheless, unequal regional (and sectoral) allocation of health resources is, of course, by no means confined only to Third World countries and is a common occurrence in Britain, Europe and North America. It is hardly surprising that countries with newer national health systems or fragmented systems are finding that regional and local inequalities in provision and access are pervasive and often worsening. In particular, the drain on resources of large cities and their facilities is commonplace.

Urban bias?

Additional factors underlie the growth and persistence of regional and urban–rural differences in access and provision. The term 'urban bias', indicating lopsided distribution in a range of resources, has become familiar in development studies, and it is sometimes regarded as the outcome of struggle between rural and urban areas (Lipton 1977). This may well account for some imbalances, but certain authors have chosen to explain the maldistribution of medical, economic and social facilities not so much in terms of urban versus rural but rather as the outcome of the class structure and alliances within (and outside) any country. In particular, Zaidi (1985: 474) suggests that 'there is no urban conspiracy against the rural population,' but rather that the various classes, whether urban or rural, have tended to strive for their own benefit. The urban bias in distribution of medical services, among others, stems from the spatial imbalance in concentration of wealthy and ruling élites. The role of the state in capitalist societies strays from the neutral, and dominant or class interests will tend to be favoured in the allocation and distribution of resources. The government reflects these power groups in deciding who gets what where. If the rich are concentrated in cities, it is in these places that political power lies, and, as a result, they are favoured in service provision.

The state and medical training

From this set of propositions, it is possible to start to explain the distribution of resources to the more powerful urban areas. The ground rules for medical training are in most cases set by the state. At the level of the individual, the decision-making process also reflects, for example, the choice of professions to follow, and the decision of where to train tends to be influenced by subsequent rewards and status. In particular, in many Third World countries, an élitist medical education patterned on Western models suits the requirements of the domestic ruling classes if not the needs of the majority. The preference for high-technology, high-status, Western-oriented medical training is evident in many ex-colonial Third World countries, particularly in the majority that have pursued a capitalist orientation to development.

Role of medical training

The reasons for an urban bias in health facilities (especially 'medical' facilities *per se*) can be traced in part to the Western orientation in training. The role of medical education is thus crucial as it favours training doctors in keeping with the values and requirements of those with income sufficient to purchase medical care (Zaidi 1985). Most of these people will require 'quality' modern care and most of them will be found in the more prosperous urban areas. Hence, this is where many doctors and specialists will practice. Apart from the possibility of higher fee earnings, there is also a better availability of medical facilities and the opportunity to practise 'modern' medicine, from a narrowly perceived medical base, in the centres near to the major and prestigious medical and academic institutions. In such locations is employment most likely for highly regarded academics. In addition, opportunities for postgraduate study (preferably abroad, with its attendant higher professional and public evaluation) are likewise largely to be found in urban settings. This urban bias goes hand in hand with the al-most universal orientation in Third World countries towards curative health services rather than preventive and promotive ser-vices. Often, well over 90 per cent of national health budgets are spent on curative services, and especially on high-technology hospi-tal services. The relatively minor proportions of budgets usually devoted to preventive, public health and community services con-tinue to foster the 'urban is best' image in health care. In spite of the alleged desire in many Third World health plans to shift resources and emphasis to rural provision, and to community and education health services, relatively little has been achieved in many cases. This is discussed further in Chapter 5 in so far as it is in-separable from comprehensive PHC strategies.

The Western orientation and urban bias in medical training of doctors and many nurses in the Third World may actually render them virtually unqualified and certainly inexperienced to deal with ailments and conditions commonly found in rural areas. This is par-ticularly true of conditions related to diet custom and practice, but even common traumas such as snakebite may be new to urban-trained professionals. In addition, the medical curricula in many Third World medical schools have tended to be medically 'traditional', with an emphasis on curative aspects and practice in hospitals, devoting less attention to prevention, public health, com-munity medicine and rural health. Ironically, many medical schools, particularly the newer, in Europe and North America now introduce all types of health students early on to community medi-cal provision, the value of PHC and teamwork.

The effects of 'high-tech' medical education and ideas im-ported from developed countries can therefore, first, increase the maldistribution of resources and give a spurious air of inappropriate 'modernity' to many Third World health systems and, secondly, result in the emigration of doctors and qualified staff abroad. This is understandable if highly trained and mobile staff see overseas opportunities for higher incomes and for professional practice using the equipment for which they have been trained. The Philippines illustrates both these points: Metro-Manila has an over-preponderance of 'high-tech' facilities such as centres for heart and lung ailments, ostensibly taking patients from all of Asia. It also, as a matter of national economic policy, fosters the emigration of trained professionals (doctors, nurses, accountants, lawyers and surveyors) to earn money abroad, with agreed amounts to be remitted home. Similarly, the dependence of many hospitals and health systems in North America and Europe, including Britain, on doctors and nurses from the Indian subcontinent is well recog-nized. The rural people of these countries might justifiably enquire why expensively trained personnel from their national institutions prefer to practise their skills for the benefit of other wealthier nations.

Unfilled vacancies and the need for rural service initiatives

The provision of medical and health education has been markedly urban-oriented both in physical location of universities and colleges and in the wider systems in which they have been set. To succeed professionally, doctors and nurses and other medical workers usually require access to post-qualification training and experience (however relevant or irrelevant to the real needs of the nation in question). This is most readily available in those places with large institutions and particularly teaching hospitals. The availability of good 'modern' facilities and technology, interesting cases and revered professors is equated with professional advancement and as such is available mainly in urban settings. Zaidi (1985) notes that this is reflected in vacancy rates for doctors and nurses in Pakistan. In the Punjab, for example, some 75 per cent of rural doctors' posts were vacant, compared with 27 per cent of urban posts; for nurses, 41 per cent of rural and 15 per cent of urban posts were vacant. In Sind, only 9 per cent of urban but 24 per cent of rural doctors' posts were vacant, and 21 per cent of urban nursing places but 60 per cent of rural posts were vacant. In Malawi, it is the remoter rural districts and health units that are likely to be staffed by un-qualified personnel. The same picture is to be seen in many other countries, emphasizing that it is unwise to rely merely on official figures for 'established' posts to indicate rural–urban imbalances. When the numbers of actual personnel employed are investigated, rural areas may be found to be even worse off than they appear on official figures.

This has led a number of developing countries to try to impose a period of rural service for newly qualified doctors and health professionals. The Philippines, for example, in the late 1970s initiated a requirement that new medical and nursing graduates undertake a period of service of 6 months in rural areas as a condition of registration (Reforma 1977). All medical graduates in Venezuela must enter a 1- or 2-year 'rural medicine' programme, which can include service in urban barrio health modules, considered almost rural because of their lack of modern infrastructure and in the characteristics of their population (Rakowski and Kastner 1985). In Jamaica, compulsory rural service in conjunction with social and preventive medicine training for medical students and graduates has actually proved popular with many who have gained their first experience of the medical problems of their rural compatriots. Here, however, distances to higher-order facilities are not as great as in many other developing countries. By contrast, compulsory rural service for medical science graduates has proved very unpopular in some parts of Nicaragua because of the dangers of rural attacks (Garfield 1989). Some countries, particularly those with socialist or revolutionary regimes, such as China and Mozambique, have attempted to go further and stress the value of rural service to national social and economic development. For the majority of Third World countries, it seems that increasing future direction of trained personnel to rural locations will be inevitable if the great rural–urban imbalances that exist (and are often worsening) are to be ameliorated.

Attitudes of medical students

In the Western world, many studies have demonstrated that medical students often have strong preferences as to where they would like to work when qualified. There is frequently a desire to work in the general proximity of their medical school, and quality of life indices and opportunities for earning from private practice also have some influence. Relatively less research on medical student preferences has been set in Third World countries but a study by Karalliedde *et al.* (1987) showed that newly qualified Sri Lankan doctors were most likely to opt for the major specialties: very few expressed career preferences for the disciplines related to PHC and few wanted to teach in medical schools. Another study by Zaidi (1986) has addressed the question of why medical students will not practise in rural areas. This study encompassed five medical colleges in Sind (which has some 44 per cent of all Pakistan's medical students) and sought information on students' professional and locatorial aspirations when qualified as doctors.

The survey showed that the vast majority (89 per cent) of students came from cities and exceptionally few from rural areas. This suggested a built-in unlikelihood of subsequently working in rural areas since most might logically choose to practise in their home towns or host cities. The majority of students were unfamiliar with rural life and, being often from the wealthier families in Pakistan, were to a considerable extent shielded from rural problems. Ironically, the few students from poorer families seemed even less likely to express preferences for working in rural areas ·as their opportunities for economic advancement would be fewer. Therefore, presumably, improving social access to medical schools will not automatically increase the number of rural doctors.

In view of the previous discussion about medical training, it is hardly surprising that 67 per cent of students expressed the hope of going to developed Western countries for specialization. On return, they will demand the sophisticated equipment for which they have been trained, both causing personal dissatisfaction when this is unavailable and increasing the urban, technology-orientation of Pakistan's health care when they are in a position to exert influence on future health policy. This is almost inevitable given the preponderance of doctors among the higher echelons of health care administrators in many Third World countries.

The Pakistan survey is of considerable interest because, whilst it supports the macro-level generalization made earlier about physicians' desires to work mainly in urban areas, it also attempted to delve more deeply into the social structure as a whole that underpins the medical system, and its élitism in Pakistan and many similar countries. Most medical students answered honestly, if unsurprisingly, and no doubt justifiably felt their aspirations for higher training and specialization to be in line with professional expectations. However, both government and social structure perpetuate this system, in allocating resources to urban rather than rural areas and confirming the latter as less desirable places for the practice of good modern care. As Zaidi (1986) concludes, in Pakistan as in most underdeveloped countries, a small, privileged class distributes resources according to its own need with little concern for the masses at large. Therefore, it is hardly surprising that most medical students express a lack of interest in rural practice because of lack of facilities, lack of opportunities, poor income and the like. Until these are improved, rural areas will not be attractive to young, aspiring professionals. The only hope otherwise may be that an oversupply of medical staff, which ironically appears even in some developing countries, may compel some to seek employment in less popular areas or specialisms (Butter and Mejiá 1987).

Of equal concern, however, is the lack of acquaintance of students with health conditions in rural, and also poor urban, areas. Overall, it is concluded that the class system in such societies, with its privileged access to health care and also to medical training, has actually predetermined the responses of these students. It is arguably the main factor that causes a dearth of medical manpower in rural areas. Certainly, these attitudes may be linked with the attitude of the modern medical sector, which frequently views traditional medicine as inferior. Since traditional medicine predominates in many rural localities, this further reduces their attractiveness for the modern professional élite, who may be sceptical of, or fear, working in close contact with traditional practitioners. Such research deserves wider replication in other Third World medical systems.

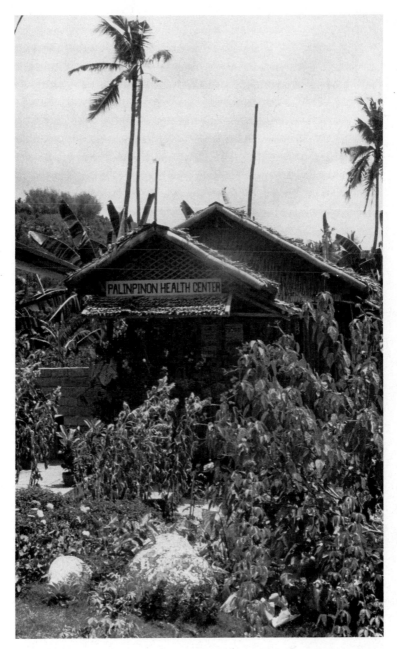

Plate 1 Primary health care post in the Central Visayas, the
Philippines; constructed mainly of locally available materials

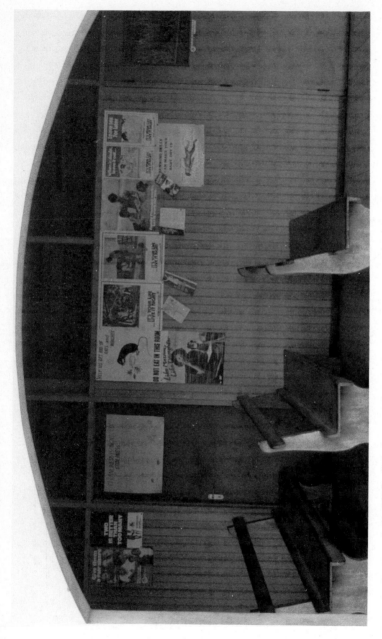

Plate 2   Purpose-built PHC clinic in rural Jamaica; note range of health and environmental advisory posters

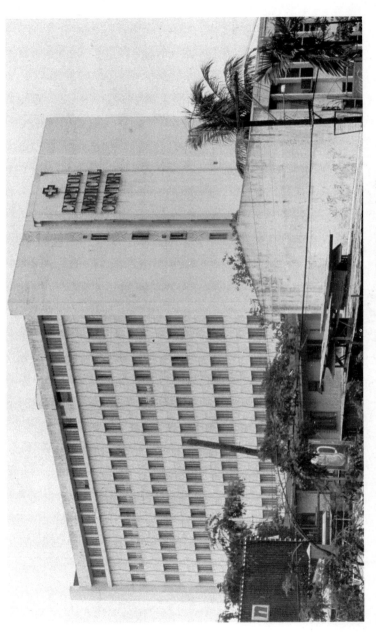

Plate 3   Metro-Manila, the Philippines; large, centralized private health care facility

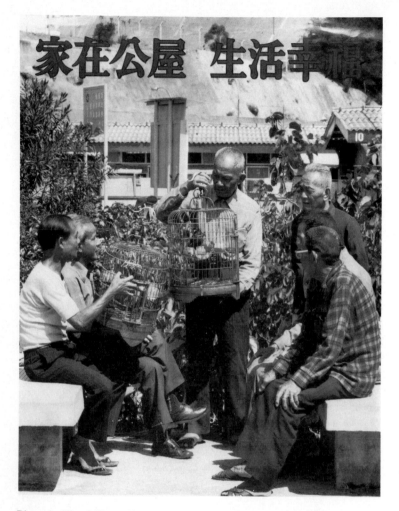

Plate 4 Hong Kong Housing Authority poster: the Authority is promoting the idea of successful retirement housing

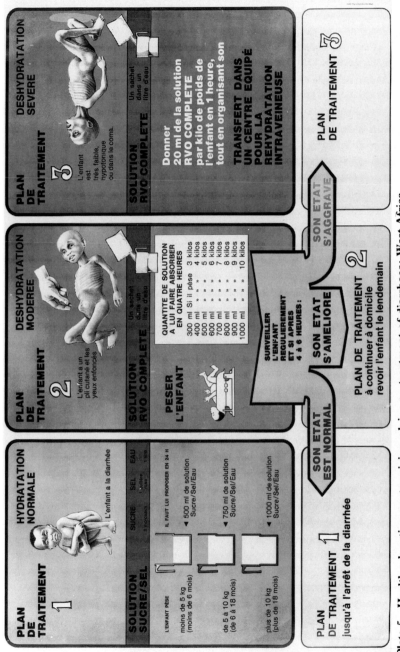

Plate 5 Health education poster giving advice on treatment of diarrhoea: West Africa.

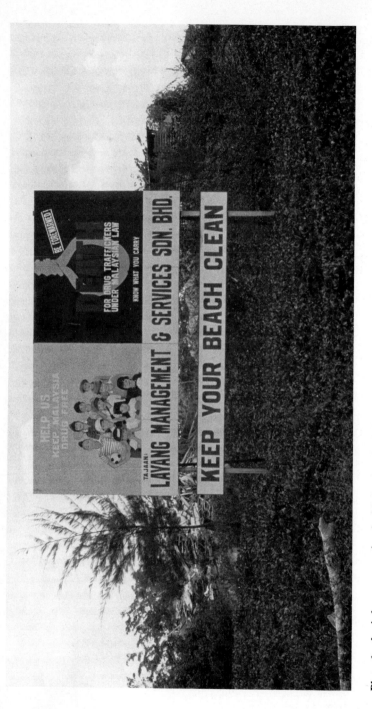

Plate 6 Anti-drugs campaign in Malaysia (the board is sponsored by a company)

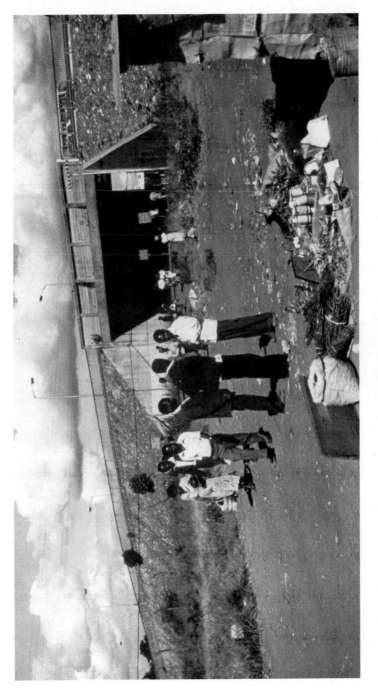

Plate 7 Traditional medical practitioner, Lusaka, Zambia; the stall has been set up near to an important thoroughfare and public building

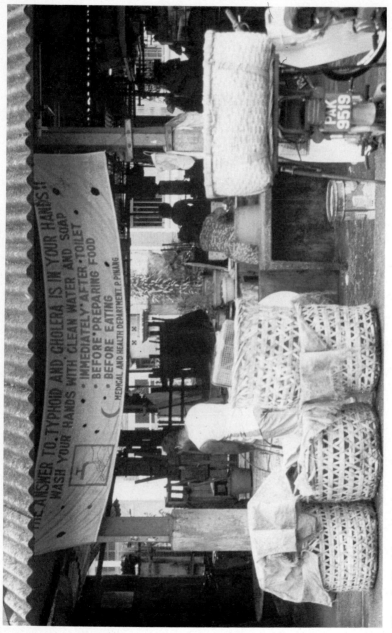

Plate 8 Health promotion and education in the market place: Penang, Malaysia

Optimizing accessibility: a Third World dilemma?

We have already noted that health care resources in many Third World countries are both inequitably distributed and inefficiently applied, although some attempts have been made to adjust such inequalities (those related to PHC and some specific sectors are discussed in Chapters 5 and 7). In general, however, the aim of much locational planning in health care has been allegedly to maximize accessibility to a given quantity of resources by optimizing spatial distributions. Various forms of spatial allocation models and spatial search have been used (Massam 1975, 1980, 1987; Massam *et al.* 1986), which, under a given set of 'acceptable' criteria, identify a number of solutions to the location of a set of health care facilities. These can be compared with the distribution of existing facilities and capacities and areas of oversupply and deficiency identified.

A practical weakness of many models for optimizing accessibility, from the point of view of the Third World in particular, is that reliable data are frequently unavailable and the models can rarely take account of all the variables that seem to influence resource allocation and health services utilization (discussed in Chapter 6). Travel costs, time, convenience, personal preference, physicians' behaviour, the nature of a facility and its reputation and the like can all be crucial. In many developing countries, local knowledge of what is available at any given facility and the length of time that one may have to wait are also crucial, as are various personal and institutional hindrances that are not easily modelled as their variables are either non-quantifiable or change from time to time. Therefore, many optimally-designed spatial health care delivery systems are not practical in the Third World.

The paucity of resources is, of course, a major constraint on the development of spatially optimal systems, particularly in the Third World. For example, a hospital, once provided, has to function for a long period to recoup the investment in it. It cannot generally be re-sited easily when population locations shift. It may, on the other hand, be much easier to open, close or move lower-order health services to take account of changed accessibility. However, in many Third World countries, not only are resources inadequate (especially for rural provision) but they are non-optimally located with respect to population accessibility (Mahadev and Thangamani 1984). Part of the problem is that health care delivery systems have often grown up in a fragmented manner, provided by public, private, charitable and aid sources, and they have frequently been non-complementary or even competing in their functions and locations. Political influence, corruption and fortuitous factors have often played their part in bringing about the present-day (mal)distribution of facilities.

Data permitting, location-allocation modelling may be used as a planning tool to assist decisions on the optimal location of a given number of facilities in a region. Alternatively, it may be used to compare the congruence of an existing distribution with a theoretically derived one, and may assist in adjusting existing location and capacity. The procedure allocates facilities to locations that will serve the most people yet minimize travel distances. However, theoretical answers do tend to neglect social and economic variation among populations, and thus can ignore equity considerations.

An application of a location-allocation model in Guatemala City indicated a quite severe imbalance in the existing distribution of primary health dispensaries, which seemed to reflect more the locational choice of local and national politicians than any objective attempt to evaluate the population's need for services (Mulvihill 1979). Guatemala City consumers, especially the poorest, were having to undertake considerably longer journeys than necessary because of the spatial maldistribution of dispensaries. In addition, a lack of confidence that certain smaller facilities could meet all a consumer's needs meant that some facilities were being bypassed and long distances travelled to larger centres perceived as more reliable. Such factors must inevitably impinge on the frequency and efficacy of utilization, with possible resultant harm to patients' health (Chapter 6). Many of the thirteen public health dispensaries studied in Guatemala City were experiencing very different levels of demand, which resulted in severe overcrowding in some and implied that others were working relatively inefficiently. Spatial maldistribution and resultant poor accessibility seem to be largely to blame for this feature; the existing pattern of health centres was based more on political motives than population need (Mulvihill 1979). However, it should be noted that aggregate modelling techniques cannot easily take account of behavioural or attitudinal variations among consumers and potential consumers. All are assumed to act logically, for instance, by attending their nearest offered facility.

Nevertheless, the application of a fairly sophisticated normative location-allocation model in the Guatemala City example suggested an improved spatial distribution that departs from the current pattern. The need for the provision of some new capacity and facilities, and also the relocation of certain existing capacity was identified. However, such a service- or facility-oriented approach to accessibility may not be ideal for developing countries. The upgrading of education, housing and sanitation are often just as crucial, although the optimizing of location, if and when new facilities or additional capacity are planned, also seems to be important to achieve the best distribution of scarce resources. The uncritical adoption of models of health care planning derived from developed countries is probably best avoided, and Mahadev and Thangamani (1984) indicate that in India, for example, experiments are being conducted into ways to optimize accessibility within realistic monetary and accessibility constraints. The modification of Western planning and accessibility models to suit local needs appears sensible although such refinements may in practice be difficult to achieve.

Simple catchment-area models to improve local accessibility

Changes in regional disparities over time may indicate improvement or deterioration of aggregate provision of health care facilities, but it is often desirable to know whether a local system is functioning or might function more effectively. A somewhat less sophisticated mode of analysis than spatial modelling may be used to identify areas that are well served or deficient in health services of various sorts. Simple measures of distance to facility and assumed catchment areas may be empirically imposed upon urban and rural settings and areas of deficiency or overlap observed. For example, in the large Pikine suburb of Dakar in Senegal, the coverage of the PHC posts was mapped and three types of areas were noted (see Fig. 4.14, p. 137): zones more than 500 m from a health facility, zones within a 500 m radius of a facility and zones covered by more than one facility (Laloe *et al.* 1986). This relatively straightforward type of cartographic analysis helps to highlight ostensibly poorly served and well-served subdistricts, in which further detailed research may be conducted on the effects of such variations in accessibility on specific types of utilization.

It should be noted that this type of approach does not generally take account of detailed variations in population density, age structure, mobility or the like. The refinement of adding a measure of population converted by facilities within a fixed catchment area can be included if local data are known. Whilst this is often difficult to identify precisely in many Third World cities, it is sometimes possible to estimate coverage in locations of wider-based facilities. An example of this is the study of proposed health care sites in Zambia, where at one time it was hoped to locate facilities so that everyone was, as far as possible, within 35 miles of a physician (Jackman 1972). When sites were identified, the type of facility (and the need for ground clinics or flying-doctor services) could then be decided in view of the number of people to be served within this catchment radius.

A similar exercise was conducted in the densely settled

Mulanje District of South-East Malawi. Here the objective was to identify under-served locations and to examine potential population catchments at possible new health centre locations. This informa-

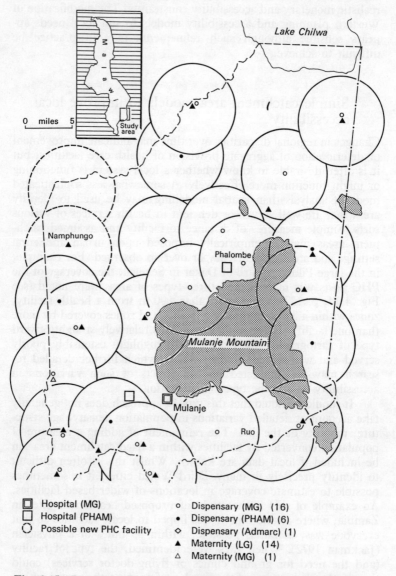

Fig. 4.15   Location of existing facilities and simple 5-mile (8-km) catchment radii to illustrate currently under-served areas in Mulanje District, Malawi, 1989 (based on author's data)

tion was to be used to decide whether new facilities (and of what capacities) could be provided within an assumed acceptable travel distance (Fig. 4.15). This was a 5-mile (8-km) radius of facilities, modified to take account of communications, and local topography and existing facilities. It is interesting to note that 5 miles is commonly being assumed to be an acceptable distance for people to travel to rural health care facilities in the Third World, but it needs considerable research into transport and travel circumstances to validate this locally.

A complementary approach to investigating health care accessibility is to derive the empirical catchment areas of specific facilities by mapping samples or enumerations of attenders. This type of research into revealed accessibility (by attendance at a given facility) may be of considerable use in the estimation of catchment-area extents, the efficiency of referrals, and whether any other facilities or locations are being bypassed. Often, especially in intra-urban situations, many services will be found to have overlapping and even competing catchment areas (Ingram *et al.* 1978; Joseph and Phillips 1984). However, mapping of catchment areas by raw attendance data does not take into account variations in population density and characteristics. Iyun (1983) found this a somewhat unsatisfactory method of defining hospital catchment areas in Ibadan City, Nigeria. When the percentage of patients from each ward (census tract) of the city going to any of the eighteen study hospitals was calculated, this type of analysis of utilization revealed a logical access to hospitals of different hierarchical rankings, namely, a higher proportion of patients was being sent from more wards to first-order hospitals than to second-order hospitals and so on. This confirms that 'standardized' utilization was following the hospital hierarchy. It did, nevertheless, enable the analysis of reasons for any decline in attendance frequency with distance from facility. This type of empirical study also enabled Iyun to identify two areas of Ibadan City that were desperately short of hospital facilities. These and other aspects of accessibility (the effects of distance on utilization) are further considered in Chapter Six.

Chapter 5

Primary health care

Primary health care

Primary health care has emerged as the dominant approach to health problems in most Third World countries. Its development has stemmed at least in part from the realization that the existing 'hierarchical' systems discussed in Chapter 4 have failed the vast majority of people. Its promotion stems from an acceptance of the proposition that health services should try to serve the bulk of people rather than a favoured few. It is also a *de facto*, practical recognition that highly facility-oriented, high-tech health care is neither appropriate for the majority of the health and development needs of most Third World countries, nor generally affordable. The principles of PHC have actually been practised for many years, although they have only been formally articulated since the mid-1970s. They have come to be the principal health care plank of many agency plans and national strategies.

The book that really first publicized the idea of the PHC approach stemmed from a joint critique by the WHO and the United Nations Children's Fund (UNICEF) of the effectiveness of existing health programmes and the extent to which they served people. The need was outlined for a shift to basic health services, not the least because of glaring inequalities in access to, and utilization of, formal health services in most countries. It was argued that fewer than 15 per cent of the rural and underprivileged populations of many Third World countries had access to modern health services. Clearly, the centralized, technological health care models of the industrialized world, unsuccessfully adopted by, and faltering in, many developing countries, were failing their people (Djukanovic and Mach 1975). The virtual revolution called for by this analysis implied changes not only in types of health care and their *location* but also in *attitudes* of administrators, providers, educators and 'receivers', who would become more actively involved not only in health but also in much wider tasks of economic and physical development. This became formally articulated by the WHO in 1978. Primary health workers were to become the foundations of health systems in developing countries; health would be 'by the people', for the people.

Primary health care has subsequently been espoused by the international health community as the major hope of solving, or at least ameliorating, the hugh health problems facing many Third World countries. True, various advocates debate points of detail and, sometimes, substance – for example, whether PHC should comprise a total package or only be selective in medical and demographic coverage – but, on the whole, the move towards primary rather than higher sectoral provision is generally accepted. Nevertheless, PHC as a concept is hardly new; it has undoubtedly existed for as long as man has sought assistance for health care and to tackle wider conditions harmful to health. In countries such as Britain, it became formalized in the years following the Second World War and, although existing earlier, it became recognized and emerged as an important effort in 'team care' at the local level, following the so-called 'renaissance of general practice' in the late 1950s (Hunt 1957; Phillips 1981b). In the Third World, it is possible to detect considerable elements of common-sense writing over 20 years which admitted that high-technology, hospital care was not only probably inappropriate for many problems but also highly unlikely to be practical in physical or financial terms (King 1966). In addition, the process of social development in many Third World countries mainly since the 1960s has been creating an atmosphere conducive to health care change: egalitarian, anti-élitist, PHC-type sentiments have clearly emerged (Gesler 1984). The most explicit formulation of PHC as a concept came in 1978, since when PHC has been identified as the strategy to move towards 'health for all by the year 2000'. This has become the WHO's slogan for the promotion of the concept.

Definitions of PHC

Primary health care was defined in the 1978 Alma Ata conference as being a mixture of curative, preventive and promotive activities of a basic nature, involving many segments of economy and society that have a bearing on health and welfare, not solely (primary) medical care. Within its broad ambit are numerous programmes and thrusts in individual countries and many of the health and health-related efforts such as FP, MCH and the like discussed in Chapter 7 are for practical purposes activities within PHC itself. More recently, selective PHC has been suggested to target and confront specific health problems in given areas. This has given rise to considerable controversy; it is especially criticized by those who suggest that, because of its selective nature, SPHC does not address the infrastructural and social problems injurious to health and, as it does not try to improve and upgrade the whole community's health, it runs counter to the spirit of PHC. This is discussed in detail below.

The underlying objectives of PHC as expressed in the 1978 declaration indicate the integration of two main streams of activities and processes. One relates to the growth and extension of basic health services; the other involves development of the local community in terms of infrastructure, education, initiatives and resources. These objectives are incorporated in the definition of PHC as:

> essential health care made universally accessible to individuals and families in the community by means acceptable to them, through their full participation and at a cost that the community and country can afford. It forms an integral part of the country's health system, of which it is the nucleus, and of the overall social and economic development in the community. (Who 1978a: 34)

Changing theories of development particularly question the ambiguous role of modernization along Western lines, and have changed attitudes to technological intervention and to social phenomena such as population growth and the role of women. These have all underlain the growth of the PHC approach. Its philosophy has often become health care policy, involving first-contact services and front-line workers within a framework of eight activities and five basic principles: equitable distribution, community involvement, focus on prevention, appropriate technology and a multisectoral approach. These principles should assist Third World countries in particular – although the PHC approach is not by any means exclusively for poorer countries – to think of ways extending health services to their often neglected rural or urban slum citizens (Walt and Vaughan 1981).

The five principles provide a framework for the basic components of a PHC service:

- education about diseases, health problems and their control
- safe water and basic sanitation
- MCH, including FP
- immunization against major infectious diseases
- appropriate treatment of common diseases and injuries
- provision of essential drugs

The totality of these components would, in varying balances in different settings, be part of a comprehensive PHC approach. Primary health care as defined above embodies the basic needs approach, and the provision of essential health services with community involvement and participation. It is wider than the institutionally oriented basic health services approach of the 1960s, as it attempts to have the front-line of daily activities carried out within the community (Ebrahim and Ranken 1988).

Many components have nevertheless been singled out and are clearly to be seen within subsequent MCH, FP or selective immunization programmes and perhaps most clearly in some SPHC approaches. However, whatever the range of cover, a basic tenet of the PHC approach should remain that services are not exclusively technocratic and provided by highly trained, technologically oriented professionals. At different levels, auxiliaries, community workers and, where appropriate, traditional practitioners will be involved within the broad orbit of health services. It is also accepted that a referral network should exist to give mutual support at all levels, and especially to provide care not locally available. Indeed, there is strong encouragement for hospitals, for example, to become involved in the overall health of the communities in which they are located and to participate directly in PHC activities. Primary health care should thus be broad-based essential care but should not be totally divorced from higher levels of the health care hierarchy. It is fair to say that the practicalities of the PHC approach are still evolving internationally, and the WHO has chosen to continue to promote the approach as the major method of stimulating services and extending them to neglected groups.

Primary health care is by definition wide-ranging and not purely a health activity, and intersectoral collaboration is a key element (Ebrahim and Ranken 1988). It involves combined health and community development, and its success depends on task-oriented activity (for example, focusing on the health problems of the community) and a process-oriented movement (involving education, improving economic and social conditions, food availability and so on). Therein lies the potential for conflict because, whilst many people will favour the improvement of services and facilities, the implementation of social change may be reluctantly accepted or even opposed in some instances. Primary health care therefore becomes not a cheap, quick, problem-oriented activity but complex and difficult to achieve, perhaps expensive if done properly, and probably slow (Fendall 1985). The involvement in addition to health of all related sectors of the economy – such as agriculture, animal husbandry, education, housing, public works and communications – may prove extremely difficult in many Third World countries, where a lack of intersectoral coordination and cooperation, not to mention a lack of resources, is often a fundamental reason for problems in the first place.

Figure 5.1 shows diagrammatically the components of the PHC approach. These include PHC programme elements (such as health education, food and nutrition, immunization, MCH and FP, and essential drugs provision) and their relationship to what will often be a loose functional infrastructure – permissive rather than excessively overadministrative – including information, manage-

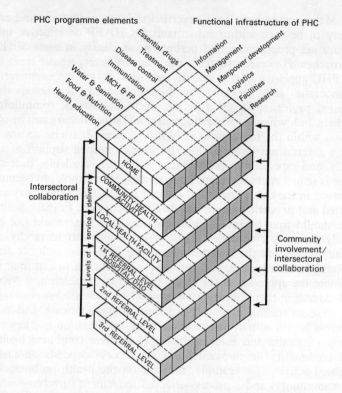

PHC programme elements   Functional infrastructure of PHC

Essential drugs
Treatment
Disease control
Immunization
MCH & FP
Water & Sanitation
Food & Nutrition
Health education

Information
Management
Manpower development
Logistics
Facilities
Research

Intersectoral
collaboration

Levels of service delivery

HOME
COMMUNITY HEALTH ACTIVITY
LOCAL HEALTH FACILITY
1st REFERRAL LEVEL HOSPITAL/DHQ
2nd REFERRAL LEVEL
3rd REFERRAL LEVEL

Community
involvement/
intersectoral
collaboration

**Fig. 5.1 Conceptual model of a comprehensive health system based
on the principles of PHC (adapted from WHO 1987d)**

ment, facilities and research. These components can and should occur and interact at various levels of 'care' (broadly defined). The
intersectoral collaboration and community involvement at all levels
provide the totality of the PHC approach.

Community participation

The reliance at local levels on health workers (trained, part-trained
and untrained personnel) can be a source of strength, although it
can also place great strain on some communities. However, with
regard to community participation in health planning itself, it is
suggested that community development is a key (Rifkin 1985). Its
success and contribution to health planning rely on activities that

do not necessarily have to be directly health related, but can include education, housing, income generation and the like. This important aspect of the PHC approach is discussed below but, within it, six critical issues emerge, relating to:

1. the role of health services;
2. views about community participation;
3. the role of the professional;
4. the role and training of CHWs;
5. evaluation of programmes;
6. financial support of programmes.

These can be viewed in a matrix model illustrating the way in which community participation in community health problems can interact (Rifkin 1985). These are obviously of relevance for the promotion and successful implementation of PHC.

Primary health care was, in its earliest specific formulation with regard to poor countries, widely seen as 'the wave of the future' (Joseph and Russell 1980). It was viewed as being a cost-effective way of saving lives at risk because of receiving no help, rather than saving fewer lives by investment in higher-technology care and health care infrastucture which would reach only a small proportion of the population. It is possible, however, to argue a case for restricting PHC to a much narrower spectrum of activities than outlined above and, particularly, for it to become selective and disease-orientated. In addition, many interest groups can compete in developing countries and arguments for the expansion of secondary and tertiary facilities are frequently advanced in the Third World as part of a 'modernization' thesis; viewed against these, PHC can be depicted by some as a lower quality, even a 'backward', option. However, in the context of many of the poorest countries, PHC should not be regarded as second-class medicine and help; it can be a rational course of action, responsive to local needs and conditions and, above all, appropriate. The reality for the vast majority of the population in many developing countries is that, in so far as Western medicine and effective traditional medicine are to be available, they will only be provided via PHC. In particular, the community improvements elements of PHC are attractive, and proponents argue that some significant advances can be made whatever the social and political context. Nevertheless, early enthusiasm for PHC has been dampened, and much research into its utilization and 'effectiveness' (however this may be measured) is required to evaluate how far it is really meeting the needs of specific populations, and how far the existence of PHC is, so to speak, a placebo.

The adoption of PHC as a national strategy faces a number of specific obstacles, which differ in their relative importance and severity between countries. These generally include financial, social and political problems. In economic terms, donor support is often associated with 'donor leverage' – the forced acceptance of the ideas of specific agencies, which often demand rapid, tangible results. Finance for PHC is frequently a major problem, even when donor aid is available. For example, at the inception of the PHC 'ideal' in 1978, it was estimated that the costs of extending PHC systems to reach the entire population of countries on a continuing basis would involve 5 year start-up costs and 10 year additional operating costs between $US20 and 33 billion in low-income countries and $US20 and 52 billion in lower middle-income countries. The populations of each group totalled about 1.3 billion, which would mean per capita expenditures in the range of $15 to $25 in low-income and middle-income countries. However, at the time, only roughly $1.5 to $3.5 per capita was being spent on health in the public sector in each group (Joseph and Russell 1980) and, in some countries such as the Philippines, even less (Phillips 1986a). Therefore, this suggests massive donor aid will be necessary to supplement national budgets to implement and expand PHC for all populations needing care by the end of the century. Such levels of aid are both problematic for receptor countries and unlikely to be maintained (Chapter 8).

Other problems are political and practical. The former relate to inadequate political commitment and informed leadership at national and international levels. In particular, the ideals and objectives of certain national health ministries will have to be altered to accommodate the breadth of PHC, as many continue to be hospital- and hierarchy-oriented. Practical problems include a lack of organizational, personnel and managerial resources, especially at the lower tiers of health systems. This can be particularly difficult to overcome if local professionals and influential community members are resistant to PHC ideas that may involve them in loss of power. Finally, the problem of replicating successful pilot or demonstration projects (of restricted population or spatial scale) more widely is often immense. Once critical thresholds of available resources, personnel and the like are reached, further expansion may be impossible. As a result, whilst many successful small-scale, pilot PHC programmes have been started, their effective spread is often some way off (MacCormack 1984). Realistic pacing of national programmes is therefore essential. The Philippines, for example, one of the first countries to adopt PHC as an explicit national strategy, has encountered manpower and resources bottlenecks and has had to rush forward training programmes for paid and voluntary personnel (Phillips 1986a).

Doubts about PHC

Primary health care has become widely regarded as a positive package, and one that will hopefully reach the majority of populations in time. However, there are growing doubts as to its real long-term potential, and these do not solely focus on the problems mentioned above but relate to more fundamental explanations of the existing patterns of inequality in health and access to health resources. These can be seen as involving the 'development of underdevelopment' debate, and many lay the blame on previous colonial systems, which undervalued the health of the masses (by neglect and by exploitation) whilst catering for the élite. Health, it can also be argued, has more 'positively' been changed in many Third World countries (Stock 1986). From such perspectives, Mac-Pherson (1982) explains that improved health is not simply, or even mainly, a matter of medical systems. Rather, a much more complex question of the relationship between health and underdevelopment, and the nature of underdevelopment, is involved.

Gish (1979) has noted that a persuasive approach was to spread scientific Western medicine to peoples considered backward and disordered; they would benefit in so far as they became like those who administered to them. To some extent, this assumption appears to have been correct and such people did prosper. However, the post-war independence of many countries has not eliminated the extremes of poverty, hunger and ill health that were developing in colonial days: indeed, in many countries, these have probably been exacerbated. The expansion of modern medicine has barely even kept pace with the needs of élite and growing middle classes in many developing countries, and the manifest incapability of 'modern' health systems to cope with the growing demands on them has led to many calls for 'health by the people', to meet the needs of the impoverished (particularly for nutrition and public health). Primary health care has become the vehicle for such thrusts, but many projects are isolated and wider impacts to date have often been limited. The approach does help, nevertheless, to circumvent some of the barriers to utilization of integrated health and other resources that can be created by a narrow technological approach to health care.

However, Gish (1979) argues that disillusion with existing health care delivery systems should not permit the persistence of an inequitable two-tier health care system (the better tier for the minority: high-technology and expensive; the inferior PHC level for the poorer: at worst meaning no care). Primary health care strategies may in fact become only a palliative; in the absence of change in the whole of the health care system, they can lead to disappointment and frustration. The major obstacles to more just and efficient health care systems are, it is argued, often not the obvious ones (limited resources, poor communications, lack of data and the like), but social systems that place a low value on the health care needs of the poor. Primary health care may have some effectiveness but improved health in the Third World is not necessarily primarily a matter of 'medical systems'. It involves better understanding of the nature of underdevelopment itself (Gish 1979), and the local and international reasons for its perpetuation.

Personnel involved in PHC

Several types of primary health workers with greater or lesser degrees of formal training have been identified. A common theme is that all need a 'wider social outlook' than the purely clinical or bureaucratic; this certainly applies to hospital staff who might become involved in PHC or its support. The community, in a broad sense, should also be involved in the total PHC approach but, in most events, and especially in the SPHC variant, the burden inevitably falls onto specific individuals. Today, the participation of relatively lowly skilled workers in PHC is often made a virtue in that it is suggested they are closer to the people, more acceptable and, of course, available in greater numbers more quickly than trained medical staff. Considerable reliance has been placed on paid or unpaid 'health aides', CHWs or VHWs in the provision of services to rural communities (the precise terms by which such PHC personnel may be known varies from country to country, as discussed below).

Some trained staff, particularly nurses, are often 'key' PHC personnel and some trained physicians are also involved. However, generally the latter are not permanently stationed in rural sites, although they may be found in larger primary health units. A crucial issue concerns the relevance of professional medical and nursing training to the needs of the localities in which PHC is set. A few countries have tried to make their syllabuses for nurses a better preparation for the realities that will confront them outside the hospital (Ebrahim and Ranken 1988). Often, a wide understanding of public health and local ecologies, and considerable skill in communication with people in their own home settings, are required.

Primary health personnel, particularly volunteers, have, however, often been regarded as peripheral health workers who have limited influence on the effectiveness of national medical services. Others argue that, on the contrary, low-level workers are in effect 'central' to PHC, as they are frequently the only formal health providers with whom the majority of the population come into contact. This realization has grown in recent years as it has become increasingly apparent that a medical division of labour based on practices in the industrial world is a barrier to the provision of basic health care services in many developing countries (Frankel 1984). A technologically oriented system based on formally qualified staff, in which care (and especially 'quality' care) is associated with referral up a hierarchy, is seldom an appropriate model for a Third World country. The upper tiers of the hierarchy on which this would depend often do not exist or are inadequate in quantity, quality or distribution to meet the needs of the population. An orientation towards PHC by all is therefore a practical and preferable approach.

Selective PHC

The comprehensive PHC strategy endorsed by the countries attending the 1978 Alma Ata conference has not necessarily been fully implemented nor is it universally viewed as the most effective means of moving towards 'health for all'. A version commonly known as *selective primary health care* has been proposed and sometimes adopted because, whilst the comprehensive approach is laudable and arguably 'ideal', its very scope and breadth often make it unattainable because of bottlenecks and shortages in finance, personnel and, perhaps, good will. Therefore, faced with a vast number of health problems of varying severity, proponents of SPHC argue that these cannot all be tackled simultaneously; some priorities must be assigned to various tasks for reasons of practicality, cost and effective use of resources. An article by Walsh and Warren (1979) introduced the concept to a wide audience, and in particular focused on the types and nature of diseases that might be tackled in an SPHC approach.

Selective PHC typically focuses on paediatric conditions, such as measles, whooping cough, neonatal tetanus and diarrhoeal diseases (Table 5.1). It has the effect of reducing priorities to those conditions which can be treated or averted at the least cost and so, cynically, it may be argued that it merely places relative costs on human lives. The typical SPHC targets, measles and whooping cough for example, have effective vaccines; neonatal tetanus is vaccinable and preventable with sterile practice; diarrhoeal diseases likewise have preventive measures, and ORT is known and available in many places. A lower priority is usually accorded to conditions such as polio, typhoid, respiratory infections, meningitis and malnutrition, a varied group of which only polio can effectively

Table 5.1   Selective PHC: some identified priorities for disease control in the developing world (from Walsh and Warren 1979)

Priority group	Reasons for assignment to this category
I High	
Diarrhoeal diseases	High prevalence, high mortality or high morbidity, effective control
Measles	High prevalence, high mortality, no effective control
Malaria	High prevalence, low mortality, effective control
Whooping cough	High prevalence, high mortality, control difficult
Schistosomiasis	Medium prevalence, high morbidity, low mortality, control difficult
Neonatal tetanus	Medium prevalence, high mortality, control difficult
II Medium	
Respiratory infections	Medium prevalence, high mortality, control difficult
Poliomyelitis	High prevalence, low mortality, control difficult
Tuberculosis	High prevalence, low mortality, control difficult
Onchocerciasis	High prevalence, high morbidity, control complex
Meningitis	
Typhoid	Control difficult
Hookworm	Low prevalence, control difficult
Malnutrition	Control difficult
III Low	
South American trypanosomiasis (Chagas' disease)	Low mortality, low morbidity, control difficult
African trypanosomiasis	Low mortality, low morbidity.
Leprosy	Control difficult
Ascariasis	Control difficult
Diphtheria	Control difficult
Amoebiasis	Control difficult
Leishmaniasis	Control difficult
Giardiasis	Control difficult
Filariasis	Control difficult
Dengue	Control difficult

Source: Walsh and Warren (1979)

be controlled by medical intervention. The lowest priorities in SPHC terms would be accorded to diseases such as dengue, filariasis and amoebiasis, as their control is difficult, largely socio-environmental and hence costly and needing continued efforts. As Fendall (1985: 312) points out, 'the complex poverty syndrome of malnutrition, gastro-enteric diseases and respiratory infection will not yield to specific programmes: the only sure answer that exists today lies in social and environmental engineering'. In this, housing, potable water and safe sanitation are at the top of the list, for otherwise even the effective treatment of many conditions (particularly diarrhoeal and respiratory infections) may only result in cured children becoming rapidly reinfected. However, SPHC does not address these broad issues.

It is its very selectivity that provides the major weakness of SPHC to its critics. Whilst few would deny the seriousness of the conditions addressed by SPHC, the major criticism is of the attack on individual illnesses without upgrading the community conditions as a whole. As a consequence, SPHC has been called a thinly disguised euphemism for the disease-approach (Fendall 1985), too technologically and cost oriented (Berman 1982) and contestable on numerous practical and theoretical grounds (Banerji 1988; Barker and Turshen 1986; Gish 1982; Rifkin and Walt 1986, 1988; Unger and Killingsworth 1986).

Selective PHC, like primary *medical* care, is nevertheless an inherent part of PHC but is not the whole of it. The diseases tackled by SPHC would feature highly on any list of health problems in most low-income countries for the simple reason they are usually the major combatable causes of mortality. However, in a comprehensive PHC package, they would be approached in a wider and community-oriented manner and their control would take place in the context of overall community upgrading. Selective PHC, by contrast, suggests that specific interventionist programmes can be aimed at identified conditions, rapidly reducing or even eliminating them. The major thrusts of selective health care would be directed towards preventing or treating the few disorders that are responsible for the greatest morbidity and mortality in less-developed areas and for which *interventions of proved efficacy* exist (Unger and Killingsworth 1986; Walsh and Warren 1979). Therefore, instead of a full health infrastructure based on a comprehensive PHC package, the SPHC approach would reduce the scope of health services to those which were justifiable in cost-effectiveness terms. This is required, it is argued, as full PHC is often unattainable because of the costs and personnel limitations identified above and because the wide provision of infrastructure entailed, especially water and sanitation, is often initially far too expensive and not practically maintainable. Critics argue against the use of SPHC both from a philosophical point of view and on the grounds that case studies cited by Walsh and Warren in support of SPHC often had dubious methodologies and ambiguous results. Certain aspects of the application of SPHC are important. For example, in SPHC, physicians tend to be confined to simple, mainly non-medical roles, including personnel management and maintenance of medical supplies. This restriction on their roles may decrease doctors' incentives to participate, and increase their urban orientation. Medical assistants are rarely required since their broader skills would not be utilized effectively in disease-control programmes that focus on a relatively narrow range of immunization and the like. The activities of SPHC are often largely logistical, involving questions of, for example, how to cover populations effectively for immunizations, and thus focus on supply, transport and personnel matters.

It is, nevertheless, widely appreciated that a large number of infectious diseases, especially among children, can be prevented by immunization or treated relatively quickly by medical intervention. The extended immunization programmes referred to in Chapter 7 bear adequate witness to this fact. However, the economic, social and environmental conditions that might have led to certain important illnesses (such as diarrhoeal or deficiency diseases) are not changed by purely medical intervention. These conditions require much broader-based environmental improvements, necessitating education and nutrition programmes. A major shortcoming of a selective interventionist approach is that patients cured of infectious conditions may be returned to environments where they will be reinfected. Nevertheless, the immunization elements do at least tend to confer a relatively long-lasting immunity to specific life-threatening diseases. In addition, as its selective nature tends to focus on problems of paediatric and maternal illness, SPHC excludes much of the adult population, especially males. It is therefore inevitable that the 'magic bullet' approach of SPHC will exclude quite large sections of the population.

Selective PHC has implicit scientific appeal as well as a cost-effectiveness attraction because its interventions appear to be determined by rational choice and, to achieve the desired effectiveness, they typically concentrate on a very limited number of health conditions (perhaps five to ten, or fewer). These are selected on the basis of prevalence, mortality, morbidity and 'feasibility of control'. As a result, the focus is on a minimum number of important conditions that affect large numbers of people, but SPHC ignores interventions known to be of low, questionable or unmeasured efficacy, or of too great cost, such as treatment of tuberculosis, pneumonia, leprosy and worm infestations. These might of course be substantial burdens in terms of community health. Unlike comprehensive PHC, SPHC services can, it is argued, be 'selectively' appended as conditions change and interventions may be chosen to suit any given circumstances. They may be regarded as a way of targeting scarce resources rationally. The implementation of selective programmes received a major boost in 1982/83 with UNICEF's declaration about improving child health through four specific advances in its GOBI scheme, discussed in Chapter 7 (Walsh 1988; Warren 1988).

Is the debate between the advocates of comprehensive PHC, on the one hand, and Walsh and Warren, on the other, therefore amenable to resolution? Walsh and Warren are not extremists in their assertions but they do claim to be making value-free choices in the advocation of SPHC. They recognize that, however evaluated, health resources in the Third World are scarce. Secondly, health problems can in practice be evaluated to assign to each a rating of importance, prevalence and tractability (Lipkin 1982; Walsh 1988). The population of a poor nation will inevitably have to make choices about how to spend its scarce resources: spreading them too thinly may mean no effect at all. Protagonists of SPHC argue their case on the grounds of objectivity and practicality, since populations may wish to attack those of the most severe problems which bear the highest probability of yielding to specific, proven approaches.

The most sustained argument against SPHC and all selective approaches (such as the Expanded Programme on Immunization: EPI) comes from the philosophical objection to the technocratic intervention by the West, which denies local initiative. Banerji (1988) and others feel this is an extension of the long use of control over access to health services as a means of perpetuating the social and economic domination of developed nations over the Third World. Comprehensive PHC represents, at least symbolically, the opportunities for promotion of self-help and democratization of health services. 'Vested interests have struck back by glorifying the work of Walsh and Warren' (Banerji 1988: 297) and, by use of political and economic strength, have imposed selective, Western-determined programmes on the Third World. This type of criticism is, of course, justifiable but is generally countered by reference to the need for judicious use of scarce resources. Many health-related professionals have wished to reaffirm the principles of comprehensive PHC and these were embodied in the Haikko declaration issued in 1986, summarized in Table 5.2 (Segall and Vienonen 1987).

It cannot be escaped that SPHC approaches do not tackle many of the numerous basic health problems (Fendall 1985; Heggenhougen 1984; Rifkin and Walt 1986). For a start, it seems that SPHC interventions involve the adoption of a narrower definition

Table 5.2 Summary of the Haikko Declaration on actions for PHC (adapted from Segall and Vienonen 1987)

Article 1. National authorities, international agencies and social activists should mount and sustain a political campaign to promote the practical realization of the PHC approach on grounds of both equity and efficiency in the allocation of resources.

Article 2. The epidemiology of health-related inequalities should be developed and the findings fed into government policy formulation. The information should be generated with popular participation whenever possible and it should be disseminated in the community in popular form.

Article 3. The need for a broad 'horizontal' social and intersectoral approach to health problems should be reasserted. Verticalism should be avoided and selection of programme priorities should be made mainly locally with popular involvement.

Article 4. More effective actions should be taken in the following four areas:
  – national health resource planning to ensure that resource allocations reflect health priorities
  – decentralization of decision-making and local planning and management
  – reorientation of health cadre training to reflect the needs of the PHC approach
  – operational research with popular involvement to adapt the general principles of PHC to local conditions.

Article 5. Actions should be taken in three economic areas to support the PHC approach as follows:
  – an international campaign should be mounted for reforms in the world economy to create better conditions in developing countries for the promotion of health and the implementation of PHC policies
  – more national resources should be mobilized for PHC using collective financing mechanisms
  – health-sector efficiency should be improved, especially in hospitals, and the savings used to support priority health services.

of health (absence of specific diseases) than the popular WHO definition of social, mental and physical well-being discussed in Chapter 1. In addition, with its alleged achievement of rapid results and its technological orientation, SPHC is possibly better suited to urban than to rural areas. However, most people in the Third World live in rural areas. Housing in such settings may often be improved at a much lower cost than in urban areas; food supplies are often available; and piped potable water can bring an immediate health boost to many. By coupling social and environmental improvements with basic health information and general education, it may in time perhaps be possible to avoid purely 'interventionist' care. In the interim, however, it seems that target-oriented SPHC programmes and wider schemes will need to go hand in hand, although resources are inevitably stretched. Whilst donor agencies and international agencies continue to support targeted campaigns and seek to justify expenditure in readily quantifiable terms such as costs per death averted, then it appears that vertical, technical (and, by definition, selective) interventions will continue.

Vertical programmes in PHC?

It has become customary to regard 'health care' as being available either as broad, more or less comprehensive provision with intersectoral involvement ('horizontal'), or in a more interventionist form, amenable to semi-autonomous provision via top-down, vertical programmes aimed at specific objectives or problems (Fig. 5.2). This duality of views often coexists within individual health care systems. It can present problems to the development of a coordinated or integrated organization and management structure; philosophically, for example, comprehensive PHC and SPHC are antipathic (Fendall 1987). The WHO has been very concerned with administrative changes from vertical to horizontal services; however, evidence of this realistically occurring is not always widespread.

The idea of integration of health services is allegedly widely accepted, although Fendall (1987) questions the validity of this assertion. However, the practical transition from semi-autonomous vertical programmes coexisting with a general health service to an integrated structure, capable of delivering both general and specialist care, has been slow to evolve in many countries. As in the PHC–SPHC debate, the wishes of donor agencies for apparently effective campaigns, and the problem-curative orientation of much medical and health philosophy, have compounded the problem. The WHO (1985) suggests that the transition to programmes such

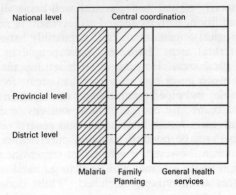

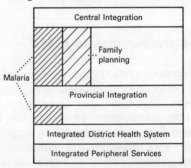

Fig. 5.2   Integrated health services infrastructure compared with a vertical, top-down structure (after Smith and Bryant 1988)

as MCH enlarges the horizontal nature of provision but this may be questionable. It is worth considering that programmes such as MCH and 'Under-Fives' clinics are as much a part of vertical ideology as are the programmes aimed at eradication of specific diseases (such as immunization and ORT). It can also be difficult to integrate such services as FP and MCH programmes into PHC even if the desirability of doing so is accepted. Indeed, PHC itself has perhaps emerged at times as a type of vertical programme with separate administrative structures, which suggests that PHC may become divorced from other linked activities. However, it should not be able to exist in a vacuum (this would be contradictory) and overall improved methods of delivery and intersectoral collaboration are the key to its success.

Nevertheless, we need to be aware that the current nature of PHC as a mixture of philosophies and activities can itself lead to a series of vertical strategies focusing on, for example, sanitation, MCH or water provision, without the emphasis on harmony of effort. Fendall (1987) feels that PHC requires a series of action principles, which should be met concurrently. In particular, the contribution of disease-control and specific socio-environmental programmes to improved health must be acknowledged, but the major issue is how to harness vertical programmes or incorporate them into a PHC framework. This question is likely to continue to exercise the skills of all involved for some time and it should be borne in mind when the health programmes and actions for specific groups are discussed in Chapter 7. The ways in which the superimposed vertical programmes can be incorporated within communities in a participatory manner are crucial. Emphasis on the dissemination of information prior to, and during, programmes seems critical. This recognition might ensure the shift from a hierarchical decision-making structure to the horizontal concept of popular involvement and collaboration.

In this context, it is worth referring to Werner's (1978) suggestion that the health care hierarchy should be turned on its side, representing the movement from vertical to horizontal, enhancing accessibility and local responsibility (Chapter 4). However, as there is little evidence anywhere of PHC having started spontaneously at a community or grass-roots level, the importance of a centralized decision-making process and a committed leadership remains until proved to the contrary. This is so even in the revolutionary and socialist regimes mentioned in this book in which health care, albeit locally and community based, has often been a major commitment of the ruling group and a priority of the regime.

Community health workers and PHC

A number of Third World countries have deployed CHWs in their PHC programmes. Indeed, considerable experience has been gained in using CHWs in national health plans and particularly in PHC, and many feel that only by the widespread use of such workers has the 'Health for all by the year 2000' goal any hope of being met. However, the nature, training and roles of CHWs vary considerably from their working full time as more or less qualified medical officers and/or assistant medical officers, to being part-time workers with little, if any, training. They have been known by a variety of names, including village health worker, health promoter, barefoot doctor (in China until 1984), trained traditional birth attendant and others (Morley and Woodland 1979). They are often voluntary or semi-voluntary, and are members of local communities who have received an elementary training in curative and frequently also preventive care relevant to the needs of the communities in which they live. In essence, they provide *accessible* primary care services to the people among whom they live (Heggenhougen *et al.* 1987). Werner (1978) and Morley and Woodland (1979) provide an interesting summary of the initially conceptualized differences in background, attitude and communication between most conventional doctors and the best examples of part-time health workers. The major differences are between the formal training and technical orientation of most doctors compared with the accessibility, shared knowledge and low resource base of CHWs. This, at least, was the optimistic view of how part-time health workers would turn the health care hierarchy to make care more accessible to ordinary people (see Chapter 4).

In considering the role and place of PHC and the more specific role of CHWs, it is useful to outline Rifkin's (1985) views of approaches that may be taken in any given programme of health and health care. Three broad approaches to community health, broadly speaking, may be identified: the medical approach, the health planning approach and the community development approach. The prominence of any particular 'approach' generally colours the attitudes of professionals and community as to *who* should be doing *what* in relation to health services, and in what form (where) services should be provided.

1. The medical approach

The medical approach considers health as the absence of disease, to be brought about by technical interventions based on modern science and technology; the community responds to directions by, and actions of, medical professionals. This has as its basis the medical model of health care, in which eradication of ill health depends on doctors and medicine (King 1966; Walt and Vaughan 1981). Health services are regarded as the means by which medical science and technology can be applied to eradicate illness in the community. High-quality, high-technology medical services are considered to be the key to improved health; community participation may be useful as a means of improving the use of such services. This approach equates 'health care' with medical care. However, it has been amply documented that improvements in health are not solely related to improved medicine; socioeconomic and environmental improvements often pre-date, and certainly have to support, better health (McKeown 1965, 1976, 1985).

It may be difficult to sustain peripherally situated health programmes when there is an overemphasis on predominantly clinical–curative infrastructure and activities. However, when VHWs have wider roles in explaining to villagers how to look after their health, housing and environment, as well as dealing with illnesses and births, this can help to sustain programmes. Village health workers have been used in this way in the Saradidi Rural Health Development project in Kenya. This project is interesting in that it was initiated by villagers themselves, only subsequently receiving external support. It also used herbalists-cum-TBAs as CHWs, renamed the Village Helpers Towards Health (Willms 1988).

2. The health planning approach

The health planning approach regards health improvements as derived largely from the appropriate *delivery* of health services. The axiom is that good delivery will be achieved by planning to ensure that poor people, in great need, will have proper care. The approach denies the assumption that medical science and technology hold the sole key to health improvements, but it couples with the technocratic in that medical advances must be integrated into a health care delivery system that allocates resources according to community and individual needs. Questions of resource allocation and, by implication, accessibility within the system are fundamental. As Rifkin (1985) suggests, advocates of the health planning approach in community health emphasize the primacy of services but particularly those which provide the most benefits for the greatest number. Such services can often use and mobilize community resources to enhance their effectiveness. This approach is inherently concerned with quantity, location and planning of health facilities and manpower, and with rural–urban differences and the like. Abel-Smith (1976), Bryant (1969), Gish (1977), Morley (1973) and others illustrate the bases to this notable orientation, which has gained considerable ascendancy in some developing countries, especially in so far as it addresses the distribution of scarce resources. This approach is arguably essential to the extension plans of the WHO and aid organizations, especially in the run-up to PHC, which can, in its most basic form, be regarded as a programme to enhance accessibility and availability of health care by effective health planning.

3. The community development approach

The community development approach derives from the tradition of community development, which sees health in the context of promotion of better living conditions and environment. Therefore, the entire range of activities, from medical services and technology, to education and agriculture, should be involved. This approach stresses that community health improvements do not stem solely from direct health-sector activities. Income generation, housing, schooling, infrastructure and general community improvements are all essential for health improvement. Importantly, this approach is underpinned by decision-making based on community wants rather than needs and objectives of policymakers. Key themes are community initiative, planning and responsibility. This is often referred to as the 'bottom-up' rather than 'top-down' orientation, for many years implemented in sectors other than health, but only relatively recently brought generally into health care. The philosophy of this approach is that health cannot be simply equated with health services and is not to be achieved merely by a well-planned, efficient and functional delivery system. It recognizes the potential for a type of exploitation of people by health professionals, especially in a 'good' system (and, of course, system effectiveness is generally professionally adjudicated). Instead, it adopts the view, now widely shared, that improvements in health in the industrial world, at any rate, have been achieved mainly as a result of general factors, including socioeconomic development. Improved access to health services and medical intervention are only part of this equation.

The community development approach, even more than health planning, is integral to many PHC programmes. It sees health services as a means by which individuals and communities can learn and develop inherent potentials. They can take control of their lives, utilize their resources and escape from over-reliance on external factors, notably intervention by state or government and outside agencies. It obviously places a high premium on personal motivation and the achievement of dignity, especially among the poor. Services, including health services, become a tool to be used in education for participation and health may be an entry point to the total development of the community. Health care systems may become developed in response to felt needs and self-help, rather than medically defined needs. This type of philosophy became familiar in fields such as housing, education and services rather earlier than in health, although today it is increasingly recognized that the use and control of health services by communities is an important way in which the goal of development of people rather than technology can be achieved (Rifkin 1985). This approach clearly implies the restructuring of the health system inherent in the widest PHC approaches discussed earlier. It is less in keeping with partial and technical variants such as SPHC, which are dependent on technical interventions imposed upon communities and aimed at specific problems.

The use of CHWs: some examples and problems

Many CHW programmes are *ad hoc*, non-governmental and often inevitably of relatively limited size and spatial coverage. Supported by various donors, small projects using CHWs have often achieved a great deal. By contrast, large-scale CHW programmes require considerable organization and resources and are therefore frequently part of national strategies. However, with a few notable exceptions, CHWs in national programmes have not achieved all they might have done. Even when part of a national PHC strategy, many CHW schemes have achieved only patchy success as, in the final analysis, they are heavily reliant on local initiative, enthusiasm and goodwill. Their nature and success have thus varied considerably from place to place. Indeed, local political interests may clash with the aims and objectives of CHWs and frustrate them. In Zambia, for example, Twumasi and Freund (1985) identify the need for traditional political institutions and chiefs to be reoriented and brought into the picture of development, so that local participation and local leadership assist rather than frustrate the developments associated with PHC. The country-wide use of 'barefoot doctors' in China was often seen as a model for CHW incorporation into national health schemes. This term was dropped after 1984: barefoot doctors who passed an exam became rural doctors; those who failed, 'health aides', like the CHWs discussed here (WHO 1989).

Tanzania, too, provides a much-quoted example of a country with a commitment to health as an integral part of national development. In particular, its attempts to train and extend the roles of CHWs have been cited as an example for other countries. However, a country-wide review of the Tanzanian programme in the late 1980s commended the commitment of the MOH but pointed to considerable difficulties in implementation (WHO 1989). Tanzania had by the early 1970s expressed the political will to improve basic health, meet basic health needs and improve access to care (Bennett 1985). When the socialist *ujamaa* village experiment was flourishing, this emphasized access to health care (to ensure less than a 2-hour walk to a health facility). Even more important was the attempt to redress the urban and hospital bias in health budget and provision, in favour of rural areas. The *ujamaa* village experiment (von Freyhold 1979) included a component of using MCH aides and creating village health posts manned by village medical workers who had primary education and 6 months' training at the district hospital. Even when enthusiasm was highest, however, many rural medical workers gave up their jobs or drifted to the towns. The PHC programme faltered because of poor health services and community support, although subsequent programmes have attempted to improve the support of CHWs and also TBAs.

Kitching (1982) explains the reasons for failure of *ujamaa*, suggesting that Tanzania's development suffered from the thorough-going egalitarianism that lay at the centre of Nyerere's populist philosophy and policies. The attempts to reduce too rapidly the differences between town and country and to avoid inequalities among Tanzanians meant that resources were spread very thinly over the country (not just in health care but primarily in agriculture and personnel). The picture that emerges is thus of a morally desirable social and health development package, but one marred by resources spread so thinly that the critical minimum levels necessary for any effective impact were nowhere obtained.

In Tanzania, the first government CHWs appeared in 1969; initially, they were regarded as a stop-gap but now their value as permanent primary health VHWs is being increasingly recognized. Nevertheless, in practice, many problems are emerging. Information on their activities has been somewhat disjointed, although Heggenhougen *et al.* (1987) provide a comprehensive review of CHW activities in that country, and their role within the larger framework of PHC and socioeconomic development.

The use of CHWs in, and following, the Tanzania *ujamaa* experiment was notable, as was, for example, the use of various health auxiliaries in Kenya during the extension of PHC. Many projects there have been, and are, community-based, with health committees sponsoring health workers, and with integration of agricultural, education and water development activities along with health. Significantly, Kenya has tried to develop a well-distributed infrastructure of training health centres, health units and smaller clinics, and to use non-government initiatives to assist small, community-based ¬rojects (Dodge and Wiebe 1985). This has, of course, been needed to redress the urban bias of formal health care provision in this country. There has, however, been a tendency to implement community-based health care programmes from the top down, with a lack of dialogue between centre representatives and community leaders. The Saradidi Rural Health Project, in the Nyanza Province, mentioned earlier, nevertheless provides a good example of local initiative and support for a health scheme using CHWs (Willms 1988). The Kenyan intersectoral approach, with its strong reliance on CHW-type service providers, is redolent of the policy extant in the Philippines since the late 1970s. Primary health care was officially adopted as a national health policy in 1979, integrated as part of a basic needs strategy, but this is perhaps something of an abrogation of government responsibility for health care provision. Non-government organizations, often with a religious base, have also been strongly involved in CHW training, and these are frequently more successful than government schemes. In both government and non-government projects, there have been attempts to define health holistically and in the context of socioeconomic aspects of society. Communities have been encouraged to seek definitions of problems and their solutions, and flexible, open-ended programmes adjustable to community needs have been sought (Phillips 1986a; Rifkin 1985).

The stimulation of people into awareness about health levels and needs is particularly visible in the Philippines. A notable reliance on voluntary *barangay* (parish or village) health workers has emerged, along with *barangay* nutrition scholars. The key 'professional' is usually the nurse or midwife, who may often work with trained or untrained TBAs (*hilots*). The extension of health care and health education has been central to the Philippines' efforts, and this includes the popular availability of FP resources and of essential drugs made through village stores known as *botica sa barangay*.

'Self-reliance' has come to be an article of faith in many CHW-based programmes, of which the Philippines is a good example. The emphasis is to utilize underdeveloped local health resources such as personnel and buildings, and the task of community-based health programmes here is often seen as helping villagers or local people to be more aware of their own resources and to maximize their use (Rifkin 1985). This may often be quite optimistic or, if adopted as the sole official (rather than non-governmental) policy, it may be regarded as a sloughing-off of the state's responsibility for providing basic health care to poor communities, who often have enough trouble providing food and shelter, let alone developing community health care initiatives, on meagre resources (Phillips 1986a).

Heggenhougen *et al.* (1987) have identified a number of critical issues relating to PHC programmes involving CHWs within Tanzania, and these probably apply to similar programmes in other Third World countries. The future of CHWs is also critical, as are their selection, training, quantity and quality. Other issues relate to their continuing education, role in the various PHC activities and community participation (see p 152). Crucially, however, their success or otherwise must be evaluated, and genuine government commitment evidenced, if CHWs are not to become the demoralized extension of professional health services (WHO 1989). Urban and rural imbalances and the role of curative versus preventive medicine also have to be addressed. If such issues are ignored, 'health for all' is unlikely to be achieved by the year 2000; some gains have been made during the decade from 1978 to 1988 but, if no real advances continue, then investment in health may give way to greater support for the so-called 'productive' sectors of industry and agriculture. Therefore, CHW and related policies must be shown to be feasible and effective.

In conclusion, many reviews have identified weaknesses in CHW programmes. Economic difficulties underline many of these, and explain why Jamaica and Colombia, for example, have suspended the training of CHWs and, in other countries such as Botswana, far fewer have been trained than envisaged. However, in some CHW schemes, the problems extend beyond economic difficulties. A WHO report on strengthening the performance of CHWs in PHC has singled out eight main areas of weakness. Space does not permit a full discussion of these but they include: hastily developed policy with insufficient integration and commitment; poor selection, training, support, supervision and finance; and lack of monitoring and evaluation (WHO 1989). A number of strategies are suggested to improve these aspects, some of which are organizational and relate to the links with district health systems and intersectoral cooperation. Other suggestions address more specifically the training and supervision of CHWs, and their working conditions and remuneration.

Hospitals and urban PHC

In rural areas, facilities such as rural health units, district hospitals, health aid posts and the like can all provide foci for PHC. In urban areas, however, whilst hospitals may often consume over half of national health budgets (and sometimes as much as 80 per cent), in many instances these have little interest in, or connection with, PHC. This is related to the weakness of social, preventive or community medicine (in its various guises) in many Third World countries and the relatively low status often attached professionally to PHC (it may be viewed as amenable for community workers, rural peasantry and the like).

Nevertheless, increasingly, PHC strategies will be essential to enhance the serious health and environmental situations of many Third World urban neighbourhoods. Housing, sanitation, availability of potable water, nutrition and effective access to health care are frequently worse in poor urban neighbourhoods, especially in slum and shanty areas, than in corresponding rural sites. Some countries, such as the Philippines, Jamaica and Senegal, have attempted practical provision of PHC in urban settings, but often projects are piecemeal and fragmented, and clinics poorly staffed and lacking medicines and equipment. Therefore, PHC clinics are frequently bypassed in favour of hospitals, which are often crowded but perceived as being the only loci at which any chance of health care is likely to be available.

What might be the answer to the apparent less successful urban implementation of PHC? The WHO has suggested that a successful health system based on PHC requires a network of supporting hospitals to be successful, to promote PHC, community health, training, education and research. In the early 1980s, hospitals were identified as having potentially crucial roles within PHC, in particular as first referral levels within a district health system (WHO 1987d). This is discussed in Chapter 8. However, strong connections and coordination with the community in which the hospital is set are necessary. Hospitals, it has been suggested, might have their images, accessibility and effectiveness considerably enhanced by being assigned a definitive catchment area within a local, 'regionalized' framework. Each might develop a department of community health to provide leadership (academic and practical) for community participation. This could form the link between the hospital's technical and medical services on the one hand and the needs of the catchment community on the other. In this manner, hospital departments under various names (community medicine, social and preventive medicine, and the like) might become involved in training of both doctors and community workers as well as in providing community-oriented programmes and research on the health status and needs of the catchment population. Such ideas, strongly developed in many countries including Britain and Australia, have been employed in places as diverse as Kingston (Jamaica), Karachi (Pakistan), Cali (Colombia) and Hong Kong.

In Chapters 4 and 8, it is suggested that such a community/PHC orientation of hospital services, providing an effective link between facilities and personnel within a catchment area, might help avoid some of the serious overcrowding and inefficient use of the hospitals themselves. This implies development and organization of an efficient referral network and system within the community, so that users will have confidence that PHC can provide adequate care and that appropriate cases will be referred on to hospital. More efficient coordination of health services should thus lead to more effective utilization. Within Cali, Colombia, for example, bypassing and underutilization of peripheral health units was leading to continuing deterioration, overcrowding and malutilization of central hospital facilities. Planned media campaigns alerted the catchment populations to the strengthening and supervision of peripheral facilities, encouraged appropriate usage, and improved attitudes of health workers and community to the use of such facilities. A main achievement of this project in the late 1970s was the strengthening of peripheral facilities, and the removal of practical and psychological barriers to their use. This would have been of particular benefit to the poor in remoter districts, where travel to hospitals is difficult (Rossi-Espagnet 1984).

Initiatives in urban PHC

The above section suggests that relatively little has been achieved in urban PHC but, more accurately, it should perhaps be said that many city administrations can barely keep pace with the scale and rate of urbanization and concomitant demands for services. Harpham *et al.* (1985) nevertheless note with cautious optimism certain evidence of community-level approaches to helping the urban poor through PHC. In particular, they suggest a useful categorization of features of urban PHC-type initiatives, which include neighbourhood health programmes, urban CHWs, community involvement, multisectoral action, extending programme coverage, and hospitals and the referral system (noted above).

This classification suggests areas for research within an urban PHC strategy. For example, urban PHC might be promoted via such devices as neighbourhood programmes (in the *barrios* of Cali, the *kampungs* of Jakarta and the *barangays* of Manila). The transferability to many urban areas of standardized national sectoral programmes for basic services, even if initially designed for rural settings, is possible if due note is taken of local conditions and needs. Community health workers, often associated with rural schemes, may be as effective in geographically more contained town localities; and the urban CHW concept has been readily adopted in various forms in a number of cities.

Community involvement has long been recognized as a major, often essential, ingredient for successful PHC, by which local communities participate in planning, implementation and use of health activities, taking responsibility for, and benefiting from, improved health and health care. At times, overoptimism has been evident as to the strength of local resources and some PHC schemes have failed. By contrast, in urban settings, a lack of social organization and cohesion has long been assumed but this has been disproved by many successful community self-help schemes in fields such as housing. Therefore, there does seem to be potential for engaging the talents and resources of local communities for PHC. Partnerships between government and community may also be enhanced by community involvement stemming from popular understanding of local problems or by solutions stemming from community initiatives (Rifkin 1985). However, examples of developments resulting from a true dialogue between the government and community in urban settings, where the respective contributions are mutually acknowledged, are relatively hard to find (Harpham *et al.* 1985), although these stemming from community mobilization based on government schemes are relatively common.

Infrastructure projects, sites-and-services schemes, low-cost housing upgrading and comprehensive redevelopment schemes all involve considerable multisectoral action. They can become entry points for PHC initiatives in low-income areas and could certainly be used for more broadly based urban environmental upgrading, including health targets. Examples of BLISS (Bagong Lipunan — New Society – Improvement of Sites and Services in the late Marcos-era Philippines) schemes for low- and medium-cost housing in Metro-Manila in the Philippines include health components via a basic needs strategy, although the poorest urban dwellers have effectively been excluded from many of these improvement schemes by cost and eligibility criteria (Phillips 1987a; Phillips and Yeh 1983). Elsewhere, at a larger scale, the upgrading of health and social services may be part of new town strategies, as in Hong Kong, Singapore, Korea, Japan and elsewhere, when PHC provision may be programmed at the design stage and facilities coordinated early on (Kim 1987; Phillips 1987b). Such all-embracing approaches as new town developments are, however, unlikely to be viable alternatives to urban squatter and environmental problems in the poorer Third World countries. They will probably be confined to the richer NICs, especially those in South-East and East Asia (Phillips and Yeh 1987), in which healthy, new urban environments may often provide enviable settings for health care and opportunities for PHC (with public and private participation).

Finally, Harpham *et al.* (1985) stress that urban PHC projects of the types noted above should not be 'one-off' actions but should be steps in a strategy for continuing, large-scale coverage for all those whose health needs have previously been ignored. However, to date, few PHC initiatives in poor urban areas have managed to extend their coverage or grow into more broadly based pro-grammes. Financial and human constraints have hindered this, and other factors have acted against extension of coverage, such as the attitude of government officials or health professionals, of the lack of community or government involvement. In addition, before attempting to extend the coverage of urban PHC initiatives, it is necessary to evaluate the effectiveness and desirability of elements within one-off projects, and to identify their wider applicability. Little work of this sort has yet been achieved.

Chapter 6

Using health services

On the face of it the matter of use of health services is quite simple: namely, either facilities are used or they are not; a service is or is not received. This simplistic assumption hides many variables and factors that can determine whether or not a service is used and, also of great importance, whether the service is used at an appropriate time and effectively. The apparently straightforward issues of who uses which services, how much, and when, have been a preoccupation of social scientists for many years and, for a shorter period, of health planners. The precursor of the modern study of health care utilization may be seen in Jarvis's detection in the mid-nineteenth century of an inverse relationship between distance from mental hospitals and admission rates. Today, the field of investigation of utilization behaviour of people when ill or when seeking to prevent illness and optimize their health is a major area of research. Whilst many studies in developed countries have identified a range of variables influencing utilization behaviour, and many regularities of behaviour according to these variables have been observed, there is still imperfect understanding of exactly how and why services are used.

In part, this relates to the enormous complexity of issues involved, the variations between specialisms in health care, and individual differences in attitudes to, and recognition of, illness and the need to maintain health – all very elusive concepts. In addition, social scientists have been attempting to identify behavioural regularities among subgroups in populations, in what is arguably a field that is dominated by individual behavioural variations. Much research to date has involved what might be called mechanistic formulations of health care behaviour. Indeed, it is difficult to move beyond these to focus on how people conceptualize health issues and how and why they decide to implement various therapeutic strategies (Stock 1987). The complexity of the field was clearly identified as long ago as the early 1970s in McKinlay's (1972) review of approaches to the study of utilization.

Today, it may be assumed to be easier in Third World settings than in many developed countries to examine fundamental issues influencing utilization: income, ethnicity, physical and social accessibility. However, there are numerous features of health care delivery systems in Third World countries that can complicate matters. These include medical pluralism (the coexistence of modern and traditional practice), the frequent lack of universal coverage of health care, and economic and mobility problems. There have been far fewer empirical studies of health care utilization in the Third World than in developed countries and there is also far less knowledge of its characteristics and influences.

A number of discrete but often interrelated variables appear to influence health care utilization. Some are service-related characteristics: type, size, location, costs and quality; others are community-wide, such as transport or the availability of financial support; yet others may be personal or family-related: age, sex, income, social status, family size, mobility, religion. Many studies in medical sociology have attempted to identify the effects of specific variables (see, for instance, Cockerham 1978; Mechanic 1968, 1979; Tuckett 1976), and Kohn and White (1976) provide a useful basis for classifying the determinants of health care. However, the merits and shortcomings of single-factor explanations of utilization behaviour are increasingly becoming apparent and a number of studies over the last 30 years or so have tried to model utilization taking account of multiple influences.

Modelling the use of health services

There have been many attempts in the social sciences and the broad fields of community medicine and public health to apply models to describe, determine and predict health services utilization. The majority of models have been concerned with specifying variables determining whether usage will occur and influencing its frequency. Some models have had a more explicitly spatial concern, attempting to identify the location of facilities that will be used, and how these may be selected. Many models can be applied to a variety of consumer behaviour in public and welfare services generally, as well as specifically in health care. The models have increased in technical sophistication and many have helped to illustrate the interrelations among variables influencing health care usage. It is useful to consider these models as an evolving group, although strictly they are not related.

Most of the models were developed in the North American context although some have been applied and tested elsewhere; relatively few have been employed in Third World settings, for some reasons suggested below. Further discussion of the models is provided by Joseph and Phillips (1984), Phillips (1986b) and Veeder (1975). The majority of the models have evolved since the late 1950s; the earlier models tended to include fewer factors, as they attempted to identify the specific variables (mainly on the population side) that might influence use rates and, indirectly, effectiveness of utilization. Many of the earlier models hold implicitly that underutilization is the main problem in social services, and that this should be a concern for health planners and providers who wish to optimize the use of facilities for their intended population; later models appear to regard underutilization as less important. Most models have attempted to identify those variables which 'predispose' or 'enable' utilization, with the explicit intention of reducing any barriers identified. One of the earliest, for example, stressed the existence of a state of psychological readiness to act, whereby a person believes himself to be susceptible to a disease that could have serious effects but that can somehow be prevented or ameliorated by action on his part (Rosenstock 1960). In addition to a psychological state of readiness to act, the environmental and cognitive elements of behaviour are also emphasized: barriers such as costs, distance, inconvenient service hours and the like should be reduced, whilst reminders from physicians or the media can serve as triggers to behaviour. The effects of physician organization and so-called 'administrative barriers' to care have long been recognized (McKinlay 1972; Wolinsky and Marder 1983) and required introduction into models.

Subsequent models have introduced additional variables or emphasized different factors. Suchman (1964, 1966) placed great reliance on social group influences and less emphasis on the psychological state of readiness. For example, he hypothesized that very different levels of knowledge and attitudes to disease and illness would exist among ethnic and social groups. In conjunction with a number of specific propositions, it was suggested that a cosmopolitan social structure is more likely to be associated with a scientific health orientation than is a parochial or local structure, in which lay or popular health beliefs will tend to prevail.

This model is of significance in that it may help to explain some differences in utilization behaviour between urban and rural residents and between various ethnic minority groups. Such a proposition might be of relevance in Third World countries. The large number of ex-rural dwellers frequently found in cities might be expected in this model to favour traditional medicine and this could be of importance to any planning of the balance between traditional and modern medical provision. The concept of the lay referral system is found in this model, in which non-professional laypersons (kin, or specially respected group members) may be consulted in preference to, or before, professional advice being sought. The accessibility of family or friends in an individual's social network can therefore influence the extent to which he or she can avail

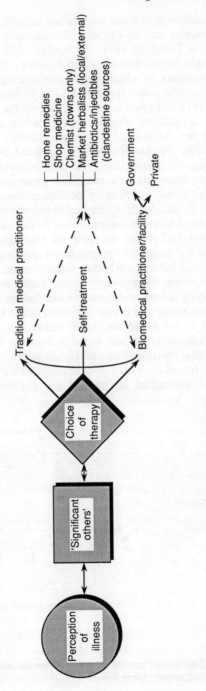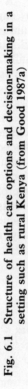

Fig. 6.1 Structure of health care options and decision-making in a setting such as rural Kenya (from Good 1987a)

himself or herself of these sometimes valuable alternative resources in health care, and so can directly influence utilization behaviour (Booth and Babchuk 1972; McKinlay 1972). This aspect of the model might be of relevance to health care utilization in some Third World countries in which laypersons perform important advisory or even curative roles. It might also be of importance in the acceptance of VHWs. Figure 6.1 outlines a possible sequence of decisions involved in deciding whether to use various sources of health care and identifies the role of 'significant others'.

A model by Andersen (1968), refined by Aday *et al.* (1980), has emphasized family life-cycle and behavioural determinants of utilization. Many models recognize groups of factors influencing utilization: those which may *predispose* towards utilization are a family's size, composition and health beliefs; certain *enabling* factors such as the family's or community's health resources may enhance or frustrate utilization in spite of predisposition to use. *Need* (measured by illness or symptoms) is the final factor in the equation, and will influence whether utilization occurs, dependent upon the predisposing and enabling factors acting together. Need may be influenced by illness and demographic factors. This model is based on common sense and makes the observation that much health care behaviour is not voluntary but is either directed or influenced by the professional (physician, nurse or dentist). Therefore, these components also warrant inclusion, although the extent of their influence for poor Third World residents is doubtful. A recent study has attempted to modify the behavioural model and to

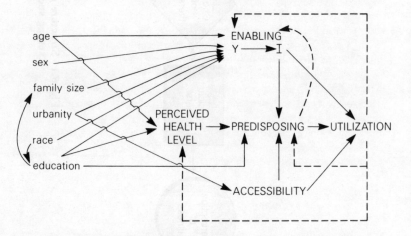

Fig. 6.2 The Gross model of major determinants in health care utilization (from Gross 1972)

refine further the measurement of the variables (Wolinsky *et al.* 1983). This focused upon health services utilization among non-institutionalized elderly people and found the model to be useful in explaining variance in health services utilization, with the most important variable being need. This suggested to Wolinsky *et al.* (1983) that the system under investigation was broadly equitable, as need was the chief determinant of the use rates in this case.

A more sophisticated and complex model by Gross (1972) incorporates behavioural components as major determinants of utilization (Fig. 6.2). A causal model is proposed that includes accessibility (something generally omitted, assumed or glossed over in certain of the earlier models):

$$U = f(E, P, A, H, X)\, e$$

where

U = utilization of various services reported by the individual or family

E = enabling factors such as income, family size, education

P = predisposing factors such as attitudes to health care, knowledge of sources of care

A = accessibility factors such as distance and/or time from facility and service availability

H = perceived health level

X = individual and area-wide exogenous variables

e = residual error term

This model obviously incorporates a wide range of variables, but their numerical expression and measurement can be very problematic. Indeed, Veeder (1975) indicates that the measurement and quantification of beliefs and attitudes, for example, has proved to be a stumbling block for most models. A number of attempts have nevertheless been made to bring the Gross model into operation although success has been limited. It is conceptually and mathematically the most sophisticated of the models developed so far but, ironically, this may prove to be one of its empirical weaknesses, since sufficiently precise data for accurate measurement of the variables are rarely available.

The majority of models today do recognize the existence of the various predisposing, enabling and need factors outlined above. However, it is also possible to envisage utilization as the product of characteristics of patient, provider and system. Aday and Andersen (1974), for example, consider a general model that provides a framework for the study of access to health services (Fig. 6.3). Broadly, health policy nationally and locally is based on the characteristics of the system and the population at risk. These may be considered 'inputs' to health services. The outputs, dependent

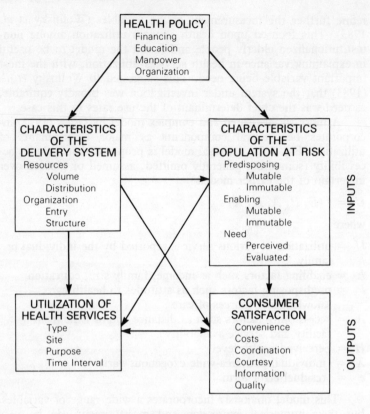

Framework for the study of access

**Fig. 6.3 A framework for the study of access to health services
(from Aday and Andersen 1974)**

on the inputs, are utilization of a given type, level and purpose,
and the resulting consumer satisfaction with costs, quality, convenience and the like. This broad framework is useful in that
national health policies in terms of nature, organization, finance and
manpower are seen as influences on utilization. The model provides
a type of blueprint for research on individual national systems
(Joseph and Phillips 1984).

The utilization models: Third World modifications?

Aday and Andersen's (1974) model relates to Dutton's (1986) formulation, which views the use of health services, both

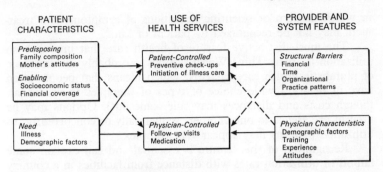

Fig. 6.4 A conceptual model of the factors affecting health care utilization (from Dutton 1986)

physician-controlled and patient-controlled, as the result of patient characteristics and the provider and system characteristics (Fig. 6.4). It is evident that such a framework might also be valuable in analysing the use of services in any given location, although the overall effect of national policy is not individually considered. In Third World countries, the distinction between discretionary (self-determined) and physician-controlled utilization may be valuable when preventive or promotive services are being introduced, and the model may help to assess their impact. Doctors are more likely to be influenced by their professional training and opinions as to the value of their treatment, whereas patients may well be sensitive to financial, organizational, spatial and cultural impediments to utilization. It is essential to recognize the relative importance of the various barriers to utilization if effective health services are to be delivered.

In addition, many of the assumptions of these models require reappraisal and perhaps modification for application in certain Third World settings. Perhaps the most important variables or factors that require reassessment relate to the effects of availability (accessibility) and the frequent existence of pluralistic health care systems (as opposed to the more or less uniform 'modern' health care systems in most developed countries; see Chapter 3), and to the effects of perceived quality of care in such circumstances. Stock (1987), for example, suggests a PEI (predisposing, enabling, illness characteristics) interpretive framework for the study of health care behaviour, a modification of the Andersen (1968) model. This can incorporate the social, economic and cultural values that may make utilization behaviour appear different in some Third World countries from how it appears elsewhere. Stock adopts modifications proposed by Wan and Soifer (1974), who suggest that the assessment of illness within a culture-specific framework is essential for the understanding of health behaviour in non-Western societies, in which modern or scientific definitions of symptoms and treatment may not be recognized by patient or kin.

The most distinctive feature of health care that impinges on utilization in many Third World settings is probably the existence of pluralistic health care systems, which means that people often have in theory a wide choice of types of therapies to utilize (although costs and distances may rule some out). Options may be used in preference to one another, sequentially or concurrently, so utilization patterns may appear very complex.

Recognition of this feature is essential and can explain some fall-off of utilization rates with distance from facilities in a country such as Nigeria. Stock (1987) found that at a distance of 5 km from a dispensary, per capita utilization fell to less than one-third of the 0-km rate. He notes that alternatives to institutional care must be serving the vast majority of needs in his study population in Kano State, and that the relative importance of these alternatives rises rapidly as distance from a Western-type facility increases. Whilst such unofficial but publicly popular sources of care may be important in many developed countries, they tend to be more so in most Third World societies. Stock stresses that Western-type care, often highly irregularly spaced and located in colonially determined distributions, is often only a theoretical option for many remote rural people. It may be too distant, too expensive or only intermittently available, and secondary- or tertiary-level care may effectively not exist. Therefore, the various options in the PEI model will vary in their spatial, economic and social accessibility. Likewise, predisposition to use various types of service will be very much influenced by cultural prescriptions (such as religious requirements or taboos) and the experience and opinions of others. In addition, many patients may regard more than one type of therapy as appropriate. For example, the Hausa in Nigeria may be open-minded about various types of treatment but certain ones may be preferred and others regarded as inappropriate. The patient may also use two or more 'appropriate' types of therapy concurrently or sequentially, as noted in 'modern' settings such as Singapore or Hong Kong (Phillips 1984).

The implied dichotomy between choice of a modern or a traditional health care source is often more apparent than real. As noted in Chapter 3, the systems sometimes abut but often overlap and, in some instances, they are integrated or moving towards integration. In addition, for certain types of ailment, a particular form of therapy, within each sector, might be felt to be appropriate. The choice of a modern therapy may follow non-success with a traditional remedy (and, of course, vice versa). The multiplicity of consumer choice thus goes beyond what has been called 'doctor shopping' in the developed world (Kasteler et al. 1976) and may consist of intersectoral choice and choice within the traditional or modern sectors. It is useful to note that four types of consumer were found in Nigeria (Ojanuga and Lefcowitz 1982): those who used either Western or traditional medicine exclusively (the majority of the population); those who used traditional medicine first, and then when dissatisfied, modern medicine; those who went from modern to traditional medicine; and those who used both types simultaneously.

Perhaps one of the main difficulties of investigating and especially modelling the use of health care in many Third World settings is this frequent need to identify concurrent or sequential use of multiple therapies. It may be necessary to consider quite long periods of time since one-off questionnaires about behaviour may not reveal accurate patterns of utilization. Some respondents may also be reluctant to admit openly to the use of certain traditional medicines because of the fear of appearing ignorant or backward. In addition, at the individual level, perceptions of the efficacy of Western relative to traditional treatments for specific ailments have great influence on utilization (both in terms of distances travelled and types selected). In Northern Nigeria, for example, fractures were felt better dealt with by traditional bone-setters, as hospitals were widely believed to amputate fractured limbs; for tuberculosis, by contrast, as traditional remedies were not effective, hospital medicines were desired (Good 1987a). This illustrates the complexity of investigating or modelling utilization, and it reminds us that, although later in this chapter (for example) the use of traditional sources is discussed independently, in reality the settings for choice and usage are varied, concurrent and also dynamic.

The need to consider the pervasive influence of state policy is stressed in some of the models. The availability or accessibility of modern treatments, in particular, will directly affect choice available locally and these are often directly provided by the state. If there are insufficient facilities, especially in rural areas, then this effectively excludes many residents from modern treatment. It is hardly surprising, therefore, to find examples of severe distance decay (see below) in utilization as alternative appropriate traditional or family health resources are used instead of distant official ones. Thus, in a Third World context, the models must be especially adaptable to a more holistic, culturally sensitive evaluation of health care behaviour and utilization.

'Spatial' models

From the preceding discussion, it seems probable that in many Third World countries, especially perhaps in rural sectors, matters of accessibility will take on greater significance than they do in the models outlined above, which are essentially products of developed country utilization research. Therefore, it is worthwhile considering a group of 'spatial' models that use location-allocation modelling and mathematical modelling to determine the optimum sites for facilities from the point of view of consumers of services. Research in this field was developed in the mid-1960s within the Chicago Regional Hospital study by R. L. Morrill and others at the University of Chicago. A number of papers made pioneering inroads into the quantification of how factors such as hospital type, size, location and finance could influence utilization or the distances people would be prepared to travel to facilities (Morrill and Earickson 1968, 1969; Morrill *et al.* 1970; Morrill and Kelley 1970). In addition, variants on normative gravity modelling were used to assign patients to hospitals of a given capacity within certain distances, to reassign patients from overdemanded to underdemanded locations and to indicate the extra travelling involved in having a spatially inefficient distribution of hospital type and capacity.

The gravity model makes use of the concept of distance decay (the 'friction' of distance, or the disincentive to utilization posed by increasing distance). Evidence for the existence of decay will be discussed later, but in its application the major weakness of models should be remembered. They are almost invariably based on aggregate, normative assumptions and it is difficult for them to incorporate individual variations in needs, aspirations, abilities and attitudes. It is therefore only possible to use them as 'average predictors' or for normative planning. It is not generally sensible to use them for 'fine tuning' of health services.

There are relatively few examples of mathematical or locational modelling of health services in Third World countries. In part, this is because of a lack of reliable and relatively large data sets (on population, boundaries and services), which the models as a rule require. However, one well-known study by Gould and Leinbach (1966) used a modelling approach to assist in the problem of deciding in which of five potential urban centres to locate three possible regional hospitals in Western Guatemala. The model enabled minimum cross-flows by adjusting the capacity of the hospitals and derived an optimal flow of population to services, minimizing aggregate travel to hospitals. At an intra-urban scale, also in Guatemala, Mulvihill (1979) used a model to overcome inequalities in resource allocation under transport-cost minimization assumptions. The model permitted the identification of PHC dispensaries that could be relocated, whilst it was able to take account of the existing largest facilities, which were for practical purposes not movable. The distribution revealed by the model departed substantially from the existing pattern of primary health centres in Guatemala City, and indicated the need for planning and rationalization to take account of population distribution and utilization patterns. Massam (1988) provides a further discussion of methods for locating health centres in Zambia (see Chapter 4).

An assessment of the models

Some of the data requirements for the models, and the associated limitations to the application of the more quantitative models in the Third World, have already been mentioned. In addition, models based on aggregate (normative) assumptions may not work very well in pluralistic health care systems in which neither the total amount of utilization nor the proportions using various types of care are precisely known. Data and assumption limitations to mathematical models, in particular, tend to be aggravated in Third World countries. Other general and specific limitations to locational analysis and modelling solutions in health care are discussed by Stimson (1983).

The non-spatial models in a way represent an attempt to specify the nature of the utilization process by means of highlighting variables (or groups of variables) that may influence it. This is a valuable function, if one fraught with frustration; the models are, for example, generally in agreement regarding the importance of availability and, indirectly, accessibility (generally in cost rather than distance terms). They differ considerably, however, in the importance that they attach to matters such as the effects on utilization of health beliefs and associated factors. In a sense, each is cumulative, building upon the preceding models, but definitions, measurements and practicality vary although increasing precision does develop as the models progress. Their rather static nature may also limit their applicability in what is essentially an evolving and dynamic area of behaviour. Perhaps their greatest value is in making the researcher aware of the great range of potential influences on utilization that may operate in any given circumstances. They do not, in themselves, provide an answer to the questions of how and why people demand or use health services.

Inappropriate utilization

Whilst much research has concentrated on how and why health services are used, and on barriers to utilization, increasingly there is recognition that not all utilization is in accordance with the needs of the individual. Techniques such as utilization review and utilization management have been developed to identify and reduce unnecessary use of health care facilities (mainly, however, at a hospital level). 'Inappropriate utilization' has come to be regarded as utilization not suitable to the patient's medical needs. In this context, this may be because of a lack of care facilities or capacity, common in the Third World, or because of the use of facilities by those who do not need them. It may be caused by physicians or other professionals deliberately or otherwise encouraging unnecessary usage or by the patient or family overdemanding or underdemanding care (perhaps because of poor recognition of what is needed).

Overutilization is defined as care that is of no benefit to the patient, such as unnecessary care, or extra days spent in inpatient care after sufficient recovery, or care that might be effectively provided at a lower level, in a less costly setting, such as an outpatient surgery, PHC unit or by community treatment. *Underutilization* is seen as care that is not of sufficient type, length, location or intensity to meet the patient's medical needs (Payne 1987). It seems that overutilization is often more likely to occur in fee-for-service, developed country systems. Underutilization, especially of hospital treatment, is, it seems, more likely to be a Third World phenomenon, because of lack of service availability or capacity. This can occur at hospital, clinic, PHC or community-care levels.

This discussion indicates that both professionals and patients can be 'at fault' in causing over- or underutilization, and that system features are also crucial: the levels of service provision (in terms of accessibility or volume provided) may be excessive or inadequate. This may be caused by relative or absolute lack of facilities or inaccessibility to users (Chapter 4). In terms of the efficiency of the

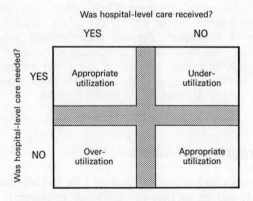

Fig. 6.5   **The relationship between need for hospital services and the services actually received (from Payne 1987)**

health care system, and its equitable and cost-effective use, both types of mal-utilization should be avoided as far as possible. Nevertheless, both do occur and they can be conceptualized as in Fig. 6.5. Patients who need the hospital services but do not obtain them are under-served, and those not needing but receiving are over-served. In the figure, patients in the upper-left quadrant are regarded as appropriately hospitalized, and patients in the lower-right quadrant are appropriately not in hospital. This type of analysis could be applied to PHC utilization and also to differences between levels of care in appropriateness of utilization. In the Philippines, for example, some suggest that as many as 60 per cent of hospital cases could medically have been dealt with appropriately in PHC rural health units (Phillips 1986a) and similar figures have been cited for other countries. This indicates an inefficient use of both levels of care, in this instance often caused by a lack of confidence in PHC by some residents, who prefer to use hospital services. If inappropriate utilization is identified in many Third World settings, then further research could be directed to pinpointing reasons for this (perhaps by attitudinal surveys of patients and professionals). Then, health education and information campaigns can be devised to increase the appropriate use of specific services at various times (see, for example, WHO 1988). In this way, utilization research in the Third World can develop from the academic to help to maximize the returns from scarce resources.

Health beliefs: utilization for varying conditions

It is important to recognize throughout the discussion of utilization of health care that actions or lack of action can vary considerably according to the nature of the illness or condition and its duration. In addition, many authors have pointed out that it is the experience of illness rather than the biological reality of disease that causes people to consult other persons about their health. In many Third World countries, not only do people's beliefs about, and experience of, illness vary considerably, but there are numerous sources that might be approached for help (see Chapter 3). Some will be considered more suitable for certain types of conditions than others and this will influence utilization behaviour considerably (Durkin-Longley 1984; Good 1987a; Lee 1973, 1980).

The beliefs of individuals and groups about the behaviour they should undertake for any given condition can be crucial in determining utilization. Whilst this point has been stressed in a number of publications, it is useful to cite a case study in Sri Lanka, which, it will be remembered from Chapter 3, has a wide range of cosmopolitan and traditional sources of care. The study involved a suburban village some 12 km from Colombo and a rural village some 15 km distant from Galle, with access to few modern health sources. The choice of therapies was investigated with regard to eight different complaints (Wolffers 1988). If the simplest case of 'fever and cough' is considered, there are many ranges of therapy options. Table 6.1 shows that in both the suburban and rural setting, self-treatment plays an important role (but it is of greater significance in the rural village). However, whilst traditional self-treatment is important in both, cosmopolitan self-treatment does not play an important role in the rural village. If self-treatment is not successful, as a second step, some 37 per cent of rural respondents said they would go to an *adura* (devil dancer) and 56 per cent would attend a cosmopolitan facility (about half of these would attend the free government hospital and the rest consult a private practitioner).

When a child is ill, or for other acute complaints, people in this study were more prepared to use cosmopolitan medicine (public or private) in either setting. The majority of rural residents in fact favour cosmopolitan health care when their child is very ill (Table 6.2), although almost 23 per cent of the suburban respondents said they would attend an Ayurvedic facility. Interestingly, as discussed below with regard to other studies, there is a striking preference for private cosmopolitan facilities for urgent attention, as the local government hospital has few facilities and supplies. Indeed, it is often bypassed by rural residents in preference for a larger general hospital at Galle.

When chronic complaints are considered, Wolffers (1988) found that some patients would use cosmopolitan medicine; others, traditional remedies. In the case of rheumatic complaints, both

Table 6.1   Therapy options of respondents in Nagar (near Colombo) and Rudagama (distant from modern facilities) in case of 'fever and cough' (from Wolffers 1988)

| | Nagar | | Rudagama | | | |
| | | | First step | | Second step | |
	n	%	n	%	n	%
Self-treatment	54	25.6	96	95	–	–
Cosmopolitan	111	52.6	4	4	57	56.4
Ayurvedic	46	21.8	–	–	1	1.0
Adura	–	–	1	1	37	36.6
None	–	–	–	–	6	5.9
Total	211	100.0	101	100.0	101	100.0

types of medicine are relatively ineffective and patients seek a variety of sources of care, traditional and modern, public and private. For a snakebite or a fracture, people seem to prefer emergency help from acknowledged local experts in the village. For the former, they go to a recognized local snakebite specialist; for the latter, they tend to patronize a traditional fracture specialist who has to be paid but whose treatment is effective (this is important for rural residents; care is available and helps their recovery for physical work). Even in the urban area, only about 10 per cent of respondents would go to the hospital of a private doctor in the case of a fracture; the overwhelming majority would go to one or two well-known traditional fracture healers. Mental illness, a difficult thing to deal with for many forms of medicine, would normally involve seeking help from the *adura* and Buddhist clergy. A total of 72 per cent of rural respondents with a family member mentally ill would consult the *adura*; only 27 per cent would go to a cosmopolitan medical facility. Similar findings were seen in the suburban settlement and only some 24 per cent of respondents would go to a Western-style doctor or hospital.

This case study has been cited in some detail because it illustrates a particular feature of health care utilization typical of many Third World countries: the selection of different therapies

Table 6.2 **Choice of therapy if a child is very ill (Nagar, near Colombo, and rural village of Rudagama) (from Wolffers 1988)**

Kind of health-care facility	n	%
Rudagama		
Modern		
Assistant medical practitioner	30	33.0
Public cosmopolitan hospital	27	29.6
Private cosmopolitan practioner	23	25.3
Total	80	87.9
Ayurvedic	4	4.4
Adura	7	7.7
Total	91	100.0
Nagar		
Modern	133	76.0
Ayurvedic	40	22.8
Home treatment	2	1.2
Total	175	100.0

(and sometimes their concurrent use). Depending on the familiarity and perceived seriousness of the complaint, self-treatment is a very likely first choice. Subsequent or alternative choice of therapy is often for the medical system that takes the least time and is the least complex to use, but there is no clear preference for a particular system in Sri Lanka, and this seems typical of many Third World situations. The choice of therapy will depend on the perceived urgency of the condition and the effectiveness of remedies in dealing with it. There seems room for at least three systems in Sri Lanka (cosmopolitan, Ayurvedic and magico-religious, plus some physical treatments). Therefore, a pluralistic health system with different utilization for varying conditions (or at different stages) is a natural consequence of the existence of varying beliefs and the inability of a single system to meet all the needs. It is important to remember that such pluralistic systems do exist in the majority of Third World countries, whether officially recognized or not, and this must be taken into account when influences on utilization are considered.

Variables influencing utilization

The preceding discussion in this chapter has tended to stress the interaction of variables in influencing the rate and timing of utilization of health services. The group of models often attempt to assess the concurrent operation of such variables but it is also useful to discuss findings of research into the effects of individual or small groups of variables. One of the earlier successful attempts to identify such groupings was by McKinlay (1972) in his discussion of approaches and problems in the study of the use of services. He identifies types of approaches that stress different variables and groups of variables as being of major influence in the use of medical services. In particular, he notes the following approaches:

1. economic
2. sociodemographic
3. 'geographical'
4. sociocultural
5. organizational or delivery-system

Other researchers have identified similar ranges of approaches and variables. However, it should be recognized that utilization is the outcome of many complex interactions among many variables and factors, visible and hidden, which act at different stages. It is impossible to observe the whole process or study it completely. As a result, few utilization studies can be anything like comprehensive; most end up focusing on a relatively narrow range of variables.

The factors emphasized in studies of utilization tend to vary from one academic discipline to another (economists stressing cost factors; psychologists, various behavioural and sociopsychological matters, for instance). However, relatively few reviews consider Third World health care usage specifically, although Akin *et al.* (1985) and Kroeger (1983) provide useful overviews. It is sometimes helpful to consider health care utilization from two perspectives: first, as a dynamic process consisting of different stages at which the patient makes decisions about usage; secondly, as the outcome of the complex interaction of determining factors (variables). However, this is rather an artificial distinction as utilization involves both perspectives: the passing through of stages *and* the involvement of complex interactions of determining factors (Fiedler 1981; Habib and Vaughan 1986).

There has also been a tendency for utilization to be considered mainly in terms of facility attendance rates or, at least, of service contact rates. Utilization is in reality more complex than this. Not only is a *quantitative* aspect involved (rates of visits or contacts) but utilization also has a *temporal* aspect (when was contact made; was

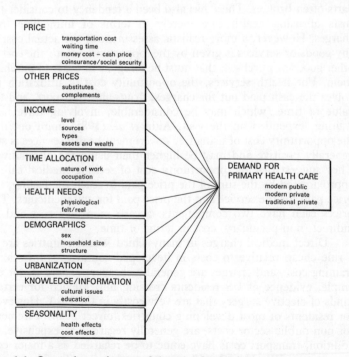

Fig. 6.6 Some determinants of demand for health services in the Third World (from Akin et al. 1985)

the time correct and appropriate?) and a *spatial* aspect (which facility and of what type and location was used?) The last two features have been less frequently researched even in developed countries but they form extremely important aspects of usage (Joseph and Phillips 1984; Phillips 1981b). Drawing on the models outlined earlier, and the discussions surrounding them, it is possible to identify major variables and groups of variables for individual consideration, some of which are shown in Fig. 6.6 (with reference to PHC in particular).

Economic factors

These tend to be stressed in all models but are particularly emphasized by economists. In some countries, in theory, publicly-funded health care is free or provided at very nominal user charges. Nevertheless, in virtually all systems, there is a certain usage of private health care and in the Third World this is particularly true of better-quality modern care or traditional medicine. Often the public-sector option provides a threadbare safety net that has in parts often broken. There has also been a tendency to consider the costs of using health care merely in terms of immediate user charges. However, a more realistic assessment of the actual cost of any goods or services is given by the 'opportunity cost': the cost of other goods or purchases that must be foregone in order to purchase them. For health services, the opportunity cost of utilization involves the cash paid out for charges, drugs and transport, and the value of time (which may be considerable, involving travel and waiting) expended on the visit. Akin *et al.* (1985) point out that the opportunity cost of using free government health services is still generally positive and may be higher than using the alternatives. They suggest that the opportunity cost of seeking medical care is approximated by the sum of the price paid to reach the facility, the price paid for the service and the price paid for any medicines. The prices each have two components: a cash monetary cost and an indirect (non-pecuniary) cost in terms of time.

Direct medical charges in many Third World countries are as a rule cheap relative to costs in developed countries (professional training costs and charges are generally cheaper). There is, for example, evidence of US residents crossing into Mexico for certain kinds of elective surgery that are very costly in the USA. However, for residents of most developing countries, direct health care costs (or non-public-sector costs) are generally regarded as expensive. In addition, transport costs have come to be regarded as a major cost component. In a Ugandan district hospital use study, 75 per cent of total outpatient cash outlays were for transport. Although the mode cited is often walking, this involves a loss of time and thereby earnings. In poorer countries, it may be only the better-off who will actually pay for transport, being able to afford not to walk.

A study in rural Kenya indicated that choice of service – free government clinic, pharmacy, mission clinic, private clinic or traditional healer – varied depending on the nature of the illness and on whether it was a first or subsequent visit. Although fairly well dispersed in the area, government clinics were used by only about 30 per cent of respondents, and about one-quarter and one-fifth went to pharmacy shops and mission clinics respectively (6.5 per cent said they attended traditional healers). The proportion using government facilities declined for subsequent visits (Mwabu 1986). This suggests that factors other than direct costs were influencing behaviour and these appeared to include quality of treatment, confidence and accessibility. It also points to the need to incorporate non-government health care, the major sector of care, into the health care system to increase the official coverage of health services.

In another paper, Mwabu and Mwangi (1986) indicate that government health services could only cover effectively about 20 per cent of Kenya's population as they were only supported in 1983 to 1984 to about $US5 per capita. As a result, a simulation was conducted of the welfare effects of introducing user fees, possibly selectively, to support the extension of services mainly into rural areas. The authors suggest that, by their effects on increasing the quality of services, user fees in public clinics might introduce welfare gains. However, if introduced across the board, these would be inequitable and user fees might thus be socially and politically unacceptable. Similar problems were encountered in Jamaica when user fees were introduced experimentally in public clinics (Bailey and Phillips, 1990). In Kenya, it was suggested that the restriction of user fees to government hospitals might help to eliminate this effect and enable more funds to be released for extending services (as hospitals absorb some 65 per cent of the national health budget). There is a general problem, however, in poorly funded and overstretched systems, that if any sector within the system becomes more efficient and of better quality, gains will soon be lost by the swamping effects of new users switching to it.

The underlying question is, of course, what can and should consumers pay for publicly provided health care in poor countries? The relative balance of costs may be very different for rural and urban dwellers, as rural transport costs may be higher and cash incomes lower than in towns. Some form of price discrimination geographically or sectorally may thus be justified. Musgrove (1986), however, points out that discrimination among consumers by income level may be of limited value in many countries, because the better-off are unlikely to be customers of the public sector and may well be covered by social security systems. Alternatively, a uniform fee (low enough not to discourage the poor consumers) could be charged per consultation and discrimination in charges only introduced at the stage of treatment. This type of practice has been employed by some mission and charitable organizations, of course, with treatment charges being based on ability to pay, even if this is difficult to ascertain.

The delicate balance in setting fees for health care (in the public sector in particular) is to reduce unnecessary or frivolous demand whilst not curtailing necessary utilization. Unfortunately, this requires a certain sophistication on the part of users, dependent on education and access to health care information, that is not present even in many developed countries. Experience in fact suggests that the pool of demand for health care is virtually bottomless and this includes 'genuine' and relatively trivial demand.

Other economic components or costs include waiting time and medicines. The waiting-time element may be considerable in many cases – sometimes a visit to a Third World outpatient clinic or an emergency room will involve several hours' wait. In addition, sick people in Third World countries in particular are often accompanied by another person, to help with travel or children. Considerable waiting periods have been identified by studies in West Malaysia, Jamaica, Guatemala and elsewhere for Western clinics or hospitals; however, Akin *et al.* (1985) comment that, in spite of their possibly greater physical accessibility, waiting times for herbalists may be almost as long although the waiting arrangements are much less formal and, to an extent, more social.

The costs of any treatment prescribed may also be an important factor in deciding whether to use a service and which type of facility to attend. In theory, for example, Western-style drugs may be free or only cost a maximum subsidized price but, frequently, the drugs will be unavailable at government outlets and patients will have to attend private shops (possibly buying black-market drugs in some circumstances) where the costs of medicines may be high and their quality and age questionable. It has been noted, for example in the Ivory Coast, that patients may be given costly prescriptions to fill elsewhere, adding to transport and time costs. Each health centre is allocated medicines to be dispensed free but these run out quickly. As a result, traditional remedies or home therapies, because of their relative cheapness and availability, may be used rather than modern medicine, especially in rural areas. By contrast, in urban settings, herbal remedies may be as expensive as some modern medicine (Lasker 1981). There is also less of an opportunity to pay for modern-sector drugs and treatment with payments in kind (in rural or urban areas), which may add to relative costs of modern medicines.

Overall, therefore, a number of hidden costs may result in the necessity for expenditure on services that are theoretically free. Costs of travel, medicines, the necessity on occasions to pay personnel (corruptly) for services that should be free, and the direct and indirect costs of waiting time all add to patients' direct and indirect costs in the receipt of health care. They may influence different groups of patients and potential patients either to use or to avoid a given facility, to repeat attendances, or to select a different facility (public or private) or even a different form of therapy. It is often assumed that the poorest patients will seek 'free' public care but this is not always so. In the Philippines, for example, Akin *et al.* (1985) note that the poorest families in Bicol often paid substantial fees for the use of private clinics for outpatient care. Free government clinics to some extent were serving many higher-income patients (especially for MCH services) as they presumably were better able than the poorest groups to deal with the various features surrounding attendance. Habib and Vaughan (1986) in a household survey in rural Iraq found that utilization of local health centres did not vary markedly according to income but that use of higher-level government health sources and private clinics did increase substantially with increasing income (see Fig. 6.7, in which the 15 to 29 dinar per month group represents those of around average income). More importantly, however, as discussed below, utilization appeared to be strongly discouraged by increasing distance, which might imply only the better-off were able to travel to more distant facilities.

Similarly, Chernichovsky and Meesook (1986), analysing household utilization data for Indonesia (covering urban and rural

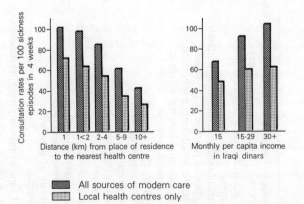

Fig. 6.7 Relationships between consultation rates and distance and income in Iraq (from Habib and Vaughan 1986)

Table 6.3 Comparison of treatment of illness by household per capita consumption level, Indonesia (abstracted from Chernichovsky and Meesook 1986)

	Java					
	Urban			Rural		
	Lower 40%	Middle 40%	Upper 20%	Lower 40%	Middle 40%	Upper 20%
Percentage of households with members who have been ill during the last 7 days	14	17	17	14	16	24
Place where received treatment (%)						
At home	58	27	12	53	41	40
At traditional practitioner's residence	10	3	1	6	7	3
At place of practice of physician	13	34	58	22	12	29
At public health centre/subcentre	19	22	15	17	37	21
At a maternity hospital or clinic	0	0	9	1	2	0
At a general hospital	0	14	5	1	1	7
Treated by (%)						
Self or family member	58	20	12	45	35	32
Traditional practitioner	10	7	1	6	10	7
Midwife or paramedic	19	23	14	34	34	20
Physician	13	50	72	16	21	41
Distance to person giving treatment (km)						
Self or family member	0	0	0	0	0	0
Traditional practitioner	0	0	5.00	0.47	13.20	0
Midwife or paramedic	0.64	1.72	2.85	2.46	2.31	1.10
Physician	1.32	1.40	2.53	5.60	10.47	11.67
Travel time to person giving treatment (h)						
Self or family member	0	0	0	0	0	0
Traditional practitioner	0	0	1.00	0	2.28	0
Midwife or paramedic	0.45	0.45	0.22	0.52	0.43	0.18
Physician	0.11	0.30	0.32	0.56	2.16	1.29

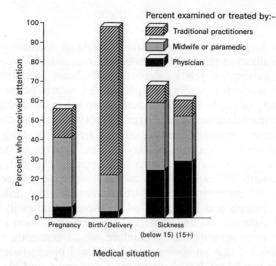

Fig. 6.8 **The proportion of people receiving medical attention for
selected medical situations, Indonesia (based on data from
Chernichovsky and Meesook 1986)**

areas, and different socioeconomic groups), found low income to
be a strong barrier to the utilization of modern primary medical
facilities even when publicly provided. The relatively well-to-do
were spending more on, and using more heavily, the services of
trained physicians. The poorest segment of the Indonesian population (the poor in Java) were mostly treated at home by family or
at a TMP's house. The rich were much more likely to have been
treated by a physician, possibly at their home (especially in urban
areas of Java) than were the lowest-income group (Table 6.3).
Public facilities were most heavily visited by the middle-income
group, especially in rural areas. Very few of the urban upper-
income group received treatment from a TMP. The same can be
said for the use of health services by pregnant women in the study
(illustrating a more standardized case of care). Only 5 per cent of
the upper-income group were examined by a TMP, compared with
29 per cent of the lower-income group. Some 80 per cent of rich
women as compared with only 55 per cent of the low-income group
had received an examination. Interestingly, practically all deliveries
were attended by a practitioner of some kind, although 76 per cent
of deliveries were by traditional midwives and only 3 per cent by
physicians. In spite of the fact that about 40 per cent of pregnant
women are seen by a midwife or physician, the actual deliveries
are predominantly conducted by a TBA (see Fig. 6.8).

Age and sex

These two important variables have long been identified as influencing utilization rates and types of services used. However, the intuitively anticipated relationships do not always hold true. For example, it might reasonably be expected that elderly people would be high users of medical services but research has often suggested that elderly populations contain large proportions of non-attenders and infrequent attenders. They are often in a relatively stable health state, in which the demands of, say, health care related to occupation, the needs for attendance for young children, or in connection with FP or childbirth are no longer directly relevant. The effects of increasing age on utilization are thus difficult to generalize (Joseph and Phillips 1984), although studies in Britain and North America do find that primary care utilization rates on average do increase with age. Therefore, at an aggregate level, it may be expected that an ageing population will place gradually increasing demands on health services (Cartwright and Anderson 1981; Donabedian 1973). Higher average consultation rates for elderly people will also be coupled with requirements for *different kinds* of health services (needs for more long-term and chronic care; more socially-related care, perhaps, relating to housing needs and the like). In the context of the epidemiological change in many Third World countries with both ageing and juvenile population segments, this is likely to be an increasingly important recognition.

There have been some suggestions that elderly people are more likely than younger age groups to use traditional practitioners (in Zambia, Nigeria and Taiwan, for example). However, whilst Good (1987a) found that the majority of TMPs' patients in his study of traditional medicine in Kenya were adults, most were in the 20 to 40 age group; women accounted for 55 to 60 per cent of consultations to healers investigated. At the other end of the age spectrum, however, results are less clear. Children under the age of 5 years have been found in some circumstances to be important clients for herbalists and spiritualists in a Kinshasha study, which was unexpected because of the numerous MCH services available. Studies in North India, rural Nigeria and rural Ethiopia have likewise noted children as important clients of TMPs (Kroeger 1983). Chernichovsky and Meesook (1986) also found a very slight increase in the proportion of people under 15 years of age who received attention from a traditional practitioner in their Indonesian study. By contrast, a Lusaka study found children to be most frequently taken to a biomedical facility and Good (1987a) found that Kenyan children accounted for fewer than 5 per cent of TMPs' patients; children under 5 years of age in particular presented very infrequently.

Age does appear therefore to differentiate somewhat whether traditional or Western-type facilities are attended. It is intuitively felt that elderly people might place greater reliance on TMPs, possibly for reasons of familiarity or perhaps costs, and it might likewise be felt that young children, being so often targeted for PHC and MCH campaigns, would tend to be users of modern facilities. However, this pattern is not consistent. Similarly, when the usage of Western-type facilities themselves is considered, in most Third World countries, age does not necessarily have a clear influence on utilization rates. This is to some extent complicated by the differences between incidence of reported illness (or need for preventive medicine) and actual utilization; of course, the two do not necessarily correspond completely.

In terms of illness patterns, two studies in 1970 and 1979 of the provinces and towns of Thailand (but excluding in 1979 the Bangkok metropolis) showed considerable age and sex variations in respondents who reported illness in the previous month (Table 6.4). The pre-school age group had the highest frequency in 1979, followed by the 65+ age group; rates were generally similar at both times for all groups except the youngest two groups. The age-adjusted illness rate for females was slightly higher than for males except in the school-age group (7 to 14 years). A refinement was to analyse the 1979 data on the basis of seriousness of illness. In this, as might be expected, major illnesses tended to be the

Table 6.4 Thailand: illness reported within 1 month of survey, by age and sex; rate per 1 000 (from Porapakkham 1982)

Age and sex		1970	1979
0–6	Total	226	441.3
	Male	–	438.7
	Female	–	444.1
7–14	Total	102	248.6
	Male	–	257.9
	Female	–	239.1
15–44	Total	114	192.3
	Male	98	185.3
	Female	127	198.9
45–64	Total	209	246.4
	Male	199	235.7
	Female	219	258.5
65+	Total	281	288.8
	Male	292	278.3
	Female	271	297.5
All ages		149	268.4

predominant causes of ill health in the older age groups; in the school age 7 to 14 group, minor illnesses were somewhat more important (Porapakkham 1982).

Age may have influence on the use of specific types of services. Family-planning services, naturally, are sought mainly by those in the younger child-bearing years, although advice may be sought by women in later fertile years also. The Narangwal Experiment, involving MCH services in rural India, focused on utilization of a range of services, including women's illness services, children's illness services and other services for both groups. Women with younger children under 3 years were using the services for children more frequently than were mothers with older children, although this was in part a consequence of the project's focus on youngsters. There were no significant differences within the 15 to 49 years married women age group in use of women's illness services. In the use of 'other services', the younger, low-caste women were receiving more attention than those over 35 and of high caste, indicating a social as well as age differential. Again, however, the targeting of services onto the lower-caste groups could have explained such a difference rather than any age-specific behaviour (Taylor *et al.* 1983).

Other variables

Many other specific variables influence health care utilization. *Education* is an important influence on the knowledge of both when to use health services and how to use them effectively; as a variable, however, its effects are strongly linked to those of income and socioeconomic status. Education also influences which types of services are used; for example, in the developing countries participating in the World Fertility Survey, women with more years of schooling had a greater likelihood of using a modern FP method and were likely to have a smaller family size (Fig. 6.9). Improved education of women in a Cebu study (the Philippines) was also found to be associated with increased use of modern prenatal care (Wong *et al.* 1987). However, as seen below, education does not always seem to advance the stage at which prenatal care is sought.

In Indonesia, less educated households were more likely to need more curative medical attention because of the likelihood of greater incidence of infectious ailments. This was, however, strongly related to home environment, household income, family size and nutrition. The independent effects of education are therefore difficult to distinguish although, today, the educational levels of mothers, and particularly female literacy rates, are generally strongly related to levels of infant mortality, effective feeding and good

Method of family planning used by women

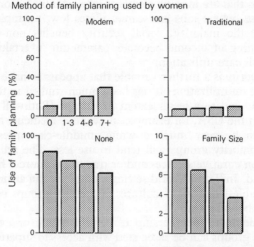

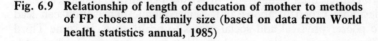

Number of years schooling

Fig. 6.9 Relationship of length of education of mother to methods of FP chosen and family size (based on data from World health statistics annual, 1985)

use of health services (higher education can mean higher and more effective utilization). Poorer education, poorer nutrition and poorer sanitation levels can all place families and children in multiple jeopardy and often result in underutilization relative to need. This is, of course, not only a feature of Third World countries but is a continuing source of concern in many developed countries (Phillips 1981b). The matter of health education for families and communities is related to this issue and is returned to in Chapter 8.

In the Ivory Coast, having some education was associated with a higher use of hospitals as a source of primary care than was having no education (although those with 'some education' appeared to have more varied sources of care) (Lasker 1981). However, not all surveys have shown that increased education leads to an earlier use of health services; for example, Marshall (1985) did not find much difference according to educational level in the timing during pregnancy of visits to antenatal clinics in Port Moresby, Papua New Guinea (although non-attenders who were not included in the survey might have had lower overall educational levels). More important in determining at what stage of pregnancy a woman attended a clinic seemed to be whether or not she was working. Those employed for wages tended to postpone their first clinic visit. This implies it is legal aspects of rights of women (in this case) to attend medical advice whilst pregnant and guarantee retention of their jobs that are missing elements in most Third World countries. Of course, where jobs are scarce, wages low, unemployment high and, for the majority, social security benefits non-existent, the safeguarding of income becomes paramount, overtaking the need for health care utilization.

Ethnicity is a further variable that appears to have considerable influence on utilization. It has been much studied in the context of the USA, and to a lesser extent in Europe (Rathwell and Phillips 1986). In the USA, for example, preventive medicine has been suggested to be very much a white, middle-class preserve, which ethnic minority groups will tend to use less. The reliance of such groups on curative services and/or traditional sources has long been suggested. In Third World settings, ethnicity can at times be a crucial variable when many cultures and ethnic groups coexist within national boundaries.

Sometimes, membership of certain ethnic or even cultural–religious groups can be associated with access to superior or inferior health care (it has earlier been suggested that this can be associated with differential utilization). In Western countries, residence in less desirable urban locations and socioeconomic deprivation can lead to poorer physical and social access to health care. In some Third World countries, this may be reflected in urban–rural ethnic differences (in Nigeria and Kenya, for example) or in different preferences among tribal groups for varying sorts of treatment (see, for example, Good 1987a; Stock 1983). Such preferences may be based on a common language or religion that leads to the patronage of certain types of healers or medical providers (Ramesh and Hyma 1981). The threshold between use of self-care and non-professional care can differ between ethnic and religious groups, and ethnic differences in symptom sensitivity may be one, but not the only, explanation (Kroeger 1983). There are also varying ethnic expectations of treatment, which may go some way towards explaining preferences for various traditional or modern health care sources. In some countries, notably South Africa, membership of different ethnic groups can affect considerably the need for use of health services, for example, because of economic, social, nutritional and political differences (Fincham 1985).

Whilst there are only a few diseases that appear to have an identifiable genetic component, there are nevertheless marked ethnic differences in the incidence of a range of disorders. Dietary, sociocultural and other explanations have been advanced. Sometimes, too, the detection of certain types of condition may lead one to suspect spatial or ethnic differences in incidence. Good (1987a), for example, notes the marked spatial variation in the incidence of diabetes among Kenya's ethnolinguistic groups. He points out that this may only reflect the way in which data have been collected and that more detailed study is required. In many countries, the true health care needs of members of certain ethnic groups may in fact be virtually unknown. The Philippines, for example, has many hill-tribe groups who are very isolated and for whom official, modern health care is virtually non-existent. This may be thought of as a form of ethnic discrimination, although the danger to the cultural integrity of groups (especially of remote, small-scale groups) from the introduction of major modern facilities has long been recognized. The dilemma of how to provide health care for them without irreparably damaging their societies frequently remains to be resolved.

Quality of service

The issue of how the 'quality' of a service (as distinct from its quantitative availability) affects utilization is complex. 'Quality' can include many facets: physical, attitudinal and socioeconomic. High-quality medical care is often considered to be that which involves an 'objective' test such as an X-ray, blood analysis or the like (Donabedian 1980). However, it also depends on many other physical and administrative attributes of the facility – space, comfort, cleanliness, seating arrangements and 'convenience' of opening hours. Finally, an evaluation of quality of service must take into account level of professional care, availability of medicines and the 'affective behaviour' of staff and ancillary workers to patients (Ben Sira 1976; Phillips 1981b). There is also an intangible aspect of quality associated with whether a service is being provided by the public sector or privately, as there may be inherent beliefs (or images) relating to care from each sector. The measurement of 'quality' is, by its nature, to some extent subjective, although minimum guidelines can be established in any setting to assess quality in a comparative (but not an absolute) sense.

To Akin *et al.* (1985), the quality issue is one of the most neglected demand issues in PHC (and probably in all health care utilization). In particular, as people become better off financially, they appear as a rule to become more willing to pay for higher-quality services. Heller (1982) illustrates that increased demand for private rather than public practitioners occurred in Malaysia with increased income, although overall quantity of demand did not increase. Mwabu (1986) sees the majority of patients in his Kenyan study seeking health care from outside the 'free' government health care system based on patient influences, nature of illness and a composite of attributes of health care providers in which quality and accessibility were all important.

'Quality' is, of course, related to costs and also to accessibility.

If 'high quality' or acceptable quality of services is not available within a local area, the potential patient may trade off the extra costs of travelling to a desired quality service further away. However, at some point, the costs to travel (including time) and the cost of the service itself may combine to deter or even prevent utilization. At this point, local or cheaper sources may be reappraised and perhaps used. However, if the accessible and/or affordable services are perceived not to be of sufficient quality to instil confidence or to be worthy of using, then either lower or no utilization may result.

Patients often tend to evaluate quality in terms of the perceived efficacy or appropriateness of treatments. When laypeople cannot judge the contribution of technical intervention to their well-being, Ben Sira (1976) suggests that the 'bedside' manner of the professional's presentation ('affective behaviour') becomes crucial. Therefore, hard-pressed public clinics may well be at a disadvantage in terms of the professionals being able to display sufficient devotion to, or to spend sufficient time with, individuals. These variables, according to Ben Sira, will affect the lay evaluation of the service (a surrogate for assessing its quality). In their Philippines study, Akin *et al.* (1985) suggest that, for illnesses perceived to be serious, there was a strong movement towards private practitioners. They view this as a quality-related phenomenon.

The question of how the quality of public care provided affects utilization of services has been investigated for prenatal care in Cebu, the Philippines. 'Quality of care' was found to be an important influence but it was differently perceived in rural and urban areas. Wong *et al.* (1987) focus on the number of visits made to the nearest public facility, the quality of care being measured by ability to see a physician and/or nurse rather than a midwife. In urban areas, if the professional providing care was normally a midwife, this tended to reduce the number of visits to the modern sector and increase utilization of TBAs. By contrast, in rural areas, the availability of a midwife seemed to be regarded as signifying good-quality care and had a significant effect on the number of public visits. This suggests that, while the urban residents consider a midwife at a public facility to provide low quality of care, she is considered to be providing a high quality of care in rural areas relative to the alternatives available. When the matter of accessibility is also included, there is something of a policy dilemma: Filipino mothers want better-trained personnel to provide services but they also want the facilities nearby. However, to make doctors and nurses available, facilities often require centralization or peripatetic staffing, distancing them from some users. These changes might be regarded as reducing 'accessibility' with concomitant threats to utilization rates.

It may be dangerous to assume automatically that publicly provided services will have a poorer image (and perceived quality) than private services. Annis (1981), as noted below, found MOH health centres in Guatemala to have a poor drawing power because of their bad image, and similar poor quality involving unavailability of public doctors, long waiting times and lack of medicines was found in rural Nepal (Dhungel and Dias, 1988). While these studies pointed to poor quality of public services, the reverse was found in Santiago de Chile. Here, 140 frequent users of a national health service system (SNSS) PHC clinic were very satisfied with the presentation and clinical aspects of care (Scarpaci 1988). The urban poor in particular claimed that, even if they had sufficient income to be able to pay for private services, they would still prefer to be treated at neighbourhood (SNSS) facilities. The conclusion is that changes in management practices might lead to such enhanced utilization and high satisfaction and that, in this case, the public sector is serving its PHC clients well and should not be cut back.

Utilization and distance

Physical distance naturally acts as a barrier or disincentive to attendance at almost any sort of facilities for good practical reasons. However, the effects of distance will vary in different circumstances: for example, where there is a good road network or good, cheap public transport, its effects will be less severe than in areas where public or private transport is not available. Distance also expresses itself as time – the time (and costs) of travel, which may well differ among facilities. It is implicit in the above that the effects of distance will vary in severity from one family to another, depending on their physical and personal mobility, their financial and other resources. The effects will also vary from community to community, because 'transport networks' are of different levels of sophistication and these 'community resources' will influence the ease with which members of the community can use services.

For medical geographers in particular, the effects of distance on utilization of health services have been of major interest. Most studies have identified a negative relationship between distance and utilization (Phillips 1986b; Stock 1987), although some show that this relationship may vary according to illness and that it is not necessarily always negative or constant. Even in systems that are allegedly free of economic or social barriers to utilization, distance does appear to have some influence on attendance rates and locations which are attended. As a rule, however, in Third World and other countries, distance is only one variable, which may interact more or less strongly with others to influence utilization. Mesa-Lago (1985) points out that a middle-class state employee or a university professor living in San José, Costa Rica, obviously has a much better opportunity of receiving quick, efficient and appropriate health care than a poor peasant living 30 km from the nearest health centre or rural post in the same country. Here, the influence of distance, accessibility, quality of care, socioeconomic status, articulateness, knowledge and many other factors combine to influence utilization.

Nevertheless, much research has been aimed at defining the effects of distance on utilization of specific levels of service or for specific types of illness. We should also remember, as noted in Chapter 4, that distance does not equate directly with 'accessibility', although in everyday speech these terms are often used interchangeably. Accessibility implies 'get-atable' (Moseley 1979), and takes account not only of physical distance but of other factors such as social distance, cost distance and opening hours (availability) of services. Gesler (1984) reminds us that the preference for traditional medicine over Western medicine may often be partly a matter of its lower 'social distance' as much as its being physically more proximate. Social distance implies some sort of comfort and acceptance in using the service; it may be that people are even willing to travel further in physical distance to use a service with which they feel more socially comfortable. In addition, in the context of health care, this may include the feeling of confidence in, or the appropriateness of, a certain type of facility for treating a specific condition. People may be willing to travel further to reach a facility in which they have, broadly speaking, greater confidence.

Distance decay in the use of health services

'Distance decay' is a well-recognized spatial phenomenon which means that as a service or facility becomes more distant fewer people will patronize it. The geographical literature is replete with evidence of distance decay in the use of services and there is not sufficient space here for a full review of this concept. Joseph and Phillips (1984) examine distance decay in the use of health services of various sorts, including hospitals, emergency rooms and primary care facilities. In general, studies tend to confirm a more or less gradual fall-off in utilization rates over distance, although the steepness of decline varies considerably from facility to facility. In the case of visits to emergency rooms in the intra-urban setting of Toronto, where there are many alternative facilities within a relatively short distance, utilization rates decline steeply and, outside a distance of 2 to 3 miles, the facility is almost ignored. By contrast, in rural New South Wales, travel rates for inpatient and outpatient care decline much more gradually as people are used to travelling further for services and have no choice on the whole other than one or two hospitals in a sparsely populated area. It is interesting, how-

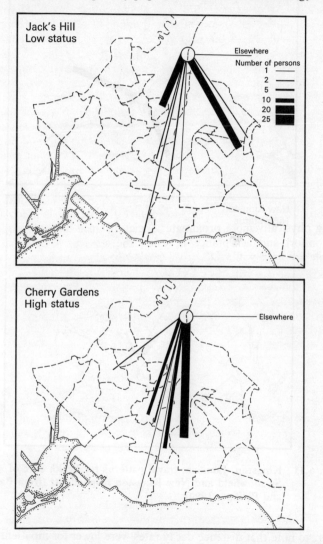

Fig. 6.10 Kingston, Jamaica: travel patterns for health care of Jack's Hill and Cherry Gardens respondents (from Bailey and Phillips, 1990). See Figs 4.11 and 4.12 for location of doctors and hospitals

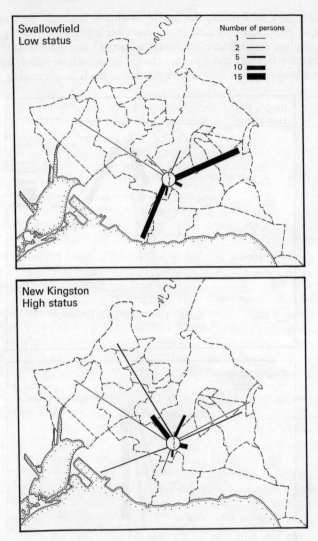

Fig. 6.11   Kingston, Jamaica: travel patterns for health care of Swallowfield and New Kingston respondents (from Bailey and Phillips, 1990)

ever, to note that distance decay rates were lower for inpatient than outpatient care (Walmsley 1978)

Distance decay rates also operate differently for different social groups. In studies of the use of general practitioner services in Britain (Phillips 1981b) and of dental services (see, for example,

Taylor and Carmichael), it has been found that better-off residents, whilst not automatically travelling further for health care, may do so in some cases. However, the converse case of less well-off people also travelling further than needed for health care has been noted, sometimes related to such folk travelling to areas in which they previously lived (sometimes to city centres for ex-city dwellers suburbanized to peripheral housing estates). These 'relict patterns' of spatial utilization behaviour are also to be seen in Hong Kong, in which some residents of the new towns return at first to facilities in their old areas of residence. Such behaviour, of course, may be expected to modify over time (Phillips 1984).

In the Third World, there is less immediately available information on the socioeconomic differentials in distance decay. However, Bailey and Phillips (1990) have noted some differences in Kingston, Jamaica, between the spatial behaviour of residents in juxtaposed pairs of survey sites, one of each pair being richer and one poorer. The residents from the high-status sites were often travelling considerable distances to reach expensive private clinics in the business area of mid-town Kingston. By contrast, poorer residents in many sites were using locally available public health centres or one of the two public emergency rooms at the university hospital or Kingston Public Hospital (see Figs 4.11, 4.12, 6.10 and 6.11). It is dangerous to generalize, however, as the better-off residents living nearer the business district of New Kingston had ready access to local private practitioners for health care whilst their poorer neighbours living close by in Swallowfield had to travel much further to the public hospitals mentioned previously (Fig. 6.11). Therefore, it is important to remember that the relative socioeconomic accessibility of services will make them more or less available (or desirable) to some types of residents. For the poor people in Swallowfield, although they were living in a medically relatively well-provided area of town, these private facilities were in effect not available to them and might as well not have existed. This serves to remind us that (in geographical jargon) spatial propinquity does not equate with social accessibility (Joseph and Phillips 1984; Phillips 1981b).

Other examples of the impact of distance on Third World health care

The reasons for distance decay can be quite straightforward (such as the lack of transport locally) but the above discussion implies that there are often complex combinations of reasons – social, economic, psychological, as well as physical distance – for the tail-off in demand and usage over distance. Stock (1987) reminds us that it is important to move beyond mechanistic formulations of how distance (as a variable) operates and to focus on the ways in which people conceptualize illness and health, how they decide upon therapeutic strategies and then how chosen courses of action are implemented. The discovery, for example, of general distance decay in health care utilization may lead to the conclusion that utilization is actually regular and easily predictable. However, when this distance decay is examined against, for example, type of illness, category of facility, age, sex or social status, then very different subcategories of influence of distance may evolve. Geographers have been concerned to fit 'exponent values' to the rate of distance decay for various facilities and illnesses, and this can appear mechanistic. It may nevertheless be a useful exercise and it can reveal interesting things: for instance, in a rural Canadian environment, Girt (1973) found that increasing distance generally did lead to a tail-off in usage but that this varied from being uniform for less serious disorders to actually being associated for some more serious conditions with an increased desire to utilize services up to a certain distance, which thereafter reduced. If such cut-off points and the 'rate' of distance decay can be identified with any certainty, this can help planners to decide where to locate facilities so that they have maximum impact, and to an extent minimize private and public travel costs and the like.

As noted earlier in the chapter, Stock (1987) has proposed modifications to a medical sociological model to analyse health care behaviour, allowing predisposing, enabling and illness characteristics to be integrated. Enabling factors in this context include accessibility, organization, financial and spatial arrangements of services, but the illness condition may also be included. The assessment of the illness is shown to be the primary determinant of health care behaviour, affecting both the decision to seek treatment and the therapeutic option chosen. Common, recognized and unthreatening conditions will in general evoke a different response from chronic, unresponsive conditions or acute, apparently serious illnesses. It is also important to look at the full range of therapeutic options available. For example, Stock (1987) found a regular distance decay in utilization of pharmacy facilities in Kano State, Nigeria, with an approximate 25 per cent fall in utilization on average for each additional kilometre to facility. However, when the action of people from individual villages within the catchment area was examined, this appeared to vary considerably from village to village. Residents of some villages within 0 to 2 km of the facility were using it only ten times per 100 people annually, whereas other similarly located villages had utilization rates six times higher. It is evident that alternatives to this source of care must have been being used by some villagers. The use of alternative sources (perhaps

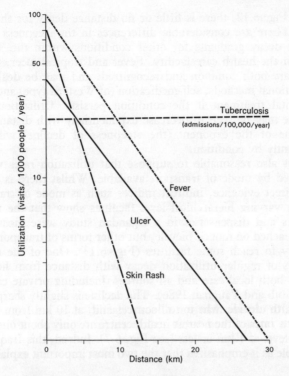

Fig. 6.12 Distance decay varies for different conditions: per capita utilization of higher-order health care facilities, for selected Hausa illnesses, Kano State, Nigeria (after Stock 1983)

traditional care) tended to increase with even greater distance from the facility under examination.

Whilst Stock (1987) emphasizes that a culturally sensitive, holistic, approach to the geographical aspects of health care behaviour is essential, statistical investigation of patterns of utilization of health facilities, such as the relationship between distance and usage, is an important beginning and arguably essential in the context of facility location. It is important to discover the use and potential usage of certain facilities for specific conditions. Stock's research in Nigeria illustrates that perceptions about sickness and specific illnesses are reflected directly in differential health facility utilization, and distance decay gradients vary accordingly. For example, fracture has already been identified as a condition for which traditional treatment is perceived to be appropriate; by contrast, *tibi* (tuberculosis) is seen as an illness for which there is no indigenous remedy and Western-style treatment is essential. As a result, as seen in Fig. 6.12, there is little or no distance decay for this condition. There are considerable differences in the steepness of the distance decay gradients for other conditions within the 30-mile radius of the health care facility. Fever and tropical ulcer, for example, are both common and recognized, and may be dealt with by traditional methods, self-medication (of Western type) and finally hospital treatment if the condition persists. Utilization rates therefore may be seen to decrease exponentially with distance but the value of the exponent (the steepness of decline) will vary significantly by condition.

It is also reasonable to suppose that utilization rates will be influenced by mode of transport available. Whilst there is not so much direct evidence, indirect indices such as mode of transport used for varying hierarchical level facilities show that the nearby aid posts and dispensaries in a Ugandan study were most commonly reached on foot or bicycle, but other forms of transport were necessary to reach some facilities (Fig. 6.13). One of the clearer examples of regular utilization decay with distance from home is seen for both local care and all sources (including private care) in Iraq (Habib and Vaughan 1986). The decline is slightly sharper for local health centres than for all sources and, at 10 km from home, utilization rates of the nearest health centre are only about one-third of their level at 1 km or less (see Fig. 6.7). Indeed, this Iraq study is valuable as it emphasizes that the two most important explanatory

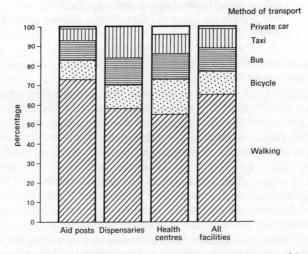

Fig. 6.13   Means of transport used to reach various types of health care facility in Uganda (based on data from Akin *et al.* 1985)

variables for utilization were perceived sickness (or need) and distance to the nearest health care facility, rather than any demographic variables. Levels of utilization were markedly reduced with increasing distance.

It is fair to say that the effects of distance on utilization have only been cursorily or even simplistically evaluated by many researchers other than medical geographers. General statements have emerged from many studies to the effect that only those close to a facility can derive full benefits from its services. Fosu (1986) points to surveys of health centre utilization in Ghana, for example, in which 70 per cent of attenders came from within a 3-mile radius, although the residents of this area comprised only 23 per cent of the health centre's catchment population. Only 27 per cent of attenders had come from beyond 4 miles, but 73 per cent of the health centre's catchment population lived at that distance. This implies that, to be used, a facility must be accessible and, conversely, that nearby residents derive disproportionate benefit from facilities. For the rural dweller, in particular, this will usually mean a maximum travel threshold and, once this is exceeded, utilization may tail off considerably. The threshold concept seems to hold true for whatever level of service is considered. This means most medical services have a relatively limited 'range' and it is important for planners to be able to identify this range in order that they can locate services so distance does not prove to be a significant deterrent. This might involve the provision of smaller-scale facilities than might otherwise be desirable or economic, or perhaps the use of peripatetic mobile facilities to extend outreach.

The rural poor and poorer peripheral urban dwellers are generally disadvantaged either in terms of physical access or in terms of socioeconomic access to health care. In urban areas of the Philippines, it has already been noted that poor people may stretch themselves to pay for private care, but in such urban areas public *barangay* health stations may substitute for traditional care and provide a network of readily accessible care, so distance becomes less of an issue (Wong *et al*. 1987). In these circumstances, quality of care and public attitudes to it might assume greater importance. Elsewhere, distance may prove to be a major additional barrier to use.

This issue of quality of care in influencing utilization is stressed in the study of rural Guatemala introduced in Chapter 4. Contrary to what is usually assumed to be the situation in the Third World, the vast majority of persons in three large departments in Western Guatemala were found to have quite good physical access to official health facilities although roads were poor and travel times slow. However, Annis (1981) found these MOH facilities to have 'minuscule geographic drawing power', which was attributed to their poor public image (the clinics were understaffed, with poorly trained personnel, were badly equipped and had low success rates). Annis concludes that raising levels of utilization in this situation depends more on achieving improvements in the quality of delivered services than on increasing accessibility by building more health posts (accessibility was already adequate) or by overcoming supposed 'cultural barriers'. Nevertheless, there was evidence that those living nearer the health posts used them disproportionately and those living further away used them far less. About 16 per cent of the population studied lived 1 km or less from a health post, but over 50 per cent of patients were accounted for by such people. Conversely, half the population lived more than 3.5 km from a post, but such people made up only 15 per cent of health post clientele. Therefore, in spite of reasonable access, there is still marked distance decay and few people travelled beyond a very short distance to take advantage of the MOH health post services. The reason people did not take advantage of the facilities on offer is their poor perceived quality, lack of treatment and poor personnel. If this occurs in conjunction with increased distance, a considerable tail-off in utilization develops. Poor-quality service therefore seems to potentiate distance decay effects (why travel far to receive bad services?). This raises a very important utilization issue for policymakers.

Many other research projects have also noted the importance of distance. Lasker (1981) in the Ivory Coast considers the accessibility of alternatives, and particularly to a range of choices, is crucial to utilization. Kroeger (1983) notes that accessibility in rural India was a dominant factor affecting use, although the strength of distance decay varied from one type of facility to another: a health centre attracted 75 per cent of its patients from within 2.9 miles, traditional practitioners 2.5 miles, and qualified allopathic practitioners had a larger catchment of 7.5 miles. Long distances and waiting times were cited as major reasons for not using allopathic dispensaries in New Delhi and, in rural Punjab, accessibility was a major factor in choice among therapies offered. In Indonesia, whilst low household income is a barrier to utilization, distance was also significant for rural people in particular and the upper-income group were able to travel more than twice the distance of the lower-income group to reach a physician. It seems that, partly as a result, fewer higher-income people were reliant on self-treatment or paramedical assistance, but here the impact of distance is being modified by the varying financial circumstances of respondents (Chernichovsky and Meesook 1986).

Distance may have the additional effect of cutting people off from their usual or expected source of care, and particularly their social networks. Marshall (1985) shows that fewer women attended antenatal clinics in Port Moresby General Hospital as distance increased (particularly it seems beyond about 5 to 6 km). However, she suggests that more women were coming from a heterogenous suburb and fewer from outlying villages as much because such women had been cut off from many of the usual village support networks during pregnancy and were more likely to have been exposed to Western-style medical beliefs. Therefore, again, the effects of distance on utilization have to be looked at in the light of health care beliefs and expectations, and with regard to the promixity of other sources of care (in this case village traditional support systems).

In rural India, Ramachandran and Shastri (1983) found little variation between socioeconomic groups in the distances travelled to Western medical facilities – a different conclusion from that evidenced in some other settings. However, they explain this by the fact that the available medical facilities were few (so choice was limited). Larger-scale farmers did nevertheless have a tendency to travel further for treatment than artisans, who tended to seek treatment within the village. There was therefore some indication in their findings that differential 'social accessibility' existed even in these circumstances and that the actual places of visits for treatment did differ among the various socioeconomic groups in a status-conscious population. In the highest status and income group, over one-third were treated by private practitioners, compared with only about 3 per cent in the poorer groups. This would naturally influence the distance that would have to be travelled for specific sources of care.

Use of traditional medicine

A deliberate decision has been made in this chapter not to segregate explicitly the use of traditional facilities from that of modern-sector facilities. In part, this reflects the relative lack of detailed studies of utilization of traditional health care in comparison to those of modern facilities, although Good (1987a) and a few others prove notable exceptions. A similar exception is the study of use of traditional medicine in Malaysia, in which interviews were conducted with 100 people who had come to visit a *bomoh* (traditional Malay healer) in Kedah in north-west Malaysia (Heggenhougen 1980).

In this study, sixty-five patients were males and thirty-five females; all except two were Malays. Some 53 per cent were under 30 years of age, indicating there was not a particular bias among elderly people to using this form of medicine. Interestingly, a wide range of complaints or problems were presented: 37 per cent were physical (and psychosomatic), 12 per cent 'traditional' illness categories, 8 per cent psychological and, possibly surprisingly, 42 per cent were involved with study, interviews and exams (anxiety sources, for which traditional therapy is often felt appropriate). Twenty-five patients had used another health source for the same problem. In terms of distances travelled, there was not marked distance decay. Some 30 per cent of patients had travelled up to 30 minutes to see the *bomoh*, but a slightly larger proportion had travelled more than 1 hour and over 10 per cent had travelled more than 3 hours. Therefore, although about three-quarters of attenders came from within 2 hours' travel, decline in attendances to this admittedly popular and well-known *bomoh* only really set in when travel of over 2 hours was involved. The reputation of this *bomoh* may account for the distances travelled to see him but, as a general point, Heggenhougen (1980) suggests that, as noted in Chapter 3, traditional resources of care are not regarded as antagonistic to cosmopolitan care but as an addition. Cosmopolitan health care concentrates on the disease; it is inattentive to the affective aspects of healing and this is why Malay traditional medicine is popular for psychological as well as physical complaints. That patients are willing to travel as long and as far as they evidently do to see this renowned healer argues against traditional medicines being used only as a local convenient alternative to Western sources of care. Perhaps this *bomoh* might be regarded as a 'consultant', providing a trusted and established mode of service. His geographical drawing power certainly seems to suggest this and one might guess that patients travel much longer to see him than they would to visit most modern PHC facilities. Here, again, perceived quality of care and faith in the provider may be traded off against considerable travel time for many patients.

Retrospect: utilization of health care in the Third World

This chapter had illustrated the difficulties referred to in earlier chapters of generalizing about health and health care in heterogeneous developing countries. Whilst the models introduced in the beginning of the chapter do provide something of a 'shopping list' of variables to be taken into account when investigating utilization, the relative weights of many variables will need to be modified in different Third World settings. For example, predisposing variables (including cultural characteristics) will have different influences, depending on local and individual attitudes to traditional medicine. Community resources will also vary very much from place to place, depending on the levels of public, private and traditional care available. Income and economic variables may take on greater significance either as barriers to utilization or as permissive factors in the poorer countries. They may especially influence the behaviour of the poorest people in Third World countries in which, almost by definition, wealth is very unevenly distributed. Similarly, for some sectors of the population, transport will be little of a problem whilst, for others, lack of money or lack of personal or public transport will mean services have to be reached on foot. The availability and price of public transport vary markedly from region to region, being generally better in Asia and Latin America than in many African countries but, again, this also varies considerably by country and between rural and urban areas. In other words, the models will have to be very flexible to explain and predict health care utilization. It may be unreasonable to expect any model to be ubiquitously functional and, perhaps, the best they can provide is a blueprint of variables for research.

Other aspects of care have tended to impinge on utilization in some Third World settings even more than they do in many developed countries. The pluralistic nature of care in many Third World societies has led to assumptions of underutilization, based usually on the observation only of the modern sector. We must not forget that Chernichovsky and Meesook (1986), Good (1987a), Heggenhougen (1980), Mwabu (1986), Stock (1983, 1987) and others have found considerable usage of traditional resources, perhaps substituting for, or used in preference to, modern-sector services. Where health care systems are pluralistic, it seems that, to reach valid conclusions, research must be broad-based and take account of all potential sources of care.

The effects of factors such as distance on utilization seem likewise to vary according to circumstances. Some researchers have stressed that accessibility and being able physically to reach services is the key to understanding consumer behaviour and choice (Lasker 1981). Others see distance as but one of a complex range of interacting variables, which may have greater or lesser influence under different circumstances (Stock 1987; Wong *et al.* 1987). A reasonable conclusion seems to be that a minimum level of access is paramount (logically) but that, once decisions have been made to utilize, the impact of distance may vary according to what people are used to and willing to put up with. The urbanite may feel that travel of only a few miles is too far, but a rural dweller may be willing in some circumstances to travel for hours or even days to reach a desired source of care. Such variability is part of the rich interest in this field of research but it does not make for neat policy decisions!

The quality of care issue as it may affect utilization has to be considered. Many aid agencies, for example, have actually stressed rather expensive and elaborate facility provision even for primary health centres. These may be attractive (if not accessible) to many but quality of care goes beyond physical infrastructure. Staff must be provided, with professional and logistical support in the form of medicines and equipment. Training needs to include ways in which staff should approach patients of varying social status and education; if the 'affective behaviour' of staff is not as anticipated or is disagreeable to certain types of potential patients, this may deter utilization and render the most modern health care facilities of little practical use. Third World health care consumers must not be assumed to be uniformly unsophisticated and, indeed, much evidence suggests directly or indirectly that the quality of care issue and its relationships with utilization must be squarely addressed in the future.

Chapter 7

Health care: special groups and programmes

This chapter focuses on health care problems, programmes and proposals for a number of specific groups and also on a range of special programmes – mainly of a 'selective' nature – that have been introduced in recent years. The reason for discussing the health of mothers and children in the first section of this chapter is self-evident: high rates of maternal and infant deaths and ill health have been a sad and pervasive feature of many Third World countries although, today, the precise situation, programmes and prognoses vary considerably among regions, countries and socio-economic groups. Many selective health programmes have focused on these two groups, often considering them jointly, under the broad heading of Maternal and Child Health (MCH) programmes. Within these, selective immunization and rehydration programmes in particular have become widespread and must be considered, whatever one's philosophical reaction to selective health care may be. In addition, wider social issues are involved in the introduction of FP campaigns and methods, which may have objectives including population control, improvement of women's social and economic position, and broader health objectives.

The chapter then discusses the fact that many Third World countries have a real or imminent 'problem' of providing for growing elderly populations. This should not be surprising in view of the demographic and epidemiological transitions discussed in Chapter 2. Nevertheless, the NICs aside, many poor developing countries are still struggling with the conjoint problems of juvenile population growth, infectious scourges and poor economic conditions. It seems doubly unfair that they are also imminently having to come to face the phenomenon of an ageing population, but this is now becoming apparent in many. Some of the more perceptive researchers in the Third World are noting this as *the* problem of the future: how to deal with an increasingly long-lived, ageing population whilst battling the old foes of infection and poverty, but without, on the whole, the support of social security systems and services for elderly people that have commonly evolved elsewhere. As traditional familial support appears to be weakening in many countries, this chapter deals in some depth with the current and future 'greying' of the Third World.

The third section of the chapter focuses on an issue of increasing importance and controversy in the developing world: the supply of pharmaceuticals, modern and traditional. The costs of drugs and medicines can be great drains on health budgets; indeed, some developed-world multinational companies have acquired unenviable reputations for profiteering, drug dumping and unscrupulous practice in the supply of medicines, which must also be set in the context of the *need* for medicines in most countries. The identification of a limited range of essential drugs has been a priority in some, and the domestic manufacture of appropriate medicines is also receiving increasing national and international attention. The chapter therefore focuses on pharmaceutical supply in the developing world, although its links with drug research, development and supply from the developed world should also be borne in mind.

Maternal and child health and related programmes

The major focus in terms of specific groups for health care in the Third World has, for some decades, been on mothers and their children. This is understandable in the case of countries with high and even rising natural-increase levels, and in those in which infant mortality has been high (Chapter 2). It is also understandable in view of the links between health of mother and child, and between child spacing, smaller family size, FP and increased expectation and quality of life. Increasingly, the role of women in development and the possible effects on health and nutrition of children of mothers working are being recognized and researched, although findings are to date often inconclusive on this topic (Leslie 1988). The interlinking roles of women as mothers and workers and the relation to health is likely to become even more important in the next decade.

Mother (maternal) and child health programmes were often initially perceived in terms of directing services towards this group (Morley 1973; Williams and Jellife 1972) to deal with medical and domestic problems rather than with people. Today, the value of involving the mother in an educated, participative way in the control of her own fertility, home circumstances and her children's health has become increasingly recognized (Bender and Cantlay 1983). To date, more attention has been paid in general to child rather than maternal health. Nevertheless, numerous children still become acutely ill, particularly with diarrhoeal diseases and other infections such as measles. Therefore, disease-oriented immunization programmes and ORT of children with diarrhoea have become and will continue as important elements of MCH. Today, MCH is also often associated with FP and health education. Indeed, health education to assist people to recognize and define health needs and develop individual and group health behaviour (diets, sanitation, immunization and the like) can often be presented in conjunction with the knowledge and means for FP, which it may be promoting along with its associated social messages. A major objective is now to develop integrated MCH services, available on one visit to a health facility. This should help overcome the frustration and discouragement often evident when mothers have had in the past to make multiple visits, frequently over long distances, to receive individual services on different occasions.

Statistics in the area of MCH are often concurrently depressing and encouraging. In its report, *The state of the world's children, 1987*, UNICEF suggests that in the 1980s, for the first time, we have the knowledge and some of the means to defeat infection and undernutrition on a massive scale at an affordable cost. It is estimated that the lives of four million children were saved in the 5 years up to 1987 by nations putting into effect at a large scale relatively low cost preventive measures such as immunization, and life-sustaining (if not strictly curative) activities such as ORT. These two methods themselves saved an estimated 1.5 million children under the age of 5 in the same period. However, the sad fact remains that there are more than fourteen million deaths of children under 5 each year, and it is estimated that half of these could be reasonably readily prevented by low-cost solutions. No 'loud emergency' such as flood or earthquake has killed 280 000 children in a week, yet what UNICEF calls the 'silent emergency' has been doing this. The first half of the 1980s showed something was possible; this continued into the late 1980s but both donor aid and national resources in the Third World were severely stretched by economic crises and recession. National and international efforts must be sustained in the 1990s as, in spite of MCH/FP programmes, the 'silent emergency' has not gone away.

There is no strictly defined 'package' of what MCH programmes should or must comprise. In many countries, they may be viewed as part and parcel of a horizontal, community-based approach. In other cases, MCH and 'Under-Fives' clinics are virtually separately run and are as much a type of vertical implant or ideology as are specific disease-eradication programmes of SPHC or similar campaigns (Fendall 1987). Nevertheless, on balance, it would appear that sentiment today tends in theory toward the development of integrated infrastructures for PHC at the local level, capable of providing both generalized and specialized care. It is sometimes claimed that the integration of MCH/FP into broad-based PHC has been a prime mover in this regard.

To an extent, the identification of MCH/FP with PHC – or even *as* PHC – is logical, given that perhaps half or more of the potential users of health services in many Third World countries will be mothers and their children. However, in the early post-war years, governments in many countries (and missions or colonial administrations before that) focused on special services for children provided by MCH teams of nurses and midwives based in urban hospitals or rural clinics and doctors either attached to clinics or visiting peripatetically. The main function tended to be diagnostic and curative ('diagnosis–treatment–referral'), in the 'medical model' mode. The last two decades have witnessed the incorporation of immunization, nutrition surveillance, FP, health education and school health programmes. Therefore, the scope of MCH has gradually broadened and so, too, have the personnel involved – volunteers, auxiliary workers and teachers. The place of care has more clearly devolved to the community level.

A number of basic characteristics of motherhood and childhood that need to be satisfied if a healthy family, community and social life are to be achieved are now recognized by the WHO and others. The role of community members as well as of professionals in MCH/FP is highlighted. The characteristics emphasize the need for healthy pregnancy and safe delivery, each child having sound growth and development in a healthy and safe environment; children having adequate social, intellectual and emotional stimulation; and each woman having a life that is socially and

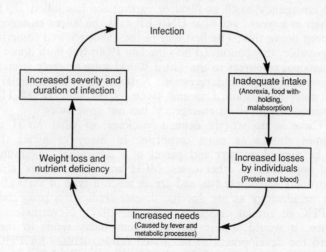

Fig. 7.1 The infection–malnutrition cycle (from Wilson *et al.* 1986)

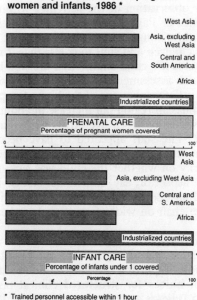

Availability of health care for pregnant
women and infants, 1986 *

West Asia

Asia, excluding
West Asia

Central and
South America

Africa

Industrialized countries

PRENATAL CARE
Percentage of pregnant women covered

0   100

West Asia

Asia, excluding West Asia

Central and
S. America

Africa

Industrialized countries

INFACT CARE
Percentage of infants under 1 covered

0   Percentage   100

* Trained personnel accessible within 1 hour
**72 countries only, excludes China, Brazil, India, Nigeria and
Bangladesh

**Fig. 7.2 Regional availability of health care for pregnant women and
infants, 1986* (from UNICEF 1988)**

emotionally satisfying – which implies the ability to control her own
fertility. It is evident that *some* of these needs can be met through
the MCH routine provided by clinic-based medical staff. Long-
term 'satisfaction', however, is much more likely to be achieved
where adequate local community participation and intersectoral collaboration exist. The need for broad-based activity to ensure a
sound educational system, good housing and a healthy environment
is obvious but important. In particular, the need for adequate nutrition for all children is being emphasized in educational campaigns
to avert the infection–malnutrition cycle to which many weaned
children are exposed (Fig. 7.1). Social-attitudinal changes may be
required to permit women to control, for example, their own levels
of fertility, or to enable wider participation in health-related activities. The availability of health care for pregnant women and
infants, and MHC in general, does nevertheless vary considerably
from region to region although, in most places, some form of infant
care is now available (Fig. 7.2).

    The example of Papua New Guinea illustrates the evolution of
MCH, since a broad-based programme now reaches an estimated

50 per cent of children under 5 years old (Reid 1984). However, even now, closer observation of the activities within MCH clinics in a single province of Papua New Guinea shows that theory and practice are not quite congruent. Over 70 per cent of interactions between mothers/children and staff took less than 2 minutes, which is perhaps acceptable if a child and mother are well but allows little opportunity for risk assessment and passing of advice. In spite of the fact that Papua Guinea has one of the highest population growth rates in the Australasian region (an increase of about 3 per cent per annum and an average of seven live births per woman), FP advice was rarely given. The staff appeared to have become very task-oriented: the time and effort the nurse spent with mother and child depended primarily on whether the child was sick or well and not on the important aspect of, say, nutritional status. Nutritional advice was given almost solely on the basis of the child's weight for age (WFA) rather than on wider factors such as health status and rate of growth.

The low priority given here in practice to FP and nutritional advice and education was thought to be the result of inadequate supervision, complex reporting systems, routine nature of work and the preference of nurses for structured clinical tasks, as well as nurses' attitudes to clients and contraception (Reid 1984). Here and no doubt elsewhere, the MCH teams could be used more effectively if they could be oriented to problems rather than tasks, and focus on families rather than (sick) individuals. Reid suggests this would give the nurses greater satisfaction in seeing the goals of their work achieved. It would require greater delegation of routine assessment tasks to health auxiliaries to free the time of the medical personnel for in-depth discussions, advice and identification of problems. Supervisors, in particular, would have to see their tasks primarily as programme development rather than administration. This might help to advance MCH more along the lines of PHC principles, moving it towards being a much more broadly based activity rather than being akin to a vertical, medical problem-oriented intervention.

Selective MCH? GOBI and GOBI/FFF

Shortly after the Alma Ata declaration on PHC in 1978 (WHO 1978a), UNICEF and other international agencies began talking of the use of specific means and measures to tackle specific issues *within* PHC. To some, this ran contrary to the comprehensive basis of PHC and aimed at technical, imposed interventions (Banerji 1988). Today, many wish to reduce dependency on such selective interventions and to re-emphasize the comprehensive form of PHC, rejecting other approaches propagated in SPHC. However, for various reasons discussed in Chapters 5 and 8, the focus of much international aid and of many national programmes has been on the use of selective programmes of 'demonstrated effectiveness' within PHC, even if this is conceptually contradictory. A major area of selective intervention has been in childhood immunization against infectious disease.

One grouping of interventions is the GOBI system – growth monitoring, ORT, breast-feeding and immunizations. Those promoting such a strategy call it a 'targeted PHC' strategy; the sceptical dub it a technocentric programme, powerfully backed, but conforming to Walsh and Warren's (1979) evaluation that 'health for all' by the year 2000 is well beyond the reach of most Third World countries and that SPHC is the best choice. Subsequently, GOBI has at least recognized the role of mothers in promoting their own health and that of their children, and expanded the strategy to include FP, food production and female literacy (GOBI/FFF). This has been included within a package entitled (euphemistically, to Banerji), the Child Survival Development Revolution. It encompasses GOBI/FFF within a major campaign of 'social marketing', which aims to make mothers and others more aware of their role in improving child health. Banerji (1988: 294) feels this is a thinly disguised propaganda campaign 'to browbeat people into accepting whatever is handed down to them from abroad'. Wisner (1988) suggests that GOBI should either be abandoned or be integrated into comprehensive PHC programmes that put parents and local workers in control and emphasize the broader struggle for health rights.

In association with GOBI come the important immunization aspects, which seek, at one level, to provide an expanded programme on immunization (EPI). An outline of the WHO's statement on the programme, discussed by Laforce *et al.* (1987), is as follows:

> A decade ago, fewer than 5 per cent of infants in the developing countries were properly immunized, despite the existence of effective vaccines.
> In 1974 the World Health Organization created the Expanded Programme on Immunization to bring six antigens to all children in the world through improved management and training for health services staff and development of an effective cold chain to maintain vaccine potency.
> The Programme has six target diseases – diphtheria, pertussis, tetanus, measles, poliomyelitis and tuberculosis. It is estimated that these diseases now account for over 3.4 million deaths a year.
> By the end of 1986 some 60 per cent of infants were receiving a first dose of DPT or polio vaccine before their first birthday. However, even at this level of coverage, the estimate of deaths averted is about a million a year, and 145 000 cases of polio are prevented. (Laforce *et al.* 1987: 214)

Even more optimistically, a programme has been initiated for Universal Child Immunization by 1990. Between 1985 and 1987,

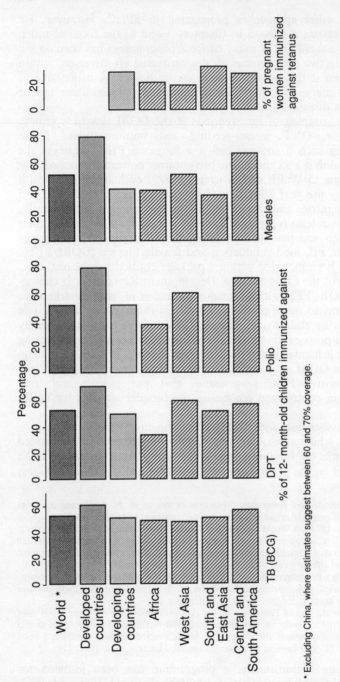

Fig. 7.3 Immunization coverage by geographic regions, 1986 (from UNICEF 1988)

* Excluding China, where estimates suggest between 60 and 70% coverage.

seventy-seven countries, with over 90 per cent of the developing world's children, declared their intention to attempt to immunize at least 90 per cent of their children by the UN target date (1990). This is unlikely to be met because, in the early 1970s, fewer than 5 per cent of the developing world's children had received even basic immunizations and, although some 40 per cent had been immunized by 1987, regional coverage varies (Fig. 7.3 and Table 2.2). The virtually full coverage envisaged will require a huge effort (UNICEF 1987), which may divert attention from wider health issues.

Immunization is very much a technical intervention that is provided to people; little in the way of their active collaboration is required. It does undoubtedly have tremendous benefits in being effective against a range of diseases and its extent can be relatively easily measured (for example, as a percentage of infants under 1 year fully immunized). Indeed, in cost-effectiveness terms, the EPI has been effective, and certain elements particularly so. Research in the Ivory Coast, for example, indicates that each case of measles averted cost $14 and the cost of each death avoided was $479. This suggests that the measles component of the EPI is highly cost-effective in preventing deaths compared with many alternative health programmes in developing countries (Shepard *et al.* 1986). Comparable data from the Gambia also suggest that their national strategy of administering measles vaccine to rural children up to the age of 15 is cost-effective, although actual coverage is less than 50 per cent (Williams 1989).

Immunization programmes do not, however, address the wider issues of health and community development. Cost-effectiveness should not be viewed as the sole, or best, criterion in comparing immunization with other health and development strategies, although it is tempting for aid donors to look for immediate 'value for money'. To critics, selective strategies such as immunization campaigns are even inhibiting community self-reliance and may be reversing historic gains by making people once more dependent on Western countries for funds, vaccine and equipment. Critics argue that there is little incentive in these programmes for people to seek socioeconomic and environmental improvement.

There is nevertheless an undeniable need for immunization, including both the 'hard' technology of supplies and vaccines and the 'soft' technology of procedures, education and record-keeping. However, the achievement of full cover can be planned and implemented in a military manner – samples can be drawn, eligible population and households mapped, community registers of households and births drawn up and the denominators of coverage rates (the 'targets') thereby identified and ticked off once immunized. In many countries, such as Sri Lanka, Tanzania, Yemen,

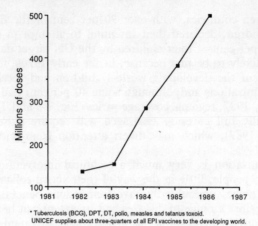

* Tuberculosis (BCG), DPT, DT, polio, measles and tetanus toxoid.
UNICEF supplies about three-quarters of all EPI vaccines to the developing world.

Fig. 7.4   Increase in the supply of EPI vaccines by UNICEF, 1982 to 1986* (from UNICEF 1988)

Zaire and the like, CHWs of various sorts have been used in this process. There has been a tendency for specialists to be involved but many survey techniques and subsequent procedures can be conducted by local personnel with little training.

The availability of vaccines has grown considerably in recent years (Fig. 7.4). Vaccines themselves have also been improved and methods of their cool storage enhanced. The improvements in the effectiveness, safety and ease of use of EPI vaccines should result in increased community acceptance and confidence, with concomitantly increasing average rates. Nevertheless, for a range of practical and technical difficulties, in June 1987 probably only about 40 per cent of infants under 1 year in developing countries were fully immunized against all six EPI diseases (diphtheria, whooping cough, tetanus, polio, measles and tuberculosis). Some 50 per cent are now receiving diphtheria–pertussis–tetanus (DPT) and poliomyelitis protection, but coverage for measles and neonatal tetanus, which cause the most deaths, is still relatively low (WHO 1987e). The external imposition of advanced technology continues to worry critics of the selective approach and, by definition, vaccines are focused on very specific ailments.

Whilst immunization efficacy has been improved, identification of children and local uptake can remain the weak link. Simple pictorial cards, or other forms of records, might be given to parents for safe-keeping in order to record child age and schedules of immunization. Cards may also be combined with growth charts and may sometimes include data from the antenatal period to the age of five, to show a full picture of the child's development. This might help to reinforce in parents' minds the need for regular visits and check-ups, and assist health workers to discern immunization status each time a child is seen. In some countries, the health recording system might be linkable to a school registration system to enhance the identification of eligible children and immunization coverage.

Decisions also have to be made as to whether to invest resources in providing booster doses before, say, 80 per cent overall coverage levels have been achieved (Laforce *et al.* 1987). The successful extension of coverage needs official endorsement and support, and the participation of a number of individuals and sectors. Naturally, UNICEF, the Aga Khan Foundation, the WHO and others advocate concerted efforts to accelerate programmes in those countries where universal childhood immunization is unlikely to have been achieved by 1990. Some countries, such as China, now have advanced and systematic procedures in place to ensure virtually total coverage. In other countries, many infants are still missed, particularly those in 'high-risk' groups (people from the poorest sectors and the worst residential districts). In addition, nomads, pastoralists and seasonal migrants are particularly likely to be missed among rural populations.

An important obstacle to increasing the uptake or success of immunization campaigns has been on the demand side: for example, a mother taking a child to a distant clinic might incur not only travel costs but lost time at work as well as the inconvenience of the journey and wait for treatment. Therefore, countries have developed various 'advertising' campaigns and techniques of social marketing. For example, between 1986 and 1988, Ecuador launched several 'pulse' campaigns, involving mass media, school songs and sermons from priests, to 'advertise' vaccinations, ORT and growth charts. On each of the 'pulse' campaigns, between 300 000 and over half a million children were vaccinated and many hundreds of thousands of packs of oral rehydration salts (ORS) were given out. This has at least increased the coverage considerably and will have reduced the number of deaths of young children attributable to diarrhoea and vaccine-preventable disease – as many as 15 000 in the early 1980s (UNICEF 1987). Similar advertising campaigns have been seen in other Latin American countries. Elsewhere, for example, in Maputo, Mozambique, schools are being widely used to teach the benefits of vaccination, although the security situation outside the main towns renders the spread of PHC-related campaigns in that country very patchy. For fear of armed attacks on health workers, advertising of the places and times of vaccination sessions has had to be surreptitious, via community organizations and schools, with volunteers visiting families to inform them only a day or two before the vaccinations are due.

It appears that over two-thirds of infants under 1 year were actually covered by 1986 in the southern province of Mozambique hardest hit by war and strife, although the maintenance of such high levels is very difficult in the conditions. As a result, the target for immunization by 1990 is 90 per cent for children in the towns but only 50 per cent for rural children.

Increasing the accessibility of immunization, either by provision of more fixed health posts or by the use of mobile teams, has been stressed. In Indonesia, the objective is that, by the end of the fourth national development plan in 1989, all children under 1 year should have access to immunization within 5 km and 65 per cent of children should be fully immunized by their first birthday. Increased access is based on a network of community or village health centres, with vaccinators travelling on scheduled visits to surrounding villages and health posts (Leinbach 1988). In Nigeria, vehicle-based mobile teams of a nurse or senior health worker and driver/cold-chain (cold vaccine storage) technician have been used with some success to provide outreach services to remote locations. However, if only one specific intervention is being delivered at a time, immunization via mobile units can be expensive and other health problems encountered *en route* will not be dealt with, which can lead to disillusionment on all sides (Kessler *et al.* 1987). Enhanced accessibility in Tamil Nadu, southern India, has been achieved by appointment of additional CHWs, increased use of peripheral and temporary clinics, concentration on underprivileged groups and public health awareness campaigns. This led to a more than doubling of immunization cover from 37 per cent to 81 per cent for DPT between 1981 and 1987 (Joseph *et al.* 1988). This example shows the large efforts needed to increase and even more to sustain the effectiveness of such selective programmes.

Oral rehydration therapy

The case of immunization as a selected intervention programme has been discussed in depth as an example of a preventive procedure. However, as noted earlier, diarrhoeal diseases are also an enormous problem in many Third World countries, being associated with about one-third of all deaths in children under 5 and causing great ill health (with children under 2 suffering from diarrhoea for 15 to 20 per cent of the time). The specific causes of diarrhoea are a number of pathogens including *Vibrio cholerae*, *Shigella dysenteriae*, *Sonnei* sp., *Salmonella typhi*, *Escherichia coli*, and others. (Many have become rare in the developed world or cause little serious illness). The *underlying* cause of the spread of these pathogens is poor hygiene: bad sanitation, poor care of food and infected water. Even the boiling of water may not give thorough protection as the water may subsequently be reinfected through storage in unclean containers or use of dirty cups, as illustrated by Lindskog's (1987) study of water sanitation and child health in Malawi. Diarrhoeal diseases are a frequent cause of malnutrition, which in turn makes children more vulnerable to other sickness and death from diarrhoea; there is also evidence of a synergistic effect in which diarrhoea interacts with other diseases, especially measles, to contribute to child mortality. Most deaths from diarrhoea itself stem from dehydration caused by abnormally large losses of water and salts from the body. Dehydration of course can occur rapidly among infants and young children, particularly in hot climates and when an individual has a fever (UNICEF 1986).

Diarrhoea can cause rapid death in afflicted children, but there is now a cheap recognized form of therapy via oral rehydration that involves the use of pre-packed sachets of ORS or various home-made solutions. The major aim of such treatment is to prevent dehydration by replacing fluids and restoring correct nutrient balance using a glucose–salt solution. Severe dehydration (more than 10 per cent loss of body weight) will still often require intravenous therapy, which is also necessary for unconscious patients or those unable to drink. The WHO and UNICEF estimate, however, that such a serious state can be avoided and 90 to 95 per cent of all patients with acute diarrhoea can be treated with ORS alone. In addition, various forms of improved, 'super' ORS are being developed, some with a rice base that is even cheaper than sugar in certain developing countries, particularly in Asia. The International Centre for Diarrhoeal Disease Research in Dhaka, Bangladesh, is a specialist institution for research on the disease and its treatment.

Whilst the specific causes and treatment of diarrhoea are now well understood, the underlying reasons for spread of the disease are much more difficult to deal with. These include individual poverty and poor daily living environments, a fact that highlights a major weakness in ORT or diarrhoeal-disease control programmes. By virtue of the focus on ORT and its administrative structure, the WHO's diarrhoeal-disease control programme is regarded as a vertical programme. It has been enlarged in some countries to include promotion of sanitation, personal hygiene and breast-feeding (to help avoid polluted artificial milk being given), but it generally does not actively improve domestic environments.

Kendall (1988) outlines a programme in Honduras and suggests a compromise in the PHC–SPHC debate in which, although selective, a programme need not be strictly vertical as it can involve a number of thrusts to tackle the underlying conditions spreading diarrhoea. Improving these via environmental upgrading will also inevitably have other health-related benefits. Kendall also suggests that a focus on issues such as donor policy (which supports programmes), health delivery, and individual aspects of utilization and barriers to utilization will provide a better framework for health improvements and the growing body of empirical knowledge on primary care than does the PHC versus SPHC debate. An additional focus might be on ways to involve traditional workers with necessary guidance and therapies in the treatment and control of diarrhoeal disease (Neumann 1988).

Extent and availability of ORT

Since the early 1980s, ORT has reached a moderate level of effectiveness and acceptance and has begun to make some national-scale impacts as opposed to those of local demonstration projects. However, availability and coverage still need extension. UNICEF (1986, 1988) suggested that, whilst almost unknown publicly at the beginning of the 1980s, ORT was reaching 12 per cent of the world's families by mid-decade although, as with immunization, regional coverage varied considerably and was proportionately lowest in Africa (Fig. 7.5). By 1990, it could potentially be used by 50 per cent of parents, to save the lives of as many as 1.5 million children per year. Within a decade, virtually all parents could be given the knowledge of ORT and vastly reduce the number of child deaths from diarrhoeal dehydration.

This is perhaps a case in which optimism, rhetoric and reality are not congruent. There is indubitably increasing local availability of ORS in most countries, although still only about 25 per cent of

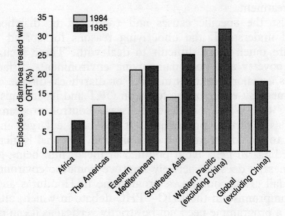

Fig. 7.5 **Estimated ORT use rates for children under 5, 1984 to 1985 (from UNICEF 1988)**

the developing world's clinics and health centres have stocks of ORS and a person trained in ORT. However, national production of ORS is gradually improving and UNICEF's contribution to world supplies has reduced from 60 to 30 per cent (1981 to 1986). More than forty nations now produce some ORS of their own (UNICEF 1986). Internationally, their distribution is still variable, although the 35 per cent mark of home-produced ORS has been passed in Bangladesh, Burma, China, Egypt and Nicaragua, among others.

Whilst is has not directly helped to remove the poor home and wider environmental conditions that favour the spread of diarrhoeal disease, ORT has at least tended to supplant other more expensive, probably less effective and even harmful antibiotic treatments. However, the support of the medical profession is not unambiguous and many health personnel still recommend withholding food during diarrhoea. Nevertheless, it seems that training workshops for health workers have increased the use of ORS treatments rather than alternatives (UNICEF 1987). Studies in Egypt suggest strong declines in diarrhoeal-associated mortality, probably associated at least in part with appropriate use of ORT in the mid-1980s, although mothers' comprehension of its role is still not always clear (Rashad 1989).

One should be cautious in extrapolating success in the extension of this effective, cheap therapy for diarrhoeal diseases, to the development of therapies for other infectious ailments, as these may not prove so simple or cheap. In addition, ORT is home-

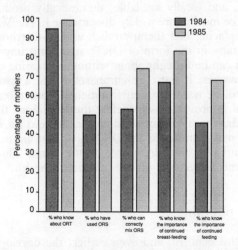

Fig. 7.6 Increase in mothers' knowledge of treating diarrhoeal disease, Egypt, 1984 to 1985 (from UNICEF 1988)

administered, whereas many other remedies or preventions may not be. Along with the increased availability and training of workers in ORT, an important factor is the growing public awareness of the use of ORS (for a Haitian example, see Coreil and Genece 1988). It is calculated that in some cities in developing countries (such as Alexandria in Egypt), whereas in the early 1980s only about 5 per cent of mothers knew of ORS and only 1 per cent had used it, in the late 1980s the corresponding figures are in the order of 90 per cent and 50 per cent, respectively. It is, however, essential for mothers to use ORS correctly. Incomplete and, at times, totally inadequate understanding of ORS was evident among over half the respondents in a survey in rural Pakistan and similar findings were obtained in Egypt (Fig. 7.6). The teaching of correct use of ORS, along with the ready availability of ORS sachets or components in the home, seems crucial, involving education as well as public acceptance. In addition, it is important for programme planners to recognize that some Third World residents might have varying explanations for diarrhoea; some traditionally based explanations require popular, folk remedies so that ORT might be considered inappropriate. Therefore, again, if potentially serious diarrhoea is to be successfully treated, mothers' attitudes to a range of illness causation must be addressed, possibly via health education. Otherwise, ORT may not be used at all, or used in an uninformed or ineffective manner, with resulting scepticism about its efficiency, and its possible abandonment (Mull and Mull 1988).

Continuing international and national professional support for ORT is therefore essential; health personnel need to accept and advocate its use, and locally available, domestically produced ORS supplies must be much more widely disseminated. The WHO point out that by replacing bad therapy (such as anti-diarrhoeal drugs) with good therapy in the form of ORT, significant improvements in child health can be brought about without increasing overall expenditure. However, it must be emphasized that a good deal of expenditure will be needed on environmental, sanitation, housing and nutritional improvements to defeat the conditions that favour the spread of diarrhoeal diseases and create the need for ORT. We should regard mass campaigns for ORT as at best an intermediate measure, essential in the foreseeable future, until Third World living environments become safer for children's health.

Family planning

For much of this century, and even earlier, the developed world has seen increasingly open debate about the need for control of population growth via FP. In some places, the debate has been on

religious or moral grounds: the justification for preventing conception by artificial methods as opposed to traditional, natural
fertility-regulating practices. In others, the legal right of families to
be able to obtain contraceptives has been debated (in Ireland for
example). In some countries, notably in the Far East and Eastern
Europe, abortion has been used as a form of population control.
This, of course, raises many additional moral issues to those of contraception, as well as often putting the mother's life or health at
risk.

There are many reasons in the Third World in general and in
some countries in particular for the existence and continuation of
high fertility. The desirability of FP as a means of regulating
population growth by reducing high fertility has only been seriously
recognized in the last three decades or so. It has been difficult, in
some cases, for governments or other organizations to introduce effective population control by fertility regulation without resorting
to Draconian measures as in India and China in the recent past but,
nevertheless, use of FP services has gradually been increasing, even
if there are vast differences in absolute levels of use of contraception
(Fig. 7.7).

The pressures on the poor in particular to have many children
have been summarized in the *World development report 1984* (World
Bank 1984) as economic (low loss of mothers' wages during pregnancy more than cancelled out by a child's earnings; low 'cost' of
children where schooling and services are unavailable, so numerous
children do not 'cost' much); demographic (persistence of high infant mortality); tradition and desire for children to take care of

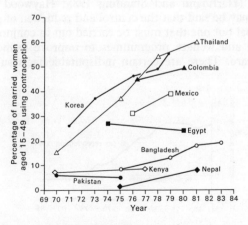

**Fig. 7.7 Trends in contraceptive prevalence in selected countries,
1970 to 1983 (from World Bank 1984)**

parents in their old age; and family systems encouraging high fertility. Finally, of course, children in every society can bring parents satisfaction and pleasure.

In the face of these factors, on what basis has FP been argued, and how is it taken up? In Europe since the 1920s, initiatives have come from two main groups: first, campaigners for women's rights (which could hardly be realized until women were able to control whether or not they became pregnant) and, secondly, the eugenists, arguing for race improvement by judicious mating and stock improvement. Whilst the former group promoted FP as a right and for health reasons, the influence of the latter group is seen more in the population control lobby. Population policies may in fact emerge with several objectives, and the three broadest categories (which need not be pursued singly as objectives can overlap) are demographic, human rights and MCH objectives.

1. Demographic objectives

A major reason for seeking reduction of fertility is to control the perceived 'population explosion'. Population policy in many Third World countries reflects both real shortages of resources and land, and also the maintenance of the status quo in the distribution of resources. The road to 'prosperity' is depicted as being through the reduction of the birth rate. This is a view held by many donor agencies and national governments. This is visible at a general level, involving global politics, and what is forced upon countries by outside bodies (Hartmann 1987), and within specific countries such as Bangladesh (Hartmann and Standing 1985; Haywood 1988). In general, it may be said that the control and reduction of population is a valid goal but one that must be carried out in conjunction with other social and welfare programmes to improve women's status and child care. There are certain indisputable facts such as that

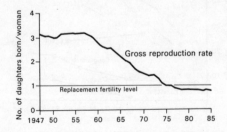

Fig. 7.8 Singapore: gross reproduction rate, 1947 to 1985 (after Singh *et al.* 1988)

only in a few developing countries have population growth rates fallen below 2 per cent per annum in the 1970s and 1980s and, in many, annual increases are in the region of 3 per cent. In general, growth has been fastest in the poorest Third World countries. Demographic profiles mean that following high growth rates and falling infant mortality since the 1960s, often 40 per cent of populations in developing countries are aged 15 years or younger. Therefore, as these enter reproductive age groups, if no population controls are implemented, potential future increase is massive. The relief valves of potential for international migration or for worthwhile movement to towns are now very small (World Bank 1984).

Demographic reasons therefore strongly stimulate the need for FP. However, the acceptance of the 'population as crisis' theme is almost forced on some countries by external agencies, and excessive concentration on reduced fertility and sterilization targets can even undermine people's access to PHC services (Feldman 1987) although, with greater equity in distribution, this need not occur (Gish 1981). Population control may seek to force down birth rate in the absence of major improvements in people's lives. Birth control can therefore be a weapon rather than a tool of reproductive choice. This is a major critique of coercive population-control programmes, especially from a feminist and civil libertarian perspective (Hartmann 1987; Hartmann and Standing 1985). Only in a relatively few developing countries, notably in South-East Asia, have FP campaigns coincided with strong economic growth and prosperity, and population increase has been reduced. Hong Kong is an example of a state where this has occurred. In the case of Singapore, the gross reproduction rate has fallen considerably and since 1975 has been below replacement levels (Fig. 7.8). The government in the late 1980s has adopted new pronatalist population policies, such as encouraging professional women to have children or larger families. In this, they have been arguably attempting to regulate the quality of the population (Singh *et al.* 1988).

2. *Human rights*

Freedom of choice in reproductive decisions has been increasingly valued not only by socialist or feminist researchers but by those interested in broad equality of opportunities and quality of life. For some time, FP has been seen as an essential component of any broad-based development strategy that seeks to improve the quality of life for individuals and communities, and was promulgated as such in the 'Jakarta Statement' of 1981 on Family Planning in the

1980s. This recognized not only the health benefits but the basic human rights aspects of FP (Rosenfield and Wray 1981).

However, as a human right, FP does not really promote reproductive freedom equally in many countries. Contemporary contraceptive research and devices are largely focused on the female reproductive system and there is a preference in the Third World in particular for systemic and surgical forms of birth control over safer but perhaps far less effective barrier methods. The concern is thus for efficiency rather than health and safety. Some feel that the nature of contraceptive technology reflects male dominance since it is women who receive the chemical and invasive methods of control (oral contraceptives, Depo-Provera, intra-uterine devices (IUDs) and sterilization). The barrier methods (diaphragm and cervical cap) are often depicted as unfashionable and unreliable, although the condom has recently been promoted for the prevention of sexually transmitted diseases including AIDS. Duggan (1986), Hartmann (1987), and others point out that the relatively inexpensive and safe barrier methods can be as effective as others when combined with adequate training and follow-up. As Haywood (1988) discusses, some writers have gone to lengths to point out the racist or at best socially biased nature of many population-control policies, which are often aimed at the poorest in Third World societies. Warwick (1982) criticizes the power-oriented bureaucratic 'machine model' of implementation of FP programmes and argues persuasively for a 'transactional' approach, in which political and cultural contexts and, especially, client welfare are fully taken into account.

3. Maternal and child health

There is considerable evidence that shows FP activities to be beneficial on balance for mothers' health and that of children. Repeated pregnancies are known to be dangerous to health and there can be many risks involved in delivery for mothers and children, especially in poorer Third World settings.

Some research suggests that an increase in FP practice can theoretically reduce infant mortality, although this is not unequivocal (Bongaarts 1987; International Planned Parenthood Federation (IPPF) 1986). This is in addition to the more obvious benefits of reducing family size and the dangers to mothers' health of multiple unplanned pregnancies. Indeed, a major aim in recent FP and health care in the Third World has been to reduce and prevent as far as possible the tragedy of maternal deaths, and the principle of safe motherhood is of increasing concern (Conable 1987; Herz and Measham 1987; Starrs 1987). It is a sad fact but it appears that a

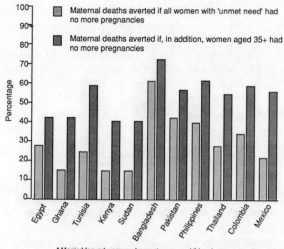

Maternal deaths averted if all women with 'unmet need' had no more pregnancies

Maternal deaths averted if, in addition, women aged 35+ had no more pregnancies

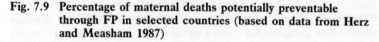

* Married fecund women who want no more children but are not using an effective contraceptive method

Fig. 7.9 Percentage of maternal deaths potentially preventable through FP in selected countries (based on data from Herz and Measham 1987)

pregnant woman in a developing country has up to a 200 times greater risk of dying than does a pregnant woman in an affluent society. As many as 1 400 women die daily in the process of carrying or delivering children, almost half a million maternal deaths a year in the developing world, and 80 per cent of them in South Asia and sub-Saharan Africa (Conable 1987). Therefore, not only is FP needed to prevent unwanted pregnancies but the whole process of pregnancy and delivery must be made much safer. If all women with unmet contraceptive need used effective contraception and had no more children, between 15 per cent (Ghana, Kenya, Sudan) and 62 per cent (Bangladesh) of maternal deaths could be averted. This is even more important for older women (Fig. 7.9). Indeed, it seems that most maternal deaths are theoretically avoidable, but major improvements in public health, care and nutrition are required to be able to effect safe pre- and post-natal care. In comparison, FP programmes may be relatively easier to deliver but are sometimes socially and psychologically difficult to implement.

Birth spacing

A child's chances of being born healthy and of surviving the first years of life are considerably reduced if children in the family are

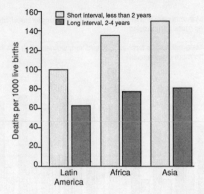

Fig. 7.10   The association between birth spacing and infant mortality in three regions (from UNICEF 1988)

born very close together in time, or if there are already three or more children in the family, or if the age of the mother is younger than 20 or older than 35 (Maine 1981). Birth spacing is increasingly recognized as an important factor contributing to MCH. When a woman has pregnancies close together, the likelihood increases in some circumstances of miscarriage or perinatal death (Figs 7.10 and 7.11). Delaying the next conception and extending the birth interval, as well as reducing the total numbers of children born per family, are increasingly being viewed as an important part of MCH.

Studies in Bangladesh, the Philippines, India and Turkey have all noted high rates of foetal death among pregnancies that began less than 1 year after a previous pregnancy. They have also documented an increase in deaths among infants born after short intervals, in particular less than 1 year or between 1 and 2 years (Maine 1981). In some instances, a longer birth interval is associated with two to three times lower mortality than are shorter intervals. Birth-spacing research suggests that increased birth intervals can contribute to a 10 to 20 per cent decline in infant mortality and that having birth intervals of longer than 2 years has a significant benefit on the health of infants and young children (Rosenfield 1986). The age and parity of mother are two other important factors, although more strongly related to maternal health. In addition, infectious diseases are often higher where there are many very young children; by contrast, longer birth spacing is associated with better school performance, better nutrition and better maternal health (Wilson *et al.* 1986).

The availability and encouragement of FP appears to be one of the major factors in lengthening birth spacing. Nevertheless, in some traditional societies, there has been an implicit recognition and understanding of the importance of birth spacing, encouraged

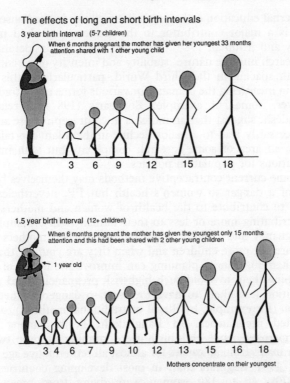

The effects of long and short birth intervals

3 year birth interval (5-7 children)

When 6 months pregnant the mother has given her youngest 33 months attention shared with 1 other young child

3   6   9   12   15   18

1.5 year birth interval (12+ children)

When 6 months pregnant the mother has given the youngest only 15 months attention and this had been shared with 2 other young children

← 1 year old

3 4 6 7 9 10 12 13 15 16 18

Mothers concentrate on their youngest

Fig. 7.11   The effects of long and short birth intervals on family life and children's upbringing (after Wilson *et al.* 1986)

by breast feeding but sometimes undermined by the availability of artificial milk substitutes.

A study of thirty-nine countries in the developing world has shown decisively the importance of birth spacing and, implicitly, of FP to child health. The dangers to health of child and mother increase dramatically with a rapid succession of births: for example, the risk of dying during the first month of life is 222 per cent greater if there had been two previous births than if there had been no births at all in the preceding 2-year interval. Whilst this research demonstrates no striking regional patterns, it seems the association between birth spacing and mortality is generally strongest in the Middle East and North Africa. As an indication of the potential cost-effectiveness of FP contributing to birth spacing, studies from Malaysia and Guatemala suggest that increasing the interval between births has about the same level of effectiveness in reducing child mortality as does giving birth in a hospital and living in a village with a PHC facility. It has greater effectiveness than 3 years of maternal education or having toilet facilities in the household; in all, it is a major contributor to the reduction of child mortality (Pebley and Millman 1986). However, there is considerable scope for research into the nature, stability and intensity of parental views on birth spacing in the Third World, particularly as this will be useful in measuring the demand for various forms of contraceptives. However, some, of example, Bongaarts (1987) in relation to Bangladesh, suggest that an increase in contraceptive use alone will not necessarily lead to a major decline in the infant mortality rate. This is an area of some research complexity but with important implications for population policies.

Some current contraceptive methods may themselves be something of a danger to women's health but FP, nevertheless, does appear to contribute to the health of women and mothers as well as contributing more or less to their human rights. Complications of pregnancy and childbirth are increased when mothers already have three or more children and when they are younger than 20 or older than 30. Family planning can improve the health of women by helping them to avoid such high-risk pregnancies, and they are in addition less likely to have to resort to dangerous methods of abortion (for example, by illegal or traditional methods) to control unwanted pregnancies. In Bangladesh, deaths among women from pregnancy and childbirth were running at over twice the rate for males from all causes for almost all reproductive age groups. Maine (1981) suggests that, in most developing countries in the mid-1970s, 40 to 180 women were dying from pregnancy or childbirth-related causes per 100 000 children born, compared with fewer than 20 maternal deaths in most of Europe. World Fertility Survey (WFS) data further suggest that maternal deaths in many developing countries could be reduced by 25 to 40 per cent if all women who explicitly say they do not want any more children were to use a contraceptive method effectively (Starrs 1987). In addition, maternal deaths increase more with age in many developing countries than they do in developed countries, again indicating the significance of availability of contraception to older women.

Availability and knowledge of FP

Many Third World people are still unable to obtain contraceptives either because of socioreligious reasons or because of local unavailability. In some countries, notably Nepal, Kenya, Mexico and Indonesia, over 40 per cent of married women did not know where to get contraceptive supplies or advice (the figure was over 90 per cent for Nepal) (Maine 1981). By contrast, other countries appear better served: in Costa Rica only about 10 per cent and in Malaysia about 20 per cent of married women did not know where to get supplies or advice. Whilst many women in developing countries *do* approve of FP, the pattern of contraceptive use of developing countries often displays an inverted-U shape: younger women anxious to start a family may not use FP, usage increases among women in their mid-twenties to late-thirties, and older women may be less willing or perceive less need to continue (Way *et al.* 1987).

Many women in Third World countries are increasingly becoming more knowledgeable about FP advice and contraceptives and approving of their use. It seems that FP promotion campaigns are having some impact and various reasons have been identified for use of contraception (Table 7.1). Nevertheless, the availability of contraception is still often insufficient; for example, a study in the Philippines found that, whilst two-thirds of women surveyed did not want another child, only 45 per cent were using some form of contraception. Accessibility is sometimes a problem here and elsewhere, but the Philippines study also showed there were considerable reservations among the women about the use of some methods (Riphagen *et al.* 1988). Internationally, the WFS estimates that some 300 million couples would like to postpone or avoid pregnancy altogether but have no access to FP services (Starrs 1987).

Certain countries have made use of personnel other than physicians to provide a variety of contraceptive services and to increase their accessibility. Thailand, in particular, since 1970 has pioneered the use of auxiliary midwives, in recognition of the urban concentration of physicians (60 per cent are in Bangkok and the majority of the remainder in other cities). Indeed, it appears that continuation of contraceptive usage may be higher when recommended by auxiliary midwives than when advised by physicians and, as noted earlier, 'model mothers' meeting specific criteria are also used to promote FP in certain villages. The concept of community-based distribution of oral contraceptives (distributed by lay personnel) has also been pioneered and, today, IUDs, injectable contraceptives and even sterilizations have been given by various grades of trained personnel other than physicians. This use of a

Table 7.1 **Married women aged 15–49 currently using a contraceptive method, by reason for use (%) (based on data from Way *et al.* 1987)**

Reason for use	Botswana	Kenya	Zimbabwe[a]
Limit family size	11	10	10
Space child-bearing	11	5	24
Undecided about whether or when to have another child	6	3	6

[a] Women aged 15–44

variety of sources to provide FP services has extended the range of contraceptive methods available at various levels of the health care hierarchy (Figure 7.12). The success in Thailand (and some other countries) in extending the availability and accessibility of FP services has been a model for the use of such personnel in the provision of a range of other curative and preventive PHC services (Economic and Social Commission for Asia and the Pacific (ESCAP) 1986). Askew and Lenton (1987) discuss some of the issues surrounding the management of an FP project that seeks to encourage community participation in its implementation.

When choice of contraceptive technique is considered, women in some Third World countries are more likely to be sterilized than to use any temporary measures, although this varies from country

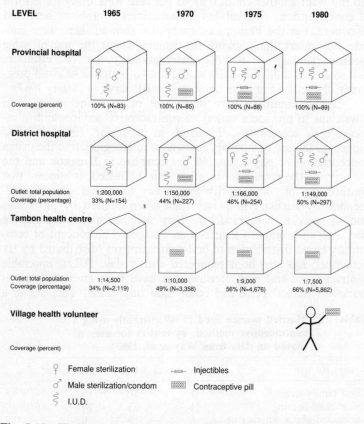

LEVEL	1965	1970	1975	1980
Provincial hospital				
Coverage (percent)	100% (N=83)	100% (N=85)	100% (N=88)	100% (N=89)
District hospital				
Outlet: total population	1:200,000	1:150,000	1:166,000	1:149,000
Coverage (percentage)	33% (N=154)	44% (N=227)	46% (N=254)	50% (N=297)
Tambon health centre				
Outlet: total population	1:14,500	1:10,000	1:9,000	1:7,500
Coverage (percentage)	34% (N=2,119)	49% (N=3,358)	56% (N=4,676)	66% (N=5,862)
Village health volunteer				
Coverage (percent)				

♀ Female sterilization   ⊨ Injectibles
♂ Male sterilization/condom   Contraceptive pill
I.U.D.

Fig. 7.12   Thailand: the increasing availability of contraceptive methods at various levels of the health care hierarchy (after ESCAP 1986)

to country. This does of course pose some health threats in itself and, also, it is not generally reversible. Injectable contraceptives, often suspect in the developed world, have been approved in over a hundred countries but their availability may be limited in practice and they are not provided by US donors. The contraceptive pill is a popular method in many countries (World Bank 1984) but fears persist about side-effects. The health of users should be monitored, although this can be difficult to do in many developing countries and some side-effects go unreported in the context of overall ill-health (Stephen and Chamratrithirong 1988).

Government activities in FP

Government support for FP is now widespread and often involves the provision of public services, frequently with assistance directly from donor countries or agencies such as the United Nations Fund for Population Activities (UNFPA) and the IPPF. External aid now pays for a sizeable proportion of all FP in developing countries, although FP activities still account for less than one-half of 1 per cent in almost all national budgets. Third World government attitudes are increasingly open to FP ideas and official support has grown. In 1965, only 21 countries supported FP; by 1974, some 102 countries reported supporting it and, by 1983, some 127 countries accounting for 93 per cent of the world's population supported the provision of modern contraceptive methods. However, in 32 countries (7 per cent of the world's population), governments provide no financial support for FP, although they place no restrictions on it; fewer than 1 per cent of the world's population now live in the 7 countries that, according to the UN in 1983, limit access to modern methods of fertility regulation (IPPF 1986). Nevertheless, some governments in Sub-Saharan Africa and elsewhere, such as Malaysia, follow pro-natalist policies in the belief that an expanding population is important for national development, security and prestige (Hartmann 1987).

Low-income countries annually spend an average of $US9 per capita on health care. Within this budget, it is calculated that a three-pronged strategy of providing prenatal care and basic health and FP services at community and first referral level can be implemented in developing countries at an annual cost of under $US2 per capita. This level of expenditure, it is suggested, should reduce maternal deaths by about a half in a decade. In the countries that cannot afford such investment, increasing annual expenditure by $US1 should still have a significant impact on mortality. This is particularly true when low-cost systems are introduced in conjunction with broader development programmes for women's income, food and education (Starrs 1987).

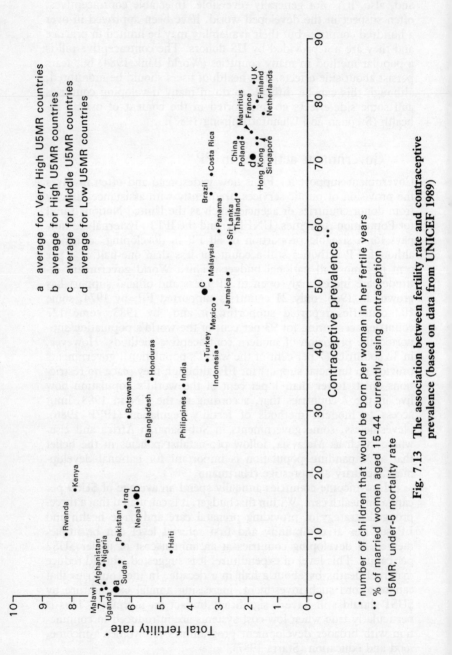

Fig. 7.13   The association between fertility rate and contraceptive prevalence (based on data from UNICEF 1989)

A note of caution should be sounded regarding the extent to which FP does actually reduce fertility, as this might also be attributable to socioeconomic improvement. There is evidence of fertility decline in the presence of FP programmes but in the absence of development; there have also been fertility declines in the absence of FP programmes. There is evidence to link contraception use with fertility but this may be more generally in line with a country's stage in transition from high to low fertility. On the whole, however, a consensus is emerging that both FP and broader development contribute to fertility decline and that the two have a synergistic effect. Figure 7.13 confirms this although, whilst the correlation between fertility rate and contraception prevalence is clearly evident, the strength of the relationship is not always constant. The IPPF (1986) agrees that there is at least a strong empirical correlation between levels of contraceptive use and fertility. Contraception is practised by approximately 70 per cent of all couples of reproductive age in the developed world and birth rates are low, at about 15 per 1 000. By contrast, in developing countries, only about 30 per cent of couples of reproductive age use contraceptives and average birth rates are about 31 per 1 000. The sharp decline in fertility levels in some, but not all, Third World countries, mentioned in Chapter 2, should be noted.

Social marketing

'Social marketing' has been applied to contraceptive use and ORT as well as to immunization campaigns. This involves both consumer research and sales promotion. In Bangladesh for example, it was felt by the early 1980s that sales of contraceptives might be reaching the limits of existing demand, in spite of social marketing since 1975. As a result, research was inaugurated to identify the major resistance points in the population. Although sceptics might consider the commercial sale of contraceptive devices to be a problem, the critical concerns identified in the research are of general interest to Third World societies that wish to increase the use of FP via modern contraceptives (Manoff 1985). Predictably, the concerns included: religious conservatism (involving interpretations that the Koran does not sanction most modern contraceptives), observance of Purdah and the seclusion of women (inhibiting the spread of new ideas); low status of women, whose attitudes are forced to mirror those of their husbands; sexual taboos, preventing contact between wives and FP workers; cultural conservatism; economic distress and the wish for male children; and, finally, but not least, the continuation of high child mortality. No doubt, similar or additional hindrances to the adoption and extension of modern FP services are to be found in other developing countries.

Integration of FP with general health care?

There have been persuasive arguments advanced in recent years for the integration of FP with other PHC services. This is not because FP is necessarily to be regarded purely as a health service but, in addition to its social and demographic aspects, it does in Third World countries in particular have important medical ramifications. For example, when FP is integrated with PHC, following the delivery of a baby by a TBA or midwife, a mother will be able to receive postnatal care and also advice as to whether, and when, she might like to have any further children. The idea that she might be¯able to regulate this aspect of her life may be quite novel and suggestions might be well received from, say, a midwife or TBA.

There are other practical reasons for pursuing integration of FP with health services. In preference to having, say, four or six workers in different categorical programmes working in the same area with the same households (as has been common in many countries), it does seem more efficient, less intrusive and probably more effective if a single, multipurpose worker can carry out several tasks, provided the package is kept relatively simple and well supervised. In addition, integrated packages can offer greater challenge and diversity to health workers, whether volunteers or paid, and they can enable families to be viewed in their totality rather than as individual components. Family planning services, equivocal at best in many societies, can perhaps be more readily accepted when seen as part of broader health care provision. Integration is being attempted in many places and a good example is the Narangwal Experiment in MCH/FP and health care in the Punjab, rural India (see Taylor *et al.* 1983).

Services and provision for elderly people

Until recently, for good reason, much of the energy of Third World health ministries and international agencies has been targeted onto health care issues that basically revolve around younger age groups, mothers, families and their needs, including FP. This has been justifiable because of the rapid population growth in youthful Third World countries, in which the prevention of as much infant, child and maternal mortality as possible is an obvious priority, as is the gradual reduction in birth rates. Children have been seen as the future and, to assure a healthy future, vast sums and huge campaigns have been directed to the younger age group.

Today, it might be said that the 'future has arrived' in many Third World countries. In some of the wealthier developing countries and the growing group of NICs, demographic change and epidemiological transition have become well established along lines seen in the West for some decades. The populations of many NICs, especially in South-East and East Asia, are ageing relatively rapidly (Chen and Jones 1988; Chow 1987; Koo and Cowgill 1986; Lee 1986) but the phenomenon of a greying Third World is also to be noted in Africa, the Caribbean, Latin America and the Pacific (Kinsella 1988). Whilst the proportional change should not be exaggerated in some of these countries in which birth rates are still high, the numbers and percentages of elderly persons in the population are gradually and inexorably rising. Sub-Saharan Africa, for example, will see major growth in its population of over-sixties early next century (Adamchak 1989). It is in the spirit of this book to reiterate that conditions are rarely static in any health care setting; the consequences of demographic and epidemiological change for the majority of Third World countries must be recognized now if any effective provision is to be planned over the next few decades. Here, we shall review briefly the experience of some countries in providing for ageing populations in the face of social and economic change. Most studies to date come from the NICs, although increasingly research is being conducted elsewhere.

Japan was one of the first emergent developing countries after the war to experience the rapid ageing of its population. Today a modern economic and industrial giant, it retains its East Asian philosophy towards age, a reverence and a desire to support elderly people in family settings, but finds increasingly that it is unable to do so. Demographic ageing in Japan has been relatively rapid. However, recent research by Palmore and Maeda (1985), following a 1975 study by Palmore, suggests that the elderly in this industrial nation are well cared for and respected by their families and their government. It is claimed that they enjoy considerable security and peace of mind, although this rosy picture of the Japanese elderly with many financial, social and health benefits and with solicitous families does not match earlier findings by Plath (1972). Lawrence (1985) also notes a shortage of trained personnel to care for elderly people in Japan, mushrooming costs of care, dependence on a hospital-oriented health care system, and lack of support for elderly people at home.

Aspects of modernization theory may be used to hypothesize that, with a movement towards industrialization, urbanization and a secular society, there will be a decline in the status and family support of elderly people. However, the extent and nature of this decline will not necessarily be the same in all societies. Cowgill and Holmes (1972) suggest that societal differences will influence this considerably. For example, a culture whose major religion is, say, Buddhism, may be quite differently affected by modernization from one founded on a Judeo-Christian basis. Equally, traditional differences in economic and political philosophies may be important. In this case, elderly people in a country such as Japan may appear to have relatively comfortable and well-provided existences but their modern conditions in terms of family and status may still be less satisfactory than in more traditional times. Therefore, modernization theory might be applied *within* cultures to investigate the changing circumstances of elderly people following the move from pre-industrial to urban-industrial times. The fundamental differences between cultures and societies might well modify the effects of development on elderly people and, hence, caution should be taken in extrapolating the nature of changes from one country to another.

Important variations have been found between developing countries in patterns of morbidity and disability among elderly populations. A WHO-sponsored project in the 1980s conducted surveys in the Republic of Korea, Fiji, the Malaysian Peninsula and the Tagalog region of the Philippines (surrounding Manila) in which the functional, health and social status of elderly people in the community were assessed (Manton *et al.* 1987). Such comparative studies are rare in the Third World and the findings enabled the identification of subgroups of elderly populations based on composites of functional and health attributes. These included a first pair of groups (types 1 and 2), who were generally healthy; type 3, who were acutely ill; type 4, who might have mobility problems; and type 5, with a wide range of limitations on daily activities and needing care to help deal with them but with relatively high health service use. The fifth group includes in effect very frail, 'older' elderly people.

The four countries surveyed seemed to have different relative proportions in each dependency category, perhaps related mainly to their levels of life expectancy, but also to the stage of epidemiological transition and nature of health care in the specific country. Interesting differences can be briefly summarized following the study by Manton *et al.* (1987). The primary pattern, for Malaysia, for example, involved types 1 and 4, who were predominantly female, representing a reasonably healthy younger and older elderly group. This is similar to findings in an earlier study in Indonesia, in which the elderly population was predominantly female with limited medical problems. The Philippines had a different pattern among the elderly, with large proportions of either healthy, older females or younger, acutely ill persons. This pattern probably reflects its lower life expectancy, with fewer 'very elderly' people, but also the urban bias of the sample in which access to modern health care facilities might support a morbid subpopulation.

Korea provided an interesting contrast to Malaysia, in that the most prevalent groups were male and either healthy or old and frail (but probably cared for in their families). It is speculated that elderly females without spouses are more likely than others to be institutionalized (Manton *et al.* 1987). Finally, in Fiji, there was a high prevalence of all types except type 1 (the healthiest). There was also a significant proportion of very elderly people (types 4 and 5) and, apparently similarly to other Polynesian societies, a higher retention of elderly persons in the community for societal reasons and, perhaps, because of low provision of nursing-home accommodation.

These comparisons found a relatively high frequency of elderly people living both with children and spouse, indicating that considerable extended family care and informal support still exist. The contrasts between the four countries do, however, emphasize that the situation and needs of elderly people in developing countries must be studied in the context of the family and health care traditions of the specific countries, and also in the light of the stage of demographic and epidemiological transition of each.

Social care, lifestyle and self-esteem

The changing lifestyle and care of elderly people in rapidly changing countries have become an important research area. De Vos and Holden (1988) discuss various measures comparing the living arrangements of elderly people, and their social care (which is wider than health care) is now increasingly being focused on. In rapidly modernizing societies, feelings of isolation, uselessness and undervalue among elderly people have commonly been noted, particularly when their families have been successful but are unable to have older relatives living with them. An economically dependent status is hard for anyone to bear but in developing countries it is often pressed onto elderly people who have aged during a time when their resources were few, pensions usually non-existent and social security networks minimal. In most NICs, distinctive changes in demographic structure have come about in a matter of two decades or so, and the socioeconomic system has yet to adjust. The esteemed position that elderly people in developing countries used to occupy in the past was often based on family headship and land ownership. In modernizing, particularly in industrializing, countries, these are of less relevance than education, income and socioeconomic status and perhaps as a result role loss is experienced. Studies in Singapore (Singapore Council of Social Service 1985), Hong Kong (Chow 1987; Chow and Kwan 1986) and Japan (Koyano *et al.* 1987), and comparing Hong Kong and US Chinese (Ikels 1983), have all indicated that both elderly people themselves and society as a whole often hold negative conceptions about ageing and the status of elderly people. These may well be erroneous but misconceptions can easily translate into fact, and public policy in many South-East Asian countries, such as Singapore, is now seeking to strengthen the traditional family system, filial piety, and general respect and reverence for old age.

Some lower-income Third World countries have yet to reach the point at which elderly people feel themselves to be, and are seen to be, a burden. If this can be maintained, then the need for remedial action will be avoided. In the Caribbean, for example, there is considerable interest in the current and future status of elderly people, from social, housing and health perspectives, and attitudes to them at present appear positive. However, 'the elderly' are often regarded as a homogeneous group as opposed to the reality of their heterogeneity, and as a medical problem rather than one involving social care and provision. Therefore, it is unlikely that all elderly people will be amenable to continued traditional support. If the Caribbean countries are taken as an example of the low- to middle-income Third World, the data in Fig. 7.14 illustrate that between 1980 and the year 2000, percentage increases in elderly folk are going to be in the region of 30 per cent (Jamaica) to 66 per cent (Trinidad and Tobago). Fortunately, this phenomenon is being looked upon fairly optimistically in this region: Grell (1987: 5), for example, states: 'in Jamaica today we have come full circle; now, having more or less taken care of the problems of persons under age five,. . .we are about to enter the era of developing parallel national programmes for the over sixty-fives'. This is an important recognition, which, whilst perhaps overoptimistic about

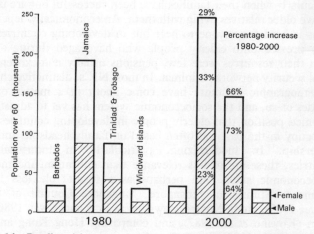

Fig. 7.14   **Predicted increase in the population over 60 years of age in the Carribbean (based on data from Grell 1987)**

having tackled the problems of childhood, at least acknowledges the need to anticipate an ageing population. Hopefully, similar positive attitudes to increasing aged populations will be fostered in other developing countries as the phenomenon of ageing becomes apparent. What has occurred in the NICs, as an exemplar for other Third World countries in this field? Hong Kong and Singapore are among the best-documented examples, although the limitations of extrapolating from compact, highly urbanized city–states to the larger, more sparsely populated, predominantly rural Third World countries should be borne in mind. The 'fact' of increasing aged populations has been recognized now for some two decades in both territories. In both places, life expectancy is around 80 years and beyond, which is the hallmark of the post-demographic transition in East and South East Asia (Leete 1987), and to be seen elsewhere in the region. As Japan was completing its demographic transition in the 1950s and early 1960s, so Hong Kong, Singapore and Taiwan were beginning theirs, with China and the Chinese in Malaysia starting a little later.

The problems of ageing populations are currently most acute in North West Europe, but the speed and size of fertility declines in East and South East Asia mean that ageing will come much more rapidly than it did in Europe. This has enormous implications for these NICs and for all rapidly modernizing Third World countries. Indeed, as noted earlier, increasing levels of dependency, skill shortages in the workforce and the like have already caused the Singapore government to pursue a pro-natalist policy after many years of encouraging FP. The same might occur in Hong Kong and will possibly be seen elsewhere in the region.

In Hong Kong, the proportion of elderly people over 60 has increased from a relatively static 4 per cent between 1920 and the 1950s to 5.4 per cent (170 000) in 1961, 7.5 per cent (301 000) in 1971, 10.2 per cent (528 000) in 1981 and to about 11.6 per cent (640 000) in 1986. This has been met with considerable activity in service and medical support provision. As in Europe, longevity among the elderly cohort is increasing: in 1961, only 13.8 per cent of the over-sixties were aged 75 years or more but, by 1986, this had reached almost 22 per cent. The 'very elderly' are those most likely to be in need of social care, medical services and/or institutional, as opposed to domiciliary, residential support. In Hong Kong, this has led to the development during and since the 1970s of support services ranging from general community care, residential care (for accommodation only or for varying levels of support) and increased institutional and community medical care (see Fig. 7.15). Hong Kong is fortunate in having had a history since the 1950s of public housing, and a fairly good and well-funded public-

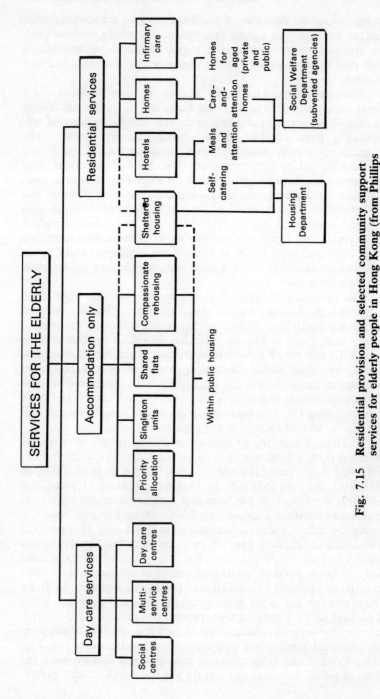

Fig. 7.15 Residential provision and selected community support services for elderly people in Hong Kong (from Phillips 1988b)

cum-charitable health and welfare system provided by a wealthy government (see, for example, Phillips 1981a, 1987b).

It is to care for the more dependent elderly people – rather than those who are able to help themselves – that Hong Kong and Singapore have had to turn their attention (Phillips 1988b). Two main types of scheme operate in Hong Kong: homes for the aged (a form of group housing, with or without meals and other social care) and care-and-attention homes, analogous in some ways to old folk's homes/nursing homes in Britain (Phillips et al. 1988). The care-and-attention home sector is where real shortages have been noted. These homes have been planned at five places per 1000 persons aged 60+, but the demand in 1988 to 1989 was still about one-third above levels of provision. The supply of infirmary beds (in old folk's wards) has been even more stretched and shortfalls in demand are predicted into the mid-1990s. Even with generous increases in provision programmed over the next decade, Hong Kong will find itself with difficulties in meeting the needs of an ageing (and more dependent) elderly population. An illustration of this increasing demand for more dependent provision is that, whereas the waiting lists for elderly accommodation as a whole increased by about 18 per cent per annum between 1983 and 1986, during the same period, the waiting lists for care-and-attention homes increased annually by almost 30 per cent (39 per cent in 1985 to 1986). The significance of such figures is that, within the high-dependency sector, costs are higher in terms of staff and buildings and, of course, there are generally fewer staff available.

Hong Kong and Singapore have mixed economies in which the public sectors have strong inputs to welfare, health and housing. However, in both, a strong tendency has evolved in the 1980s for the private sector to move into provision of care for elderly people. Whilst this may not in itself be a bad thing, it raises issues of quality monitoring and the potential exploitation of elderly folk for private gain. Hong Kong has been persuaded to introduce a code of practice in 1987 for private-sector old folk's homes and it is anticipated that legislation on standards may also be necessary. Other NICs and the poorer Third World countries might be tempted to follow the route of reliance on private provision but, without rigorous standards and enforcement procedures, there is always the danger that low-standard geriatric ghettos will be created. In Hong Kong, for instance, the number of private homes for elderly people increased from some 80 known in early 1986 to over 200 in March 1988, an increase of 150 per cent in 2 years (Phillips 1988b). In Singapore, a similar if not quite as rapid growth seems to have occurred in the private sector, although there current plans are to focus services onto the 97 per cent of elderly people who still live in the community (Singapore Council of Social Service 1985). In both territories, this has been largely a phenomenon of the 1980s, and the governments recognize the burden and potential burden of the increasingly aged populations on their health and social care.

Urbanization, industrialization and social trends towards nuclear rather than extended multigenerational families are felt to have undermined the security and prestige of a growing proportion of elderly people in some African countries. In Zimbabwe, for example, the socioeconomic pre-eminence of some elderly people has been eroded and there are evident, for the first time, numbers of destitute elderly people, particularly in urban areas. Pension schemes, day-care centres and residential sheltered accommodation have proved to be vastly inadequate for today's needs. In particular, surveys in homes for the elderly in Zimbabwe have emphasized that the provision of physical facilities – accommodation, services and food – is insufficient to create overall feelings of well-being among aged residents. Some feel that socioemotional support is needed, to show elderly people they are still valued (in tribal society, for instance) and that they can help in running the places in which they live (Nyanguru 1987). In future, Third World countries developing residential care facilities might emphasize opportunities for self-help, self-expression and maintenance of the individual's sense of dignity and worth if such policies are to be successful and, importantly, affordable.

Issues of cultural acceptability of institutional care have been considered in some developing countries, although of course this sector is often very small in overall terms. Western Polynesia had opened its first home for the aged, established in 1975 near Apia, and cultural acceptance may influence the continuation of such schemes. By contrast with the situation in many other countries, residents at the Apia home seemed to be there by their own choice and relatives frequently wished them to return home to live, perhaps because of the disapproval they were encountering about letting others care for their elderly relatives. Some elderly folk undoubtedly liked the prestige of living in a religious home and the medical care was good for many. However, surprisingly, a reduction in demand for places was found over time, and this was not due to a lack of elderly people (who comprised in 1981 about 5 per cent of the population) (Holmes and Holmes 1987). Possibly only the most frail were now attending the home, as its novelty for others had worn off, and care in the villages and communities by relatives was continuing. This may be welcomed if appropriate care is being provided in the community, but it certainly is a contrast to what seems to be occurring in many other Third World societies today.

Family support

The varying levels and extent of family support available for elderly people in different Third World settings are important underlying reasons for different patterns of overt dependency and need for residential care. Whilst variations between societies in the impacts of 'modernization' on attitudes to family care of the elderly have been stressed, there is often an assumption that family care is in sharp decline. Evidence does not always support this, and the family does appear to remain a crucial source of support and care. In many developing countries, there is a strong reliance on family care, and many governments wish to maintain and extend existing systems of such support. This is true in many South-East Asian countries such as Indonesia (Chen and Jones 1988). Even in Hong Kong and Singapore, many elderly people still live with their families and both governments wish to encourage proper care by the family (Lee 1986; Phillips 1988b). Chen (1987) also notes that 72 per cent of elderly Malaysians in a survey were living with their children. Indeed, 95 per cent of elderly Malaysians do not live alone (but with a spouse, child or some other relative), although living alone there does increase with age and is more prevalent among women. Some 81 per cent of urban elderly compared with 67 per cent of rural elderly residents in the survey were living with their children. The rural elderly folk might, however, be living in close proximity to their offspring and hence continuing to receive support. In addition, the main source of income for elderly Malaysians is the family, who provided for over 60 per cent of respondents. Pensions were relatively unimportant and formed the main income of only 14 per cent of elderly people. Overall, however, housing policies in most Third World countries have rarely responded to the needs of multigeneration extended families, and this has reduced the ability of families to support their elders.

In Hong Kong, although one-quarter of a sample of 441 low-income elderly people were living alone, the majority were living with spouse or children. Chow and Kwan (1986) did, however, find that lone elderly persons were more likely to be living in poverty and to have a poor image of themselves. They therefore suggest that priority should be given to the needs of the lone elderly, as do Chen and Jones (1988) for other South-East Asian countries. Many do, it seems, receive public assistance and other support, but the deficiency of such provision means that domiciliary services, in particular, are not widely available to those who are living with families. This may be a cause for domestic strain and certainly the implication is that families are substituting for proper care in the community. Sufficient resources have yet to be made available to help support people as members of the community, in particular those living with their families.

Elderly people in developing countries tend to remain working for longer than they might elsewhere, and for many the concept of retirement with financial security has little meaning. Family financial help is therefore important; the Hong Kong survey, as in Malaysia, showed the family to be the major source of financial support for many elderly folk, with children supporting 52 per cent of respondents. Formal pensions were of very limited significance, although this might be expected, given the low-income family focus of the research. Public assistance helped 16 per cent of respondents and a further 16 per cent were still receiving wages from work (in comparison, 20 per cent of the Malaysian group were likewise in receipt of wages). This highlights the potential problem of the welfare of elderly people in other Third World countries: they may have no pension and often no formal social security scheme to support them financially; if they have no children or none locally, the problem may become acute. Indeed, in rural South Asia, elderly people without surviving children, especially women, have been found to be at greater risk than others of higher mortality and loss of property (Cain 1986). If, as some suggest, family support will decline with modernization, then other sources of income as well as care will have to be provided. For the poorer developing countries, this burden will be considerable in the future.

Pharmaceuticals: use, abuse and dumping

The availability of pharmaceuticals in many Third World countries has for long been a source of concern, for a number of reasons. Absolute shortage of essential, basic medicines (curative and prophylactic) is a common phenomenon; however, there is also a problem of easy availability of sometimes dangerous drugs, which should be, but are not, regulated. In addition, many medicines of dubious efficacy, or that are even dangerous, remain on sale in many developing countries after they have been withdrawn from sale in their countries of origin. To these features may be added the sale of out-of-date, adulterated, improperly stored or incorrectly dispensed drugs, which occurs widely in the Third World.

Drugs are generally a major source of expenditure in the health systems of developing countries. For example, in Tanzania in the late 1970s, about 22 per cent of the health budget was allocated to purchase of drugs but the total purchases amounted to some 40 per cent. This proportion is actually low in comparison with that in some developing countries, which spend as much as 50 or 60 per cent of health budgets on drugs (Taylor 1986; Turshen 1984). It is hard to believe that value is being achieved for such proportional expenditure, and national-level action is often needed to rectify this. Steps include adoption of the essential drugs listed by the WHO (see below), generic rather than brand prescribing, controls on purchases, education of physicians, and the extension of local pharmaceutical production (with appropriate quality control).

Drugs are essential components of much Western medicine, whether curative, or as part of some treatments (chemotherapies, analgesics and anaesthetics), or as prophylactics and vaccines. However, whilst modern Western society is now to some extent alerted to the dangers of over-reliance on drug treatment and pill-popping, and recognizes iatrogenic illness (Illich 1976), in the Third World, many drugs are presented as cure-alls, and marketed with few, if any, checks.

Indeed, the utility and potential of drugs are often misrepresented by doctors, drug companies and sellers in certain Third World countries. They may be promoted as cures or preventives for conditions in which they are only marginally effective or totally ineffective. Consumers are often left at the mercy of the pharmaceuticals industry and it seems that many professionals play along with consumer demand and prescribe or recommend inappropriate or even dangerous drugs. There has been considerable research into issues concerned with the promotion, distribution and inappropriate use of many types of drugs in the Third World. This has highlighted the dubious promotion of drugs and exaggerated claims by pharmaceutical firms and medical professionals, which often give incomplete disclosure of side-effects and dangers, and misleading information about the use of drugs. In addition, numerous cases of dumping of dangerous, banned or 'stale' drugs into poorly regulated Third World countries have been documented or suspected (Stock 1985). Perhaps the most comprehensive surveys of the impact and nature of drugs usage and abuse in Third World countries are to be found in the publications by Melrose (1982), Patel (1983) and Silverman and Lee (1982).

Certain countries are developing domestic capacity for pharmaceutical production, but quality controls may be poor and many countries remain important markets for multinational drug companies. There is also considerable doubt whether local manufacture actually produces cheaper drugs, when costs of capital investment and the like are taken into account (Peretz 1983). Nigeria, in spite of increasing its own drugs production, remains about 90 per cent dependent on imports and continues to be the largest drug market in Africa. It is still a major profit area for multinational corporations, even with a declining turnover since the mid-1980s (see, for example, Stock 1985). However, by contrast, some countries such as Brazil and Egypt produce most basic drugs locally, although the precise cost savings may be questioned even if economic dependency is reduced. In Bangladesh, the adoption of a national essential drugs policy in 1982 and a concentration on locally produced drugs have led to nearly 90 per cent of drugs marketed there being formulated locally, and the national pharmaceutical industry is growing steadily (Hye 1988).

Pharmaceutical abuse by companies, professionals or individual consumers (whoever is to blame) is obviously a major problem as it may lead to damaged health and a build-up of resistant pathogenic strains. However, curative and preventive drugs are also absolutely crucial to many Third World countries battling with infectious and chronic ailments and poor environmental conditions. The financial and human cost of having inappropriate drugs is often accompanied by an absolute lack of drugs, but the problem in the past has been to determine which drugs are required, at what cost, and how they should be controlled. The organization of an effective, secure and reliable supply system in both urban and rural areas also has to be addressed. It appears that double deprivation often exists: not only do the poor suffer disproportionately from ill health, but they have no access to life-saving drugs, and neither the public nor private drug-distribution systems by and large cater for their needs. Drugs are wasted and misused worldwide but, in developing countries, the social consequences of wasteful drug purchases and inefficient and corrupt distribution are acute. They ultimately serve to perpetuate existing inequalities in economic and health conditions in which the poorest and most ill have little power to redress the inequitable access to required medicine. Whilst widespread environment and sanitation improvements within PHC frameworks are doubtless crucial, Melrose (1982) also considers there is little doubt that, if the poor has access to even a small number of essential drugs, the unnecessary suffering and premature death of millions could be averted. This emphasizes the need for comprehensive national drug policies to rationalize both public and private sectors and improve the availability of essential drugs.

Essential drugs programmes

Whilst there is a shortage of safe, effective and reliable drugs in much of the Third World, it is still possible to question the assumption that pharmaceuticals are good for health. However, the development of health services along, say, British and American lines has meant a considerable reliance on modern drugs and growing perceived need for them. In India, for example, many people equate 'more drugs' with a better situation and medical practice has become equated with drug prescription (Stoker and Jeffery 1988). This situation obtains in many countries and makes even more necessary the identification and efficient provision of basic drugs, in which supply, prices and profits can be reasonable but balanced. In the late 1970s, the WHO (1977, 1979) was already drawing up a list of 200 essential drugs, based on the prevaleñce and severity of diseases and the cost-effectiveness of available therapy (the links to selective PHC will be apparent). In 1981, a special action programme on essential drugs and vaccines was introduced by the WHO, which attempted to bring together selection of drugs, use of generic names, efficient procurement, supply and distribution, and comprehensive training of staff in rational prescription. By 1987, more than 100 developing countries had prepared essential drug lists suitable for their own circumstances and considerable amounts of public and private money had been invested in the purchase of drugs.

Criteria for identification of essential drugs are generally pharmacological and attempt to exclude those known to be ineffective or even harmful. Often, too, economic criteria are included, such as the prohibition of foreign companies from manufacturing simple products such as antacids and vitamin preparations. Foreign imports are often banned if local equivalents can be produced. Since developing countries are generally short of foreign exchange to purchase essential drugs, it is important that generic rather than brand names are specified, so that the best-value sources may be tapped. Some drugs are identified for PHC use, others for secondary and tertiary use (approximately one-third of Bangladesh's 150 drugs for most therapeutic purposes have been selected for PHC).

However, it seems that the implementation of essential drugs programmes (EDPs) is meeting serious problems in most developing countries and that 60 to 80 per cent of their populations still do not have access to even the most essential drugs. Reasons for this are interlinked and include political, organizational–managerial and financial factors. Indeed, at the time of writing, the EDP is under review and evaluation.

Political problems include resistance of the pharmaceuticals industry and other private-sector participants (wholesalers, retailers) to EDPs, as they stand to lose vast profits on other proprietary drugs. Sometimes government lack of will or obstruction may be a problem (for example, by insistence that certain personnel distribute drugs). In pharmaceuticals, it is suggested that six countries control almost three-quarters of world drug production (and also contribute 50 per cent to the WHO's budget), and companies are unwilling to see the market in Third World countries eroded because, although relatively small, their expenditure accounts for 20 per cent of world spending on drugs. There is still a need for certain essential drugs to be imported, despite attempts by many countries to build up their own manufacturing capability. Drug import costs are often further eroding chronic shortages of foreign exchange (Wang'ombe and Mwabu 1987).

Organizational problems in EDPs include inadequate storage; poor packing and labelling; corruption and illegal sales to the private sector; fraud; pilfering; and poor transport, quality control and inventory control (Soeters and Bannenberg 1988). In addition, there may be considerable practical difficulties in deciding the quantities of each drug to purchase in a given country. However, Soeters and Bannenberg suggest that the use of recently available microcomputer programs can, with improved availability of essential drugs, enable such calculations to be made with an efficiency unimaginable only a few years ago. In Gabon, for example, they estimate a saving of 45 per cent may be made in the drug budget. If such savings can be used either to purchase more drugs or to be spent elsewhere in the health system, improved quantification of essential drug requirements (by reference to standard treatments and estimated cases per disease) is clearly very worthwhile.

Essential drugs programmes are frequently in place at a national level, but the introduction of community-based schemes to ensure local availability of low-priced essential drugs has often met with problems. Many are similar to those outlined above (organizational and political), and relate to the gains and losses for various interests. Sometimes cheap supplies 'leak' back corruptly into the private sector, to be sold at high prices (Smith 1987). In addition, if official prices are set above people's ability to pay, schemes will not succeed; if set too low, costs will not be recovered and the schemes also may founder (Foster and Drager 1988). Figure 7.16 illustrates the options, problems and considerations to be taken into account at various times and places in a community EDP – note the complex links and potential pitfalls between supply and consumer. A good example of such a scheme is the Philippines *Botica sa Barangay*, in which shopkeepers in villages retain a small profit on the sale of drugs to encourage them to stock and supply selected medicines.

Traditional medicines

A majority of Third World citizens may have recourse to traditional forms of medical advice, either solely or in conjunction with modern medicine, and many also use various types of traditional remedies. These may be prescribed by TMPs, or purchased or acquired by the consumer, based on experience or recommendation. As may sometimes occur in Western medicine, the traditional

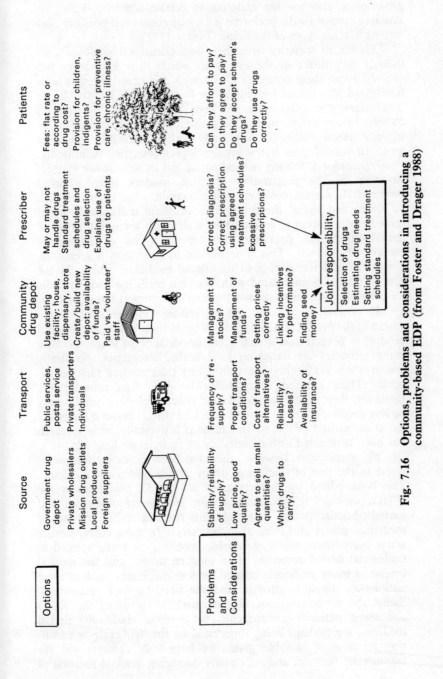

	Source	Transport	Community drug depot	Prescriber	Patients
Options	Government drug depot	Public services, postal service	Use existing facility: house, dispensary, store	May or may not handle drugs	Fees: flat rate or according to drug cost?
	Private wholesalers	Private transporters	Create/build new depot: availability of funds?	Standard treatment schedules and drug selection	Provision for children, indigents?
	Mission drug outlets	Individuals	Paid vs. "volunteer" staff	Explains use of drugs to patients	Provision for preventive care, chronic illness?
	Local producers				
	Foreign suppliers				
Problems and Considerations	Stability/reliability of supply?	Frequency of re-supply?	Management of stocks?	Correct diagnosis?	Can they afford to pay?
	Low price, good quality?	Proper transport conditions?	Management of funds?	Correct prescription using agreed treatment schedules?	Do they agree to pay?
	Agrees to sell small quantities?	Cost of transport alternatives?	Setting prices correctly?	Excessive prescriptions?	Do they accept scheme's drugs?
	Which drugs to carry?	Reliability? Losses?	Linking incentives to performance?		Do they use drugs correctly?
		Availability of insurance?	Finding seed money?		

Joint responsibility

Selection of drugs
Estimating drug needs
Setting standard treatment schedules

Fig. 7.16 Options, problems and considerations in introducing a community-based EDP (from Foster and Drager 1988)

prescription may include undertaking certain activities, eating or avoiding certain foods, performing various rituals and possibly consuming certain types of medicine (Foster 1983).

Almost all societies have their own traditional medicines, although they differ in the extent to which their knowledge has evolved about these remedies. Sometimes this knowledge has been formalized into herbal formularies or homoeopathic handbooks; at other times the information has been handed down by word of mouth. In any event, today, the gathering and preparation of the ingredients for traditional (especially herbal) medicines constitute an enormous occupation in many developing countries. Admittedly, its organization is usually not industrial and its scale is not factory-based as is the preparation of most modern pharmaceutical products. In China, however, and in certain other countries such as Korea and India, the preparation of some traditionally based remedies does occur at an industrial scale, with some factory-based manufacture and packaging of certain types of commonly prescribed products. This is dependent to an extent, it seems, on a more formal recognition of traditional medicine, which, in the case of China, is integrated with Western medicine and, in India for example, exists with its own training and support infrastructure.

In general, large profit and big business elements are mainly absent in the production of traditional medicines, but consumers and producers nevertheless attach great importance to them. Because many remedies are based on local herbs, sometimes specifically grown, their availability is usually wider than modern pharmaceuticals. Their cultural acceptability is also often considerable. However, their chemotherapeutic and pharmacological benefits may be less predictable than those of standard drugs, because many are based on natural products. In addition, historically, little research has been conducted into the efficacy of many remedies.

For some years, however, there has been increasing formal interest in the role of traditional drugs within traditional medicine. The book edited by Bannerman *et al.* (1983), produced by the WHO, includes a substantial section on herbal medicines and herbal pharmacopoeias, and highlights the availability and use of medicinal plants and local plant resources. In some cases, similar active ingredients, albeit of variable potency, are being applied in traditional herbal remedies as in modern drugs, and the natural origins of many artificially created modern medicines, such as some antibiotics, digitalis, atropine and the like, are well recognized. Sadly, the initiatives from various quarters, including the WHO and some national governments, to promote traditional herbal medicine are perhaps being threatened by the deliberate or unwitting removal of valuable plants by large-scale deforestation for commercial reasons, and by equally damaging gradual removal of vegetation for fuel, and by the over picking of specific medicinal plants themselves (Ayensu 1983). Overhunting also endangers some types of reptiles and animals such as the rhinoceros and musk deer, which are believed to provide some form of medicinal benefit. The overexploitation of natural resources may thus inadvertently remove irreplaceable plants and animals before their curative values have been established.

Anything from 25 000 to 75 000 species of flowering plants have been estimated to have been used in traditional medicine, although only about 1 per cent of these (250 to 750 species) have been scientifically acknowledged to have human therapeutic value. Some might act through placebo effects; others, through active ingredients. However, full research into rarer species, particularly in the tropical regions of the world, which contain some two-thirds of all organisms, has yet to be systematically completed. A computerized data base NAPRALERT (Natural Products ALERT) is being developed on the chemistry and pharmacology of natural products. It includes reviews of the literature and computerizes original information as it becomes available. Whilst acknowledged to be incomplete, it provides a valuable resource in data retrieval and problem-solving in traditional medicines, particularly for specific remedies and geographical variations in availability (Farnsworth 1983).

In the developed world, increasing recognition of the dangers of continued intake of artificial chemicals has prompted a widespread search for natural cures and a 'return to nature'. Phytopharmacology and phytotherapy (the study of pharmacological properties of plants and their use as treatments) are increasingly important research areas. In developing countries, phytotherapy has persisted in the practice of traditional medicine, which has often preserved and extended the large number of components of many traditional medicaments (Attisso 1983). The incorporation of such medicines into Third World EDPs is beginning in a small way in certain countries; in some, such as China, it is well advanced. Research into the chemotherapeutic value of traditional medicines is also under way in numerous countries in Asia, Africa and Latin America, and will no doubt be a strong influence on future use and extension of such medicines.

Availability and cultural acceptability have frequently been cited as reasons for the consumer popularity of many traditional medicines (Joseph and Phillips 1984; Neumann and Lauro 1982; Ramesh and Hyma 1981). In addition, it is sometimes alleged that the cheapness of traditional medicines is also attractive, although whether this is actually so varies considerably. In some cases, the cost of traditional medicines may be as high as, or higher than, Western drugs, and the cost of herbal medicines is very variable, as evidence from various African countries such as Malawi (Morris 1986) and Nigeria suggests. Indeed, the price of both consultations and medicines may be varied according to the perception of the practitioner as to what the client can afford. Ironically, in wealthier countries such as Singapore, some clients claim to use traditional Chinese medicines as they are 'cheaper', although objectively the prices of many such remedies have soared in the 1980s (Ho *et al.* 1984). Supply and demand can cause considerable fluctuation in prices and often highly sought-after substances such as ginseng and rhinoceros horn in the Far East can make prices rise very substantially.

The outlets for traditional products are also varied, ranging from formal shops, stocking solely traditional remedies in India and many South-East Asian countries, to shared modern pharmacies, and to market stalls in African countries. Frequently, the client or patient will see little or no contradiction in using traditional and modern medicines either sequentially or in combination: as noted in Chapter 3, the segregation and differentiation between many forms of traditional medicine and modern systems can be exaggerated. In Singapore and Hong Kong, for example, many ordinary people regard certain Chinese and Western medicines as performing equivalent or complementary functions (Ho *et al.* 1984; Lee 1980; Phillips 1984; Quah 1981). The same applies in many other regions of the world. Lee (1980) notes that about half the respondents in a Hong Kong survey felt that, for most diseases, the joint effort of both Chinese and Western-style practitioners would be more effective than either type alone, and over 95 per cent felt that both styles of practitioners should learn the practices of the other.

A note of caution should be added about the interpretation of the use of traditional medicines solely as medical therapies. In many instances, their use is ritualized; dosages can be imprecise and, in practice (in Africa in particular), there may be relatively little consistency in use of identical plant preparations even for the same malady. Good (1987a) cites evidence to suggest that many Africans do not necessarily expect to be healed by medication alone, but that the ritual associated with the treatment of the practitioner and the client's subsequent behaviour are all crucial. These may be less significant in some other Third World situations, although the evidence from a review of different regions by Bannerman *et al.* (1983) suggests cultural and psychological factors are important in most traditional medical consultations. Good (1987a) points out that the focus of many Western observers on the nature, content and efficacy of African pharmacopoeias has led them partly erroneously to characterize traditional medicine largely in terms of clusters of practices related to 'herbal remedies'. This oversimplifies African and many other therapeutics, and leads to inaccurate interpretations in particular about the role of plant medicines. 'The use of herbal medicines is thus inseparable from the art of healing' (Good 1987a: 265). It is intricately tied up with diagnosis, beliefs and rituals, and this should be borne in mind particularly when studying the prescription of medicines of various guises in traditional systems.

Charging for drugs and health care: the Bamako Initiative

A greater threat to health care extension and EDPs than organizational problems has emerged in the deteriorating economic situation in many developing countries during the 1980s. Many African and Latin American countries have large external debts and are being forced to accept IMF economic recovery packages. These generally entail a reduction in budgetary proportions spent on social and health sectors. However, whilst allocations have been shrinking, there is the struggle to meet increased demands for health and social care. In the late 1980s, many donors had begun requiring the introduction of some kinds of cost recovery as a condition for supporting health care programmes. The World Bank has called for charges to be introduced for some types of government health services; yet more controversially, UNICEF has proposed the 'Bamako Initiative' of September 1987. In this, it was suggested that the drug supply and MCH problems of sub-Saharan Africa would be solved by cost recovery. The initiative aims to introduce a pragmatic solution of supplying poorly-served rural areas in particular with drugs which would be sold for two or three times the cost price and the proceeds used to establish a revolving fund for the repurchase of drugs and as income for local PHC and MCH activities. UNICEF has issued operational guidelines for the Bamako Initiative which have been widely endorsed by African nations as a possible means of supplying essential drugs and health care (Garner 1989; Kanji 1989).

Whilst it is recognized that there is often not enough money allocated to health care and drugs, the Bamako Initiative has raised several important practical and ethical issues. Whether people will be able to pay, and at what cost to their families, is in doubt. Whether really needy people will be exempt from charges will also be difficult to ascertain (Garner 1989). The need to institute cost recovery in health care is often at odds with many political manifestos guaranteeing its free provision and there are important problems in starting cost recovery at community level whilst more specialised levels of health care might remain free. Few doubt the financial difficulties facing many Third World countries and the effects of economic recession and adjustment on health, but the Bamako Initiative is by no means universally accepted as their solution. It poses serious questions related to equity and the implementation of fee systems, and it might have deleterious effects on the health of the poorest, especially women and children. In so far as the initiative also purports to support GOBI-FFF and their essential drugs elements, it is favouring selective interventions and sacrificing comprehensive PHC. The Bamako Initiative rests on the belief that people will pay for drugs but many factors, chiefly poverty, may render people unable to do so. Economic evaluation of demand therefore appears to be replacing the criterion of need in health care. UNICEF's (1989) strong stance on the effects of debt and poverty on the health of the poor in the Third World appears to be at odds with its support of the Bamako Initiative which in practice may well undermine access to health services for the poor (Kanji 1989). Whether there should even be an attempt to recover health care costs in the Third World and, if so, from whom and how they should be recouped, will no doubt be a major debate in the decade of the 1990s.

Conclusion

The provision of health care services for mothers and children and the development of safe environments for them have been major emphases in Third World health programmes for two or three decades. However, elderly people are one of the Third World's problem groups of today and the future. Whilst many poor developing countries are still struggling with maternal and paediatric priorities, NICs in particular, but also others, are already having to cope with a significant increase in numbers of elderly people. It is essential that lessons are learned from the experience of many developed countries that have had belatedly to recognize the needs of their elderly population. Perhaps by judicious planning and fostering of any family systems that will help to care for elderly people in the future, Third World countries can avoid the social and financial difficulties that many European countries are now facing.

This chapter has been selective in focusing on special groups and issues: the young, their mothers and the old; the availability or lack of pharmaceutical supplies and the importance of developing EDPs suitable to the country's needs, incorporating traditional medicine where appropriate. A considerable time has been spent looking at population issues and the availability and extent of FP methods. These are of pressing concern, but other topics, perhaps equally important, have not been touched on directly because of space constraints. For example, another growing concern for many developing countries is mental illness and services for mentally (and physically) handicapped persons. The Third World has, on balance, an unenviable history of dealing with mental ill health and the needs of most handicapped people have not been high priorities. With epidemiological change and higher survivorship rates, such groups will increase in number.

This issue of mental health in particular is likely to become increasingly pressing as the whole process of modernization reduces the stability of life, disrupts family routines and living, and introduces the types of Western diseases often associated with stress noted in Chapter 2. In China, for example there is concern about the impacts on mental health of policies such as the one-child family, the stresses on families unable to cope with the growing numbers of elderly people, and of the pressures to succeed economically in modernization. Providing mental health care by modern and traditional means for one billion people in China is a formidable task (Lin and Eisenberg 1985). This area of health provision will undoubtedly also increase in significance elsewhere (Higginbotham 1984). The urban environment and life in many Third World cities is not only distinctly stressful but often acutely dangerous in terms of pollutants, vehicles, drugs and alcohol. Research in Pikine (Senegal) and Ibadan (Nigeria) shows there are many environments in Third World settings potentially injurious to mental health (Dieng and Hanck 1986; Iyun 1989). There is also some interesting work on, for example, the use of traditional healers in mental illness and on the place of traditional medicine in psychiatry, as noted in Chapter 3 (see, for example, Coppo 1983; Koumaré 1983).

There are, however, relatively few detailed studies of the ecology of mental ill health and distribution of caring facilities in Third World cities. Iyun (1989) points to the data and definitional problems involved in undertaking such research, and her study of Ibadan points to certain important distributional patterns that differ from those in many cities in the developed world. Interestingly, men and women seem to be almost exactly equally prone to mental illness as a whole, although there were slight differences by diagnosis. In addition, Iyun notes that both inner- and outer-city zones in Ibadan seem to suffer from environments likely to be associated with high rates of mental stress. Different forms of blight and environmental degradation tend to predispose individuals to mental stress in the inner core of the city. This is similar to findings in many Western cities but, whereas in these, suburban settings tend to have displayed lower incidence of mental ill health, in the Nigerian city, socioeconomic frustrations (stresses of modernization perhaps?) have been felt to be responsible for the relatively high incidence of mental disorders in the outer zone of the city. The economically active who had recently been hurt in trade depressions added to the numbers vulnerable to mental illness. Other speculative aetiologies of some mental illnesses are not considered here but, in so far as these are related to demographic change and modernization, then the Third World is likely on this basis as well to witness considerable future increases in mental ill health.

Chapter 8

Health care: the end of the century and beyond

So far, this book has considered mainly the evolution and current status of health care in developing nations. There are many encouraging features, but even more discouraging ones in many systems. Demographic, epidemiological and economic factors seem to unite to make the current prospect of providing 'Health for All by the Year 2000' increasingly elusive and illusory. The *annus mirabilis* in global health care appears increasingly unlikely to occur in the near future.

Some moderately optimistic reviews of progress towards the goals of health for all, or at least of setting out the field for the goals, are identified in the review of the years 1978 to 1984 by WHO member countries (WHO 1987b, c). The seventh report on the world health situation shows frankness on the part of WHO member states in declaring advances and weaknesses in their health care plans and achievements. General global trends have been identified as harmful to their plans: inflation, fluctuating exchange rates, insufficient aid or aid cut-backs, and debt-servicing problems. The increase in global population – now past the 4 800 million point – has largely occurred in Third World countries, as has hyperurbanization. Rising tides of young and old folk have also been seen in many countries. The precise impacts of these factors have differed from one country to another but, as usual, the poorest countries and people have had the narrowest margins of survival and have been hit hardest.

The world is smaller at the end of the 1980s in terms of communications than it was at the beginning of the decade, but it is still fragmented in terms of health care. There are, however, many encouraging signs. Community commitment to, and participation in, PHC programmes has been evident in many countries, and numerous governments have declared in favour of PHC (of various modes). Yet many weaknesses remain: in particular, measures to achieve effective intersectoral action and cooperation are still absent in most countries. National and local conflicts of interest, bureaucracies and tangled responsibilities have often worsened this decade. Many NGOs are nevertheless increasingly cutting through and across red tape, but there is still a need for stimulation of individual responsibility, not easily achieved by top-down programmes.

It can be argued that the developed world this decade has been a source of poor examples in health care for many Third World countries. The principles of self-reliance in health being promoted by Thatcherite–monetarist policies in many countries downplay the role of the state in providing the infrastructure for health for all. This might be acceptable to many wealthier residents in rich countries but, even in these, there is far from universal approval of the ideas of gradual government withdrawal from universally provided health care. The reduction of public-sector funding for many types of programmes, which are left to stand on their own financial feet, is a persuasive example for poor governments to follow, as it minimizes their need for expenditure on what is regarded as an infinite demand for health care. This example may prove to be one of the worst exports of the decade from the developed to the developing world. Other major difficulties, largely exported from North to South, include the cost explosion of health care goods and products; an increasing dependence on technology and drugs when public health reforms are more important; and support for, and imposition of, dubious prestige facilities for health when fundamental communications and infrastructure are lacking.

Not all is negative, however. If the realities are congruent with the propaganda, then most pregnant women and infants in developing countries now have access to health care, although the proportions do vary considerably regionally (see Fig. 7.2) and even more so locally. Selective programmes such as ORT and vaccination are now quite widely available, but political will to carry these campaigns to their logical conclusions is not always evident (and, of course, not all agree with selective interventions). A major weakness remains the difficulty of deriving sensible, affordable local comprehensive programmes to sustain health for all once selectivity has been applied. However much criticized, selective and targeted campaigns are probably here to stay.

In this concluding chapter, it is only possible to highlight some of the issues that will influence the possibility of health for all by the end of the century and beyond. These include the provision of clean water, the underlying issue of health education (crucial to PHC) to improve chances of correct diet and healthy behaviour, and the potential impacts of various trends in health care delivery, such as the emphasis on hospitals as first-level referrals in PHC. The proclivities of donor agencies cannot be ignored either, as these often quite directly shape short-term health care activities in particular, and even longer-term strategies may be strongly influenced by the levels of aid support anticipated.

Some foci of 'health for all' campaigns

Whilst the ultimate success of the 'health for all' strategy should be measured in terms of the improved health status of the population, it is generally too soon to identify this clearly in many developing nations. It is also sometimes difficult to attribute health improvements to specific health campaigns. However, it is still instructive to summarize some examples of key issues pursued in specific countries, to illustrate the nature of policies in progress. Table 8.1 summarizes major issues and problems noted in the quest for 'health for all' in ten selected countries. The issues raised so far in this book surface clearly, such as collaboration between traditional and modern sectors, intersectoral cooperation requirements, accessibility and acceptability problems, the use of volunteer workers and community participation.

Table 8.1 Some major foci, issues and thrusts in health-for-all campaigns (after WHO 1987c)

Country	Important issues pursued	Remarks/ organizational factors
Sierra Leone	Provision of the same amenities for rural as urban folk. Via: a comprehensive rural development strategy, emphasis on coordination of activities	Three-quarters of the population is rural, but incomes are only one-third those of towns
Tanzania	Creating more rural health centres. Shift of resources to develop small rural health facilities and train their staff	Change in budgetary balance; now somewhat less than 50% to curative services
Togo	Assist rural people to realize their health needs, via health education, community participation and increasing health awareness/ motivation	Community participation in defining problems and priorities recognised as essential

Table 8.1 Cont.

Country	Important issues pursued	Remarks/ organizational factors
Sri Lanka	Revival of traditional values and confidence in traditional medicine; attempt to reverse lack of confidence in the traditional medicine system, change public and professional attitudes	Focus on decentralized teamwork for annual district health development plan formulation. Central synthesis into national health plan
Thailand	Creation of health volunteers in villages: villagers to become initiators and actors in health efforts; health volunteers in 90 of all villages; 'model mother' campaigns for FP	Staff briefed on community participation, social preparation, use of local resources
Botswana	Traditional and modern health practitioners meet and work together – joint workshop, agreed referral practices between sectors in some cases	Some TMPs members of village health committees
Saint Lucia	Nurse practitioners in health centres (district nurse/midwife)	Upgrading skills of these nurses to help diagnosis and prescription
Papua New Guinea	More trained midwives; more transport to increase coverage. Emphasis on trained health	About two-thirds of births are unsupervised. Emphasis on TBAs and modern health practices

Table 8.1 Cont.

Country	Important issues pursued	Remarks/ organizational factors
	workers and outreach to improve MCH accessibility (improve transport management and provision)	
Tanzania	Reorganize the MOH to overcome its tendency to operate vertical programmes, compartmentalized administration	Trend to develop intersectoral cooperation, horizontal programmes, review of PHC conducted
The Gambia	Identify and overcome obstacles to change, to increase intersectoral cooperation, clarify objectives; improve team concepts	Change often resisted; why? how to overcome? Obsolete hierarchies

Health education: a way forward?

It has been widely recognized for a decade that childhood survival in developing countries (as an indicator of health status) is remarkably sensitive to the length of formal schooling of the mother (Caldwell 1979, 1986; Cleland and Van Ginneken 1989). For example, even after adjustment for economic factors, 1 to 3 years of schooling are associated with a 20 per cent fall in childhood risk of death. This has been noted in all developing regions and in countries with both accessible, effective services and in those with weak PHC systems. Therefore, improved general education for mothers, in particular, is crucial. However, education oriented to health is also important. No one is born with a perfect knowledge of how to live his or her life and develop his environment in the most healthy manner; indeed, there is not complete agreement even among trained professionals as to how to achieve such an end.

Nevertheless, many individuals and communities can be equipped with the knowledge and skills to achieve better living conditions and health status, which are central themes to PHC. In recent years, many have recognized that the achievement of improved health for all through the PHC route will be as much a matter of health promotion and education as of providing the wherewithal and professional skills to prevent and cure illness.

Whilst some elements of health education are overoptimistic and fall in the category of 'something being better than nothing', informed participation by the community and individuals can vastly enhance the chances of improving public and individual health even where there are few medical resources. Health education can be directed at groups (communities) or individuals (and families). Governments can foster and facilitate more community involvement in decision-making and implementation of health-promoting schemes and, secondly, individuals can be taught their potential for improving health by their own activities (sensible diets; avoidance of harmful substances; increased sanitation and cleanliness). The first strand involves an initial political decision but the involvement and education of communities then becomes a matter of communication. This is particularly so when individuals are to be reached: this becomes an education issue as people need to be informed of what practices and activities, within their grasp, are likely to benefit their own and their family's health. As such education is more likely to be possible than realistic health care provision, the WHO (1988) has become a great proponent of health education as central to PHC in particular. It has produced a practical manual for training health educators and others whose role may bring them into such positions. Werner's (1977) book on essential medical care and health practices, *Where there is no doctor*, was an earlier recognition of the value of sensible and informed medical self-help. Today, health education has to an extent gone beyond this to focus on the means of effective communication of how to prevent illness, promote good health and deal with individual and community health problems.

Health education activities involve pointing out dangers to health (things to be avoided) and healthy versus unhealthy behaviour (activities to be encouraged or avoided). Dangers to health include: disease-causing organisms such as bacteria, viruses, fungi and parasites; vectors such as certain insects and molluscs; inorganic but toxic substances found naturally in the environment and as a result of man's activities (pollution); natural events and disasters such as floods and earthquakes; man-made environmental dangers such as house fires, vehicle accidents and industrial injuries; and, finally, certain hereditary or genetic diseases. Such things can be identified and, if not totally avoided, health education can at least alert people to these dangers and start to create levels of awareness which will lead to their eventual reduction.

Health education can be the means of informing individuals of what constitutes healthy and unhealthy behaviour. Correct diets, beneficial cooking and correct food- and water-storage practices, simple personal hygiene such as hand-washing, avoidance of insect bites, and good child care can all be taught. Many such things can be improved by personal or family attention, although enhanced environmental sanitation and the provision of a reliable water supply, for example, might be beyond a single family and require wider community participation. There are also notorious difficulties in evaluating the impact that improved water supply, sanitation and health education projects have on community health, since control groups are often not available or researched and research methodologies not explicit. Indeed, as Lindskog *et al.* (1987) point out, some weak methodological studies may give a false impression of the success of such programmes. The exact contribution of health education to such improvements is also very difficult to quantify.

Nevertheless, it is generally accepted that health education programmes that promote healthy behaviour are effective in improving health levels. In MCH, for example, the promotion of child spacing, breast-feeding, infant nutrition and immunization does seem to help to raise community health levels by improving the health of the bulk of the population (the young and mothers). It is easy, however, to suggest what might be effective sounding health education programmes but which never really have a chance of success. This is because most practices in health relate to long-standing beliefs, attitudes and even local taboos, many, if not all of which, are often rooted in sensible actions. Therefore, in order to promote healthy behaviour, research is required into why certain behaviours persist and to suggest practicable ways of modifying them to make them safer. Unless understanding of the basis of behaviour is achieved, the best presented of health education programmes might have little impact.

Many people might become involved in health education: trained professionals and local individuals. The WHO identifies the functions of health education as being the responsibility of everyone engaged in activities related to health and the community; it should not be purely the preserve of professional health educators, although such trained personnel can act as specific *promoters* or stimulators for health education. Health professionals, ancillary staff and schools all have to set good examples in communities for health-related activities. However, coordination, communication and the basic knowledge of those involved must all be sound.

Health education may be with *individuals*, and this is particularly the concern of counselling, through which individuals are encouraged to think about their problems and potentials for improving their circumstances. Counselling may be focused on families, or on specific members such as the mother or children (via schools or clinics, for example). Home visits may be possible but often the counselling may take on a more formal, 'taught' role in a health care setting. In the Third World, particularly in rural situations, the counsellor will often be a CHW or a nurse/midwife, whose role will be broader than that of specific health provider and certainly will not focus purely on curative functions. Health education may also be appropriately aimed at *groups*. This is increasingly becoming a major activity as many environmental and community health problems are, almost by definition, best tackled collectively.

Health education for groups can be aimed at existing formal groups, such as farmers' cooperatives, various village associations, youth clubs or the like, or it may be with informal groups. In the case of formal groups, there will generally be an organizer or committee to approach, and health education might be arranged via regular meetings or by talks or displays set up specially for the group. Informal groups such as friends meeting together, some family or social gatherings, or the like may be less easy to target but equally important. If their common interests can be identified, such as a family gathering for children, then this can be turned to good effect and members invited to attend then or later for health education purposes. In both cases, a wide range of media activities may be used for the promotion of health education: talks, posters, simple stories, active participation, demonstrations and songs (widely used in Latin America). The personnel involved have to be sensitive to the levels of knowledge of, and reasons for, existing behaviour among the group, and they may, if skilful, be able to promote discussion to highlight aspects (such as beliefs, knowledge or superstitions) that could be improved for better health.

Health education may also be focused on *communities*; these, as such, generally share a common set of values, and have spatial and social links. However, health education 'in the community' may be rather difficult to achieve if no set meetings or identifiable focus is evident. Quite often, for example, attenders at an MCH session in a primary health unit may receive a group talk on some health-related issue (such as malaria prophylaxis, or the local availability and use of ORS). The WHO (1988) discusses in some detail the difficulties of identifying a 'community' for health education purposes as these usually cannot be easily drawn on a map without some detailed household investigations. The need to identify community leaders who help to shape opinion can also be crucial and their involvement can very much influence the success of health education efforts (the passive or active acceptance by 'significant persons'). One way suggested to achieve community involvement might be the establishment of local health committees, and this is particularly relevant when wider involvement (community participation) is required to put some health education or PHC elements into practice.

Therefore, health education, which seems on the face of it a simple objective, actually involves a great variety of aims and methods. It may be more or less successful depending on the care and tact that has gone into its planning. Health education may occur within PHC; individuals, groups or communities need to be given skills, confidence and motivation to help themselves, and this depends on effective communication with and between community members. The WHO suggests that, once local health problems have been noted, more or less formal sets of priorities, objectives and actions should be set out. For example, the most serious problems should be identified, the possibilities for improving them discussed and potential obstacles (financial, resources, personnel) should be noted, perhaps the key person being a coordinator with a formal health education training. Once these aspects have been dealt with, individuals, groups and community sources must be identified and included. Methods for encouraging follow-through and for evaluating results and achievements should also be set up.

Health education thus forms an important package and is an integral part of comprehensive PHC. It can be the stimulus that encourages community participation and mobilizes popular support for all sorts of health activities. Selective PHC programmes act 'on' people or 'for' people, with relatively little need for their further actions. By contrast, comprehensive PHC requires improved levels of personal and community knowledge about healthy behaviour and of dangers to health. Many aspects of environmental health improvement can only be achieved by concerted common effort – for example, good sanitation and non-infected water sources must be encouraged by all. A few careless or unknowing people may be able to spoil the provisions for the community. Therefore, health education should be an essential component, necessary not only to the 'health for all' type thrusts, but also if any reasonable levels of community health are to be achieved and maintained.

Access to clean water

Diarrhoeal diseases, and malnutrition and undernutrition associated with them, have been consistently recognized as major causes of high infant mortality and general debility, especially in the poorest

Third World countries. There are numerous links between water and health, and interactions are complex. Water is a 'vehicle' for water-borne diseases and it can provide a breeding ground for some vectors of disease; however, it also serves as a medium to prevent water-washed diseases (Learmonth 1988). Many Third World water supplies have been and are heavily polluted, to well above WHO safely levels (especially for faecal coliform counts). Nevertheless some improvements may reduce these counts to acceptable levels even in very poor social settings (Feachem *et al.* 1977, 1983).

The health impacts of water are often assessed via study of the incidence or prevalence of diarrhoeal diseases or specific pathogens. However, often the practical outcome in health terms is a change in infant or under-5 mortality, because this can often be directly attributable to diarrhoeal diseases and/or malnutrition. Child growth may also be an indicator of water-supply quality. Child mortality being so important, UNICEF (1988, 1989) is now ranking countries according to under-5 mortality rate (U5MR). It notes over thirty countries with a very high U5MR of over 170 per 1 000 born alive, and over sixty countries with a high U5MR of 95 and over. It is scarcely surprising that, in many of these, the percentage of the population with access to drinking water and/or health services is low (Fig. 8.1). In spite of the major attempts made during the decade of the 1980s to extend access to clean water to as many individuals as possible, many are still without supplies. The percentage of the population with access to drinking water varies considerably, with rural populations often being 50 per cent or more unserved. It also appears that many traditional water supplies remain polluted, as they were in the early 1980s (Feachem 1980). Quality varies among traditional supplies, both by type (springs, for example, are often better than wells, which can become contaminated) and seasonally. Water quality often deteriorates during rainy seasons, especially in wells, a fact that has been confirmed by studies in Nigeria, Sierra Leone, Malawi and elsewhere (Lindskog and Lindskog 1988).

The global effort to extend water to all and to solve domestic water-supply problems is very laudable but relatively few attempts to provide safe water have proved successful. Indeed, in six cases from three countries, Ethiopia, Malaysia and Liberia, Roundy (1985) found failure or projects in jeopardy. The reasons for failure or potential failure vary from case to case, and lead to the suggestion that there are *no* general answers to the provision of safe water. Technical reasons, such as the problems of siting of a water pump too far away from homes for access during the rainy season, were seen in Ethiopia. Potential contamination of the water supply permitted by the poor design of a well (in which excess water could become contaminated on the surface and percolate unfiltered back into the supply) is another problem.

Percentage of total population with access to drinking water, 1983 - 86

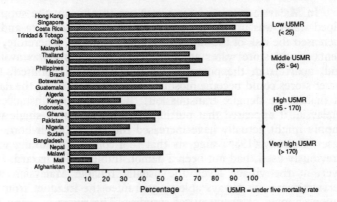

Percentage of urban population with access to drinking water, 1983 - 86

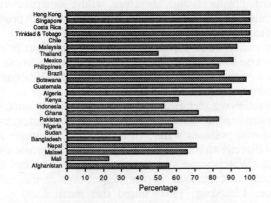

Percentage of rural population with access to drinking water, 1983 - 86

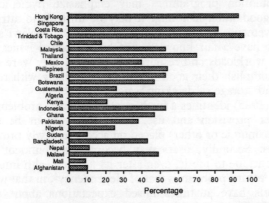

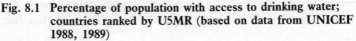

Fig. 8.1 Percentage of population with access to drinking water; countries ranked by U5MR (based on data from UNICEF 1988, 1989)

In Malaysia, variations in water pressure meant the supply of piped water was unable to satisfy demand in a rural area and also increased the risk of the supply becoming polluted. Therefore, residents would store water at home when the supply was available and, apart from the potential for this becoming polluted, these water stores could become mosquito breeding sites (with the danger of malaria or dengue transmission). In certain circumstances, in Malaysia, it appeared that putting all villagers onto a single water supply might actually have increased the risk of water-borne diseases. Roundy (1985) suggests that roof-collected drinking water, previously used, had not been a demonstrable health hazard. However, at the village level, the usually reliable Malaysian water services were not always able to guarantee the freedom from pollution (human or chemical) of supplies. The rivers in many parts of this country have been becoming increasingly polluted from agricultural toxic chemicals and, therefore, whilst sometimes reducing communicable disease hazards, domestic water-supply provision might inadvertently increase toxicological exposures.

Therefore, once water-supply systems have been put in place, there is an onus on local people and on water authorities to maintain the flow and to ensure water quality. In both the Liberian and Ethiopian examples discussed by Roundy (1985), systems broke down quickly following technical and maintenance problems. Once fractured, for instance, a water-supply system loses its integrity and may merely spread polluted water. In addition, if the water is not actually piped directly to the point of use in people's homes, storage problems arise. Water-borne and water-related diseases can therefore be encouraged if unclean storage exists, even if the water is pure at source. Lindskog (1987) found this particularly to be a problem in rural Malawi. In addition, whilst health education and sanitation-promotion programmes may emphasize hygienic behaviour and good water-handling, it may be difficult to attribute health improvements to them. Many people in the Malawi study did appear to have a fair knowledge of health-related issues but, due to heavy workloads and resource constraints, they were often unable to accomplish their good intentions, especially with regard to the care and storage of drinking water.

Roundy (1985) identifies a further set of 'human' problems related to water provision and use. First, there might be some restrictions (economic or other) placed on access to newly provided water systems. Secondly, users may become overconfident in a supply and continue to use it, even after its public-health integrity is destroyed. A third problem is that of 'dependency', in that water-supply projects have at times raised expectations about other developmental activities that cannot be met with local resources. The failure of, or inability to maintain, water supplies has been seen at times as an indicator of the inability to provide, say, other agricultural improvements. Unmanageable breakdowns of externally sourced projects can thus be costly not only to the project in question but also to people's future confidence, and willingness, to innovate. A population with a poor experience of past initiatives may well be highly sceptical of, and unlikely to support, other modernization schemes. This might be particularly problematic if water-scheme failures were to discourage participation in PHC programmes.

The use of local resources, based on realistic appraisal of social data, must therefore be taken into account by engineers and planners of low-cost water and sanitation systems. This is equally true in rural water-supply programmes or in the extension of sanitation in squatter communities (Hasan 1988). Importantly, however, whatever techniques are used to provide water, effective health education about how to store and use water (boiling it shortly before use, for example) has to be undertaken. As Narayan-Parker (1988) points out, unless women in particular become convinced of the need to change the way they handle drinking water in the home, it will continue to be polluted, regardless of improvements at source.

Extensive education intervention for altering water-sanitation behaviour has been investigated in urban Bangladesh. The involvement of community members as trainers to improve hygiene knowledge and behaviour has been useful, but technical support for communities, to provide the facilities for sanitation, clean water and storage, has often been inadequate (Stanton *et al.* 1987). Nevertheless, this study provides a good example of the formulation, delivery and presentation of education intervention related to water, sanitation and hygiene, and indicates the strengths and weaknesses of some health education methods in this context.

The importance of supplying good, potable water to all households is readily acknowledged. However, for technical, financial and physical reasons, the success of the International Drinking Water Supply and Sanitation Decade (to 1990) has been only moderate. For these and for various other reasons noted above, some initial gains have even been reversed in specific areas. Indeed, complete global service of safe water by 1990 was recognized from the outset as unattainable and the desire was to achieve the supply of clean water to 90 per cent of urban areas, with a lower, unspecified target for rural areas. In addition to the problems discussed, conflicts in many parts of the globe have meant the disruption of supplies and, in some circumstances, access to water is still provided only to a favoured few or as a reward for economic payments or political support.

Aid and international health agencies

A multitude of health and health-related projects and programmes – selective, comprehensive or administrative – have been initiated in Third World countries over the past three to four decades. Many of the projects have been funded totally externally; others, on cost-sharing bases with national governments. Projects have varied in their use of local resources (personnel, infrastructure and the like) and of external specialists and consultants. They have certainly varied in the extent to which they have been suited to the social and cultural realities of life in the countries in which they have been established.

There are scores, or hundreds, of organizations working in the international field with some input to the health sector directly or indirectly (almost all development projects have some health effects!) In brief, Foster (1987) places them in a fourfold classification:

1. *Multilateral organizations*, which are exemplified by the UN specialized agencies such as the WHO and UNICEF; membership is open to all countries; members set policy and their goal is to improve the health levels of member nations.

2. *Bilateral government agencies* such as the United States Agency for International Development (USAID), whose basic structure involves working agreements between the aid donor organization and the MOH of specific countries. Donor agencies largely set the basic policy within the broad objective of health improvement, and broadly determine the main areas and types of activities they will support. They are a foreign-policy arm of their governments.

3. *Private–secular organizations*, such as Rockefeller, Ford and other large and smaller groups, depend on charitable foundations or donations. Often these have stressed preventive and promotive health measures rather than purely clinical activities.

4. *Private–religious organizations* such as medical missions have provided important practical health care presence in many Third World countries since the early nineteenth century. Often, their provision of health care has been part of wider aims to gain and serve converts. Medical missions and private secular organizations have been generically termed private voluntary organizations or non-governmental organizations (NGOs). International NGOs such as Christian Aid, Oxfam and Save the Children Fund have a distinctive record in supporting local health-related efforts. As they are not encumbered by policy or ideological requirements, they can

both test models of social and service action, and provide often substantial support (Ebrahim and Ranken 1988).

Today, many international health programmes, especially on the part of the multilateral and bilateral organizations, conform more or less to a 'donor–recipient' model, in which representatives of technologically advanced countries work with those of less developed countries to improve health services. The prevailing pattern has emerged in the past 40 years and has evolved as a major arm of foreign policy of donor ('rich') countries with broad fields of technical aid, including health, agriculture, education and others. As Foster (1987) points out, the idea of foreign aid, a twentieth-century phenomenon, arose in part from American activities in Europe after the two world wars but, especially with regard to today's Third World, it has become increasingly institutionalized.

There is some feeling that increased size and institutionalization of foreign aid have resulted in a loss of sensitivity to needs of receptor countries. Certainly, it can be argued that either 'cost-effective' or 'high-profile' (i.e. immediately enacting) programmes might be favoured by donor nations wishing to see rapid, short-term effects of their contributions. This, it is argued, has influenced the orientation towards selective PHC, in which efficacious and cost-effective remedies or interventions are applied. These make a greater immediate impact and, cynically, make portrayal of success on the part of donor agencies easier than does the gradual development of public health, comprehensive PHC strategies that require considerable local, grass-roots involvement and cooperation. Certainly, selective sectorally, spatially or demographically targeted interventions are easier to implement on a 'one-off' donation basis than are the much more complex, long-term, comprehensive programmes.

An important limitation to the efficacy of aid can be that it is assumed that the health strategies that have served the West are universal and equally applicable in all Third World settings. This belief persists in spite of much country- and culture-specific research showing that the diversity of problems and characteristics of developing countries almost certainly defies universal solutions (in health or other sectors). As Naipaul (1986) points out, for example, what works in pragmatic, omnivorous China may well not work in fastidious, vegetarian Indian communities.

Nature and role of aid in the health sector

Health-sector aid specifically provided to the health sector may not have any direct (or even indirect) impact on health. Its definition excludes other forms of assistance, in money, personnel, advice, technology or physical donations of equipment, which accrue to other sectors but which might in practice have greater effects on health. Surprisingly, there has been relatively little published research on aid and assistance to the health sector internationally and most of that which exists has focused on the suppliers rather than on the recipients of aid (Jeffery 1986; White 1977). This contrasts with research on other forms of aid and assistance (the terms are debated but may be used for simplicity) to other sectors, particularly the effects of large-scale development projects. Such official development assistance has attracted a considerable amount of hostile criticism but this has not, in general, been focused on health-sector aid. Jeffery (1986) suggests that the aura of disinterest that surrounds the doctor and nurse has carried over to the aid programmes that support, train, equip or employ health professionals. There is, however, some feeling that it is wrong to focus solely on health-sector aid since this may have a lesser impact on health than other aspects of economic development, in which context it should therefore be set.

Nevertheless, whilst few people have argued for the cessation of health-sector aid, its form and function have increasingly been debated. We have already referred to the general issue that aid, even health-sector aid, comes with strings attached. For example, some religious bodies may wish to spread their particular brand of evangelism; certain countries may give aid only to those who are politically acceptable. Some agencies and charities, adopting disease-eradication programmes, may ignore the social and environmental contexts of these and support selective interventions that have quick, apparently short-term cost-effective outcomes. Such criticisms can be fitted into a broader debate that focuses on three potential problems of health-sector aid (Jeffery 1986):

1. The extension of dependency relationships
2. Inappropriateness
3. Malthusian intentions?

1. The extension of dependency relationships

It can be argued that health-sector aid can benefit donor rather than receptor countries. For example, the training of medical personnel in the Indian subcontinent who have subsequently worked in the United Kingdom and Europe, or of Filipino doctors and nurses who depart for the United States, benefits the developed countries. These links, it may be argued, are only maintained because of foreign support for medical educators abroad. Another feature of a

Western-oriented medical training that tends to perpetuate dependency relationships is that the professionals are generally expected to use, and buy, foreign-manufactured medical technology and drugs, which are often not produced locally.

There is a need to be specific in this type of dependency analysis about the period under consideration. For example, a period shortly after independence may illustrate very different levels of training and demands for equipment and medicines than might a later date when domestic training and manufacturing capability might have grown. As most aid is perforce channelled through the state (if it is to be officially accepted), this increases the resources of the state and tends to focus more power into the hands of the ruling élite. In addition to their other resources, they can in effect ration the direction and receipt of health provision, even that provided by relatively strong agencies. The modern-sector orientation of much aid and of many members of the bureaucracy in most countries will also tend to disparage or minimize the contribution of the traditional sector in health care. This could as a result tend to militate against the active integration of traditional medicine with the modern discussed in Chapter 3.

An important plank for critics of aid has been its effect of reducing the capability of communities to care for themselves and utilize indigenous resources. Critics point to new hospitals, equipment, health centres and vehicles that become run down and poorly maintained because of a faith that new goods will keep rolling in from abroad. This level of critique is of the millenarian variety that encouraged cargo cults in the Pacific: the belief that riches would continue to flow in from some unknown benefactor, reducing local drive and initiative. Whilst examples of the misuse and non-maintenance of health care facilities and equipment are unfortunately quite common, perhaps the fault lies as much with a lack of selection of appropriate models and goods on the part of donors as with local inabilities to sustain maintenance schedules. In addition, as noted earlier, there may be some reluctance, albeit unrecognized, to make large-scale health aid projects work in a self-sustaining manner. The wholesale upgrading of the health of the poor might threaten established power groups. Of course, effective health projects can liberate large numbers but they could also help raise economic efficiency.

2. Inappropriateness

This strand of criticism holds that much aid has been, and continues to be, inappropriate in nature and scale. For example, much assistance has gone in the past to large-scale, prestige projects, especially hospitals and related services. Maintenance costs for these are often beyond the budgets of poor countries and staffing levels cannot be maintained. In addition, their benefits touch relatively few of the population. Care has thus tended to be focused on urban élites and not to be relevant to the needs of the bulk of the people.

This criticism is increasingly recognized and, in the late 1980s, many countries have been requesting assistance in the primary and public health fields. The Malawi Second Family Health Project, for example, is an integral part of the National Health Plan (1986 to 1995). Whilst this still concentrates some 80 per cent of health expenditure on hospitals, the Family Health Project is much broader in scope and aims to extend a network of primary health facilities with associated activities to improve the health of mothers and children, and promote child-spacing services within an MCH programme. Both the International Development Association and the European Community are involved in the Family Health Project and, whilst much of the budget is to improve and expand hospital facilities, a significant element will be for spreading PHC-type services to unserved and under-served rural areas. This is not an isolated example of an attempt to orientate assistance to larger numbers of needy people but, in the poorest countries, the costs of maintaining essential hospitals are always competing with extension programmes and frequently knocking them from priority. The relative costs of maintaining hospital care and pressures to support high-level facilities will in fact be likely to grow in view of the professional and technological 'cost explosions' in health care (Joseph and Phillips 1984). Aid agencies need to be very aware of the relative benefits that might accrue from orienting their assistance to different forms of health care.

The narrow technical base of many health care assistance projects has been a continuing source of discussion. This has focused particularly into the PHC–SPHC type of debate. Where Western-oriented technological assistance has been applied uncritically, it has sometimes failed, for rather obvious logistical reasons (such as lack of running water for sanitation in hospitals or clinics, or a lack of reliable electricity supplies to maintain refrigerators, lighting, air conditioning or radiological equipment). This has led to the development of more appropriate equipment (such as the UNICEF 'cold-chain' fridges for use in immunization programmes). However, there is a continuing and increasing need for the careful introduction of Western-type technology and practices into the poorest countries in particular. There is evidence, albeit rather infrequent, that aid agencies are becoming more ready to sponsor training in local appropriate medicines and techniques and to regard this as worthwhile expenditure.

3. Malthusian intentions?

Much aid has in the past focused on population programmes and, associated with these, there is often the assumption that social and economic problems of developing countries stem largely from uncontrolled population growth. As Jeffery (1986) notes, from the mid-1960s USAID and the Ford Foundation became involved in assisting many population programmes, but support for them has been influenced by changing attitudes to birth control (especially to abortion) on the part of US governments in particular. There is considerable ambiguity in this area of critique: many argue that it is a basic human right for women to be able to control their fertility but this has to be finely balanced with policies that force them to control the number of children they have.

Sources and destinations of aid

It is sometimes difficult to trace exactly the source and destination of aid, either geographically or even by specific projects. Many aid and assistance projects also have capital and revenue elements built in, but the relative balance of these can be crucial. For example, if the majority of aid is capital intensive, this might provide (say) new clinics and hospitals, but this may demand new expenditures on roads, electricity and communications that the host (recipient) country is unable to provide. Commonly, newly provided facilities are unable to be staffed sufficiently or continuously provided with supplies. This feature of aid is particularly poignant; donor agencies are frequently unable or unwilling to provide medium- to long-term support to run and operate facilities, whereas they may be readily willing to support short-term capital projects, even if expensive.

The main sources of aid vary considerably from one receptor nation to another. Many socialist regimes, for example, would be likely to receive Soviet, Eastern European or Cuban assistance. Capitalist countries tend to look to the United States or Europe although, in the Third World, aid is often received from both sources. For the period 1947 to 1979, Jeffery (1986) identifies the main donor sources to India, in order of total health aid given, to have been the United States, UNICEF, WHO, UNFPA, World Bank, Ford Foundation, Sweden, Norway and the United Kingdom. However, the relative importance of each changed over this period as did the specific foci of assistance. In addition, the nature of aid has differed at times, including unilateral and bilateral aid, extending credit, equipment donations and overseas training fellowships. All these matters make the impact of aid in the health sector difficult to judge in either the short or the long term.

Funding for population programmes is one area in which it is possible to be more specific about international sources (domestic contributions are, however, frequently difficult to assess). Some 93 per cent of external assistance committed to population programmes in developing countries comes from the public sector, from the governments of seventeen developed countries or indirectly through the UN (Nortman 1988); 7 per cent comes from the private sector. Assistance has increased steadily, adjusted for inflation, by about $US2 million annually since 1971 and in 1985 stood at some $US513 million. Whilst the USA and Japan are the largest total donors, Norway, Sweden, Denmark, Finland and the Netherlands are highest in proportion to their GNP. It is estimated that approximately one-third of population aid goes respectively through each of bilateral programmes, UN agencies and organizations in the private sector (whose intermediary agencies may channel public and private donor funds). The Asia and Pacific region has consistently received the largest amount, followed by Latin America, Africa and the Middle East (on a per capita basis, Latin America, then Africa receive the most).

Programmes to slow population growth in developing countries began some decades ago, but only since the mid-1960s have international governments and the UN been adding their support to FP. At first, external support was purely from private philanthropy although this is now proportionately much smaller. The UNFPA attempted to obtain an unduplicated picture of who gives what to whom, where, for the period 1982 to 1985. Some

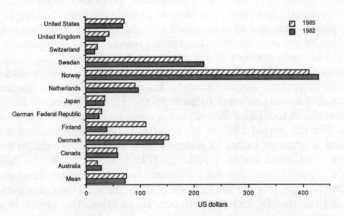

Fig. 8.2 **Top twelve donor nations and the dollars per million dollars US of GNP committed to population programmes in developing countries, 1982 and 1985 (based on data from Nortman 1988)**

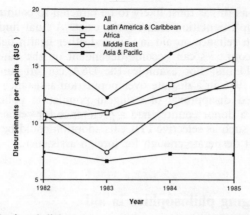

Fig. 8.3 **Regional disbursement of international funds for population programmes in dollars US per capita (based on data from Nortman 1988)**

results (proportionate to the GNP of countries concerned) are summarized in Fig. 8.2. These funds reach developing-country programmes via the three main routes noted earlier. An important feature to note in the analysis is that Africa's share of total disbursements increased steadily over the period in absolute and per capita terms (Fig. 8.3). This is perhaps some practical recognition of the population-pressure problems noted in many countries on this continent (see Chapter 2). Senegal, Kenya, Nigeria and Ghana received the largest absolute amounts.

Reliance on foreign assistance for population programmes, as for other activities in the health sector, can be problematic for receptor countries. For example, developed countries have shown considerable variability over short periods in the channels used to distribute aid. In 1977, for example, approximately 44 per cent of total commitment for population policies was in the form of bilateral agreements. This had fallen to 26 per cent by 1983, as developed countries channelled more of their assistance through the UN, an attractive route as the developed countries do not have to identify needy countries and monitor project implementation. This can therefore render developing countries open to pressure to conform with certain requirements of international agencies. Similarly, the existence of a fairly substantial body of professionals and administrators is usually needed to run a population project in any country, and this varies considerably. Historical, cultural and social factors and the level of development can therefore influence levels of aid received. Consequently, there is a positive correlation between effectiveness of FP effort and the amount of foreign support, presumably as this is most likely to be targeted to countries where adequate implementation frameworks exist. A final limitation associated with reliance on aid in this and other health fields is that developing countries can become dependent on the whims of the developed donors. For example, the USA cut off funds to the UNFPA in 1986 in a dispute over population assistance to China. This followed disapproval of stringent population policies there; similarly, if a donor country had a preference for certain types of health care, such as selective PHC, its adoption could be forced on a recipient if desperate enough for foreign assistance.

Changing philosophies in aid

A watershed in thinking about aid can be identified around 1970. Prior to this, much of the old development orthodoxy defended policies and programmes that promoted modernization along Western lines (Jeffery 1986). A wide range of technologies, allegedly embracing the universal best practices in health (and in other sectors) were exported to Third World countries. Some excessively large, urban-based metropolitan hospitals were built under such programmes and long-distance referrals for specialist treatment assumed. After the mid-1970s, a new orthodoxy began to emerge, which recognized that technology should be related to needs, cultures and levels of development. It accepted that existing aid patterns of provision often concentrated on urban, relatively affluent groups. Vast majorities of rural dwellers and the urban poor were excluded. In health care, the new philosophy began to focus on PHC, use of community and paramedical workers, and providing appropriate popular levels of care. An underlying principle became the provision of simplified techniques, and to make health care more accessible to the masses. Community participation was often sought and broader campaigns were introduced to upgrade maternal and child health (although many specific programmes persist). The value of indigenous practitioners began explicitly to be recognized.

In the decade of the 1980s, some of these newer, worthy philosophies within aid and assistance have been promoted but not all have developed as much as might be hoped. Meetings, workshops and seminars of the international aid bureaucracies have nevertheless flourished. Employment in international agencies such as the WHO or UNICEF has become greatly sought after by many professionals in developing countries (Foster 1987); many are now involved in an international circuit far removed from the practical needs and problems of their countries. For some observers, there is a growing feeling that the bureaucratic context of international health has rendered many PHC programmes ineffective, adapting them to the needs of the bureaucracies involved rather than to those, in particular, of the village recipients of services. Justice (1987) cites examples from Nepal and other South Asian countries that support this contention.

There does also remain a tendency for programmes to focus on disease-oriented, Western technology. Banerji (1988) and others feel that there is hidden menace in programmes such as that for universal child immunization. Indeed, severe criticisms have been voiced of selective programmes even if they focus on crucial issues. Today, certain 'free-market' supporters may have gone beyond the philosophical underpinnings of aid as assistance to view it as one means of promoting economic and popular health so that countries are able to interact more strongly in a world market system. There is still much evidence to suggest that aid programmes bear little direct correlation to the real needs of many countries but that they reflect more the 'high-points' that developed countries would like to see assaulted. Once attacks on specific problems have begun to have realistic impacts, aid can often tail off at a crucial time. This occurred with malaria programmes in South Asia and will no doubt occur with many other pressing problems in the future.

Other changing philosophies: a revised view of hospitals in health care hierarchies

Much current thinking in developing countries today suggests a necessity to focus on the PHC level and broad-based health care needs of populations. Does this leave any role for higher-level institutions? Economic constraints are shifting philosophical emphasis from hospital care, making it only a resort when no appropriate alternative exists. This is occurring in theory if not yet in practice.

Nevertheless, hospitals continue to be the apexes of most national health care hierarchies and their influence should spread into and beyond their immediate environs. As discussed in Chapter 5, in urban settings in particular, it is felt that hospitals may be able to strengthen their involvement in PHC. However, to do this successfully they must understand the philosophy, values and components of PHC. An Expert Committee of the WHO has recently attempted an analysis of PHC and the means of incorporating hospitals as first referral levels in support of PHC within a district health system (WHO 1987d). The intention has been to highlight examples of effective interaction of hospitals and PHC, from which general lessons may be learned. The 1986 World Health Assembly emphasized the importance of the district as the grass-roots of national systems (Ebrahim and Ranken 1988); if PHC is to grow within communities, it is felt that professional and managerial support needs to be developed locally, or at least as close to the periphery as possible.

An important philosophical shift has been the identification of the major preoccupation of hospitals with (curative) care of the individual, while the PHC approach advocates promotive and preventive treatment and is oriented to the needs of entire populations. A sensible use of existing resources and technology can make these two approaches more compatible. The hospital often believes the improvement of health is beyond the power of the individual, whereas the PHC approach sees individuals and communities as central to, and responsible for, their own health, with the professional and technician as a 'facilitator'. Figure 5.1 (see Chapter 5) shows the crucial role of a hospital in PHC. Whilst the diagram is drawn with neat lines and solid edges, it does illustrate that it is not wise to consider hospitals as separate from other levels of the health service. Their knowledge, expertise and services can be turned to wider community benefit. The arrows in the figure indicate flows of resources and ideas in all directions; components should not be isolated. Figure 8.4 illustrates various elements that may be incorporated even in hierarchical systems to enhance PHC and hospital links.

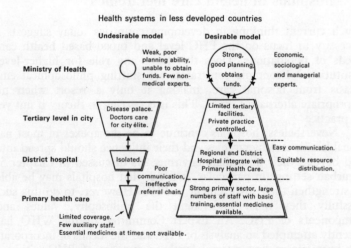

Health systems in less developed countries

Undesirable model   Desirable model

Ministry of Health — Weak, poor planning ability, unable to obtain funds. Few non-medical experts. / Strong, good planning obtains funds. — Economic, sociological and managerial experts.

Tertiary level in city — Disease palace. Doctors care for city élite. / Limited tertiary facilities. Private practice controlled.

District hospital — Isolated. / Regional and District Hospital integrate with Primary Health Care. — Easy communication. Equitable resource distribution.

Poor communication, ineffective referral chain

Primary health care / Strong primary sector, large numbers of staff with basic training, essential medicines available.

Limited coverage. Few auxiliary staff. Essential medicines at times not available.

Fig. 8.4 Towards appropriate structures for PHC systems in less developed countries (from Morley and Lovel 1986)

The district health system

The concept of a district health system emerged whilst the Expert Committee examined the implications of the role and function of hospitals at the first referral level (WHO 1987d). This is worth outlining briefly since it highlights many issues of service accessibility, areal and population coverage raised earlier in this book. In essence, a district health system as envisaged would be based on PHC, with the key feature being the serving of a well-defined population, living within a clearly delineated 'catchment area'. This would probably be an administrative and geographical area, urban or rural. Therefore, the means of defining such a catchment is crucial. This might include concepts of local identity, locality, travel time and service-usage patterns. It is an inherently geographical planning task, which needs considerable research to clarify the appropriate scale and distances that are acceptable to the residents in *any given setting*.

A district health system not only will be locality-serving but will include numerous interrelated elements that contribute to health at home, at school and in the workplace. It therefore has a strong multisectoral orientation and is clearly in line with the comprehensive, inclusive philosophy of health care discussed in Chapters 1 and 5. It consists of self-care as well as formal health services, and incorporates both publicly provided and non-governmental services, up to and including the hospital at first referral level (with associated laboratory and diagnostic provision). The district health system brings together the elements in the locality and it therefore needs to be managed as an entity, so that comprehensiveness and complementary functioning are achieved. Promotive, preventive, curative and rehabilitative activities would be provided, with the system being monitored to enable progress and change as necessary.

The achievement of a district health system seems to be a highly desirable target because many Third World local health systems are currently fragmented and haphazard. Such a system would utilize and capitalize on local resources (for example, in some developing countries, traditional medicine might be used if it is popular and trusted). The dominant role of the hospital is de-emphasized. The system will be 'people-centred' in jargon terms, focusing on the needs of the local population and recognizing local social and physical environments. The system can comprise many elements: public, private, modern and traditional. It should also have considerable managerial autonomy within a national health framework in order to use local resources most effectively to meet district needs.

The WHO (1987d) report gives considerable attention to the

definition of 'district', which can vary in size depending on circumstances. It may incorporate, for example, only certain villages
or a deprived urban area; it might focus on a specific section of a
population (such as the young or the old) or it might involve an
existing or redefined hospital service area. There is thus little
rigidity in the definition of a district, although the coverage of a
whole geographical district is felt to be preferable as this makes
comprehensive and collaborative activities easier (especially in a
clearly defined district with recognized administrative boundaries).
The coverage of a clearly defined catchment population can also
help to estimate local risk and need for specific types of service,
and some correlation of care with needs may be attempted. The
major feature of current health care provision in many Third World
countries is, of course, the mismatch and maldistribution of care
and provision relative to need. Availability of care has had a strong
spatial differentiation and is generally positively correlated with income rather than need. As a result, from the point of view of
resource allocation, neither the poor nor the rich tend to receive
optimal, appropriate care; the poor usually receive too little and the
wealthy can receive too much. If the work of the hospital at the
district level is closely coordinated with broad community needs and
resources, this can go a considerable way to harmonizing services
and moving towards appropriate treatment for all.

Nevertheless, we should not be overoptimistic about the ease
of achieving such a reorientation of the activities of hospitals to the
specific needs of their served populations. No sector of a health
system or sections of the populace will readily give up resources or
power. In addition, where hospital resources are small, and the
population dispersed, coverage will inevitably be thin. The WHO
(1987d) provides the example of the Patan Hospital in Nepal, which
serves over 200 000 people and finds it very difficult to provide for
those living up to 2 days' journey away. It is equally difficult to
avoid becoming wholly involved in providing for those who live
nearby, even if they have relatively lower need for hospital care.
Recognition of the phenomenon of distance decay in utilization discussed in Chapter 6 is of paramount importance if the aim is to
spread services to all relatively equally or on an equity basis (of
need). The justice of serving distant, peripheral folk must always
be borne in mind. By contrast, the heavy local demands on hospitals in urban settings (such as in Kingston, Jamaica, or Manila),
where hospital emergency and outpatients departments are used as
a surrogate for PHC is equally to be guarded against. This tends
to reinforce the image of the hospital as the pinnacle of health care
quality and excellence, and to support the notion that the community has little to do with its own health care. The movement

towards a district philosophy can perhaps help to modify both these extremes.

These is no single, 'ideal' district system as yet. Economic, social, geographical and political settings are too varied for this to be practical, although models do exist in China, India, the USSR and also in the United Kingdom, where support for 'locality planning' has been growing (Haynes 1987; Joseph and Phillips 1984). In urban areas, several hospitals may need to be involved in 'consortia', when there is no clearly defined catchment for any single one. Some higher-level hospitals may also become involved in PHC, especially through teaching or research functions. The overall philosophy is that, where PHC is weak, hospitals may have a role in reaching out to strengthen or even to help create it. Thus, community involvement, central to the Alma Ata declaration, applies as much to hospitals as any part of the health system. This philosophy may be accepted but its expression is not simple to achieve. Many efforts to promote community participation have ended in disappointment as rhetoric and reality have not been matched when initial enthusiasms wane. Neither do all cultures place a high value on participatory approaches to decision-making in health care (Brownlea 1987) or in other sectors. In addition, where there are limitations on democracy or on rights to information, where the medical model is strongly dominant, or where positions and privileges are entrenched, it will be difficult to achieve the participation and intersectoral collaboration necessary to develop a practical district health system.

Conclusions

Much of this book has been involved essentially with identifying issues in health care in the Third World. It has attempted to highlight some common themes, phenomena and problems, and it has also stressed the *diversity* of experience and resources that exists between and within countries. In conclusion, it might nevertheless be instructive to attempt to draw together some characteristics of Third World health care, which Meyer-Lie (1987) feels represent the 'political abuse' of medicine (using the term 'political' in a wide sense to refer to public policy and government administration).

Many obvious abuses of medicine and health care personnel exist (not exclusively in the Third World, of course). However, beyond these, there are underlying indirect abuses that often relate to the maldistribution of resources and power imbalances in many countries. An obvious example is the devotion of relatively small proportions of national budgets to health and welfare when compared to other sectors, especially the military. It is estimated, for example, that the cost of one half-day's spending on arms could pay for the immunization of all the world's children against common infectious diseases. This type of misuse of resources, reflecting decisions at national and international levels, is widely recognized and condemned but little if anything has yet been done to redirect resources (indeed, evidence exists to show the reverse is happening).

A second example of misuse of resources is the continued dominance of high-tech medical care and particularly the building of hospitals, with strong curative orientation, which can consume 80 per cent of poor nations' health budgets. The majority of the population have no access to such facilities, which are, strictly speaking, irrelevant to most of their health care needs. A third area of criticism may be directed to the medical and political establishments who perpetuate such resource allocations. Indeed, the role of medical training and the orientation of much overseas aid have arguably maintained this type of imbalance favouring the 'white elephant' facility. The activities of multinational pharmaceutical companies in encouraging developing countries into a modern drug dependency constitute another example of this type of misdirection of resources and knowledge.

Perhaps more problematic is the wider attitude of professionals to their fellow citizens. Universities and training hospitals in the developed and developing world have in part been a cause of this. Well-qualified, generally wealthy students are trained for medical degrees and thereby earmarked for positions of authority and importance. However, as frequently pointed out, these students are prepared in great depth for scientific approaches to Western diseases. Many courses have a highly scientific, academic orientation to research but barely remember or even ignore the pressing needs of today. The nature and content of much medical training require considerable reorganization to focus on the current problems practitioners and health workers are likely to encounter. This requires not only considerable national confidence but also international encouragement. Werner's (1977) book *Where there is no doctor* and Morley and Lovel's (1986) *My name is today* are still relatively unusual in promoting practical, popular health care for commonplace Third World health and environmental conditions. Unless their orientation is more widely accepted, it is quite probable that the health care needs of the majority of people in developing countries will continue to receive little more than token attention.

References

Abel-Smith B (1976) *Value for money in health services*. London, Heinemann

Abel-Smith B, Leiserson A (1978) *Poverty, development and health policy*. Geneva, WHO

Adamchak D J (1989) Population aging in sub-Saharan Africa: the effects of development on the elderly. *Population and Environment* **10**(3): 162–76

Aday L A, Andersen R (1974) A framework for the study of access to medical care. *Health Services Research* **9**: 208–20

Aday L A, Andersen R, Fleming G V (1980) *Health care in the US: equitable for whom?* Beverly Hills, CA, Sage

Akhtar R (ed) (1987) *Health and disease in tropical Africa*. London, Harwood

Akhtar R, Izhar N (1986a) Inequalities in the distribution of health care in India. In: Akhtar R, Learmonth A (eds) *Geographical aspects of health and disease in India*. New Delhi, Concept: 437–60

Akhtar R, Izhar N (1986b) The spatial distribution of health resources within countries and communities: examples from India and Zambia. *Social Science and Medicine* **22** (11): 1115–29

Akhtar R, Learmonth A (eds) (1986) *Geographical aspects of health and disease in India*. New Delhi, Concept

Akin J S, Guilkey D K, Griffin C C, Popkin B M (1985) *The demand for primary health services in the Third World*. Totowa, NJ, Rowman and Allanheld

Andersen R (1968) *A behavioral model of families' use of health services*. Report no. 25. Chicago, IL, Center for Health Adminstration Studies, University of Chicago

Annis S (1981) Physical access and utilization of health services in rural Guatemala. *Social Science and Medicine* **15D**: 515–23

Antoine P, Manou-Savina A (1988) Les conditions d'habitat en milieu urbain et leurs incidences sur la mortalité des jeunes enfants. In: *Enfants et femmes d'Afrique Occidentale et Centrale: Bidonvilles, l'urbanisation et ses incidences sur la vie de l'enfant*. Abidjan, Côte d'Ivoire, UNICEF

Ashley J, McLachlan G (1985) *Mortal or morbid: a diagnosis of the morbidity factor*. London, Nuffield Provincial Hospitals Trust

Askew I, Lenton C (1987) *Community participation in family planning: some suggestions for organization development and management change*. London, IPPF

Attisso, M A (1983) Phytopharmacology and phytotherapy. In:

Bannerman R H, Burton J, Ch'en W C (eds) *Traditional medicine and health care coverage.* Geneva, WHO: 194–206

Audy J R (1971) Measurement and diagnosis of health. In: Shepard P, McKinley D (eds) *Environ/mental: essays on the planet as a home.* New York, Houghton Mifflin: 140–62

Ayensu E S (1983) Endangered plants used in traditional medicine. In: Bannerman R H, Burton J, Ch'en W C (eds) *Traditional medicine and health care coverage.* Geneva, WHO: 175–83

Bailey W, Phillips D R (1990) Spatial patterns of use of health services in the Kingston metropolitan area, Jamaica. *Social Science and Medicine* **30** (1): 1–12

Banerji D (1979) Place of the indigenous and Western systems of medicine in the health services of India. *International Journal of Health Services* **9**: 511–19

Banerji D (1988) Hidden menace in the universal child immunization program. *International Journal of Health Services* **18** (2): 293–9

Bannerman R H, Burton J, Ch'en W C (1983) *Traditional medicine and health care coverage.* Geneva, WHO

Barker C, Turshen M (1986) Primary health care or selective health strategies. *Review of African Political Economy* **36**: 78–85

Barrow C (1987) *Water resources and agricultural development in the Tropics.* Harlow, Essex, Longman

Basta S S (1977) Nutrition and health in low income urban areas of the Third World. *Ecology of Food and Nutrition* **6**: 113–14

Beaver S E (1975) *Demographic transition theory reinterpreted: an application to recent natality trends in Latin America.* Lexington, Lexington Books

Behrhorst C (1984) Health in the Guatemalan highlands. *World Health Forum* **5** (4): 364–72

Beijing Review (1983) *Facts and figures: health service* **26**, November No. **46**: 23–5

Ben Sira Z (1976) The function of the professional's affective behavior in client satisfaction: a revised approach to social interaction theory. *Journal of Health and Social Behavior* **17**: 3–11

Bender D E, Cantlay C R (1983) Mothers as resources for community health in the Third World: a Bolivian example. In: Morgan, J H (ed) *Third World medicine and social change.* Lanham, MD, University Press of America: 29–40

Bennett F J (1985) A comparison of community health in Uganda with its two East African neighbours in the period 1970–1979. In: Dodge C P, Weibe P D (eds) *Crisis in Uganda: the breakdown of health services.* Oxford, Pergamon: 43–52

Bennett F J (1989) The dilemma of essential drugs in primary health care. *Social Science and Medicine* **28**: 1085–1090

Berman P A (1982) Selective primary health care: is efficient sufficient? *Social Science and Medicine* **16**: 1054–9

Bernstein H (1983) Development. In: *Third World studies*, U204, Block 1B, The Third World and Development. Milton Keynes, Buckinghamshire, Open University Press

Bhardwaj S M (1980) Medical pluralism and homeopathy: a geographic perspective. *Social Science and Medicine* **14B**: 209–16

Bianco M (1983) Health and its care in greater Buenos Aires. Paper presented at joint UNICEF/WHO meeting on Primary Health Care in Urban Areas, July, Geneva, WHO

Bibeau G (1985) From China to Africa: the same impossible synthesis between traditional and Western medicines. *Social Science and Medicine* 21 (8): 937–43

Bongaarts J (1987) Does family planning reduce infant mortality rates? *Population and Development Review* 13 (2): 323–34

Booth A, Babchuk N (1972) Seeking health care from new resources. *Journal of Health and Social Behavior* 13: 90–9

Bradshaw J (1972) A taxonomy of social need. In: McLachlan G (ed) *Problems and progress in medical care.* Oxford, Oxford University Press: 69

Brandt W (1980) *North-south: a programme for survival.* London, Pan Books

Brockington F (1958) *World health.* Harmondsworth, Middlesex, Penguin

Bromley R, Gerry C (eds) (1979) *Casual work and poverty in Third World cities.* Chichester, Sussex, Wiley

Brown A W A, Deom J (1973) Health aspects of man-made lakes. In: Ackermann W C, White G F, Worthington E B (eds) *Man-made lakes: their problems and environmental effects.* Geophysical Monographs Series, Vol. 17. Washington, D C, American Geophysical Union: 755–64

Brownlea A (1987) Participation: myths, realities and prognoses. *Social Science and Medicine* 25 (6): 605–14

Bryant J (1969) *Health and the developing world.* Ithaca, NY, Cornell University Press

Bulatao R A, Lee R D (eds) (1983) *Determinants of fertility in developing countries,* Vols 1 and 2. New York, Academic Press

Butter I, Mejiá A (1987) Too many doctors! *World Health Forum* 8 (4): 494–500

Cai J F (1987) Towards a comprehensive evaluation of alternative medicine. *Social Science and Medicine* 25 (6): 659–67

Cai J F (1988) Integration of traditional Chinese medicine with Western medicine – right or wrong? *Social Science and Medicine* 27 (5): 521–9

Cain M (1986) The consequences of reproductive failure: dependence, mobility and mortality among the elderly of rural South Asia. *Population Studies* 40 (3): 375–88

Caldwell J C (1979) Education as a factor in mortality decline: an examination of Nigerian data. *Population Studies* 33 (3): 395–413

Caldwell J C (1982) *Theory of fertility decline.* London, Academic Press

Caldwell J C (1986) Routes to low mortality in poor countries. *Population and Development Review* 12 (2): 171–220

Caldwell J C, Caldwell P (1987) The cultural context of high fertility in sub-Saharan Africa. *Population and Development Review* 13 (3): 409–37

Carlstein T, Parkes D, Thrift N (eds) (1978) *Human activity and time geography* London, Edward Arnold

Cartwright A, Anderson R (1981) *General practice revisited.* London, Tavistock

Chapman M, Prothero R M (1983) Themes on circulation in the Third World. *International Migration Review* **17** (4): 597–632

Chen A J, Jones G W (1988) *Ageing in ASEAN and its socio-economic consequences.* Singapore, Institute of South-East Asian Studies

Chen P C Y (1981) Traditional and modern medicine in Malaysia. *Social Science and Medicine* **15A**: 127–36

Chen P C Y (1987) Family support and the health of the elderly Malaysian. *Journal of Cross-Cultural Gerontology*, **2** (2): 187–93

Chernichovsky D, Meesook O A (1986) Utilization of health services in Indonesia. *Social Science and Medicine* **23** (6): 611–20

Chiwuzie J, Ukoli F, Okojie O, Isah E, Eriator I (1987) Traditional practitioners are here to stay. *World Health Forum* **8** (2): 240–4

Chow N W S (1987) The urban elderly in developing East and Southeast Asian Countries. In: Schulz J H, Davis-Friedman D (eds) *Aging China: family, economics and government policies in transition.* Washington, D C, Gerontological Society of America: 93–103

Chow N W S, Kwan A Y H (1986) *A study of the changing life-style of the elderly in low income families in Hong Kong.* Hong Kong, Writers' and Publishers' Cooperative

Cleland J, Hobcraft J (eds) (1985) *Reproductive change in developing countries: insights from the World Fertility Survey.* Oxford, Oxford University Press

Cleland J, Van Ginneken J (1989) Maternal schooling and childhood mortality. *Journal of Biosocial Science*, Suppl. **10**: 13–34

Cockerham W C (1978) *Medical sociology.* Englewood Cliffs, NJ, Prentice-Hall

Colbourne M J (1976a) The pattern of disease in Hong Kong. *The Bulletin: Journal of the Society of Community Medicine of Hong Kong* **7** (1): 7–26

Colbourne M J (1976b) Mortality trends in Hong Kong. *The Bulletin: Journal of the Society of Community Medicine of Hong Kong* **7** (2): 18–42

Collier J (1989) *The health conspiracy.* London, Century Books

Conable B B (1987) Safe motherhood. *World Health Forum* **8** (2): 155–60

Conyers D (1982) *An introduction to social planning in the Third World.* Chichester, Sussex, Wiley

Coppo P (1983) Traditional psychiatry in Mali. *World Health*, June: 10–12

Coreil J, Genece E (1988) Adoption of oral rehydration therapy among Haitian mothers. *Social Science and Medicine* **27** (1): 87–96

Correa H, El Torky A (1982) *The biological and social determinants of the demographic transition.* Washington D C, University Press of America

Corruccini R S (1984) An epidemiologic transition in dental occlusion in world populations. *American Journal of Orthodontics* **86**: 419–26

Cosminsky S (1933) Traditional midwifery and contraception. In: Bannerman R H, Burton J, Ch'en W C (1983) *Traditional medicine and health care coverage.* Geneva, WHO: 142–62

Cowgill D, Holmes L D (eds) (1972) *Aging and modernization.* New York, Appleton-Century-Crofts

Crow B, Thorpe M *et al* (1988) *Survival and change in the Third World.*
Oxford, Polity Press

Crozier R C (1968) *Traditional medicine in modern China.* Cambridge,
MA, Harvard University Press

Dando W A (1980) *The geography of famine.* London, Arnold; New
York, Halstead-Wiley

De Vos S, Holden K (1988) Measures comparing living arrangements of
the elderly: an assessment. *Population and Development Review* **14**
(4): 688–704

Dhungel B, Dias H D (1988) Planning for rural health services in
Nepal. *Third World Planning Review* **10** (3): 239–54

Dieng I M, Hanck C (1986) Santé mentale et environnement urbain.
Paper presented at a Conference on Urbanization and Health in
the Third World. Dakar, Senegal, ORSTOM

Diesfeld H J, Hecklau M K (1978) *Kenya: a geomedical monograph.*
Berlin, Springer-Verlag

Djukanovic V, Mach E P (eds) (1975) *Alternative approaches to meeting
basic health needs in developing countries.* Geneva, UNICEF/WHO

Dodge C P, Wiebe P D (eds) (1985) *Crisis in Uganda: the breakdown of
health services.* Oxford, Pergamon

Donabedian A (1973) *Aspects of medical care administration.* Cambridge,
MA, Harvard University Press

Donabedian A (1980) *The definition of quality and approaches to its
assessment*, Vol. I. Ann Arbor, MI, Health Administration Press

Donahue J M (1986a) *The Nicaraguan revolution in health: from Somoza
to the Sandinistas.* Cambridge, MA, Bergin and Garvey

Donahue J M (1986b) Planning for primary health care in Nicaragua: a
study in revolutionary process. *Social Science and Medicine* **23**
(2): 149–157

Duggan L (1986) From birth control to population control:
Depo-Provera in Southeast Asia. In: McDonnell K (ed) *Adverse
effects: Women and the pharmaceutical industry.* Toronto, Women's
Press: 159–66

Dunn F L (1976) Traditional Asian medicine and cosmopolitan
medicine as adaptive systems. In: Leslie C (ed) *Asian medical
systems.* Berkeley CA, University of California Press: 133–58

Durkin-Longley M (1984) Multiple therapeutic use in urban Nepal.
Social Science and Medicine **19** (8): 867–72

Dutton D (1986) Financial, organizational and professional factors
affecting health care utilization. *Social Science and Medicine* **23**
(7): 721–35

Dyson T, Murphy M (1985) The onset of fertility transition. *Population
and Development Review* **11** (3): 399–440

Ebéné R T (1987) Health risks to the population of Gezira/Sudan
following irrigation of cotton fields. In: Akhtar R (ed) *Health and
disease in tropical Africa.* London, Harwood: 293–303

Ebrahim G J, Ranken J P (eds) (1988) *Primary health care: reorientating
organisational support.* London, Macmillan

Elson D, Harris L, Sen G (1989) The international setting. In: *Third
World studies*, U204, Block 4A-C. Milton Keynes,
Buckinghamshire, Open University Press

ESCAP (1986) *Multivariate areal analysis of the efficiency of family planning programme and its impact on fertility in Thailand.* Asian Population Studies Series No. 68. Bangkok, ESCAP

Evans-Pritchard E E (1937) *Witchcraft, oracles and magic among the Azande.* Oxford, Clarendon

Fabrega H (1977) The scope of ethnomedical science. *Culture, Medicine and Psychiatry* 1: 201–8

Farnsworth N R (1983) The NAPRALERT data base as an information source for application to traditional medicine. In: Bannerman R H, Burton J, Ch'en W C *Traditional medicine and health care coverage.* Geneva, WHO: 184–93

Fassin D, Fassin F (1988) Traditional medicine and the stakes of legitimation in Senegal. *Social Science and Medicine* 27 (4): 353–7

Feachem R G (1980) Bacterial standards for drinking water quality in developing countries. *Lancet* ii: 255

Feachem R G, McGarry M, Mara D (eds) (1977) *Water, wastes and health in hot climates.* Chichester, Sussex, Wiley

Feachem R G et al. (1987) *Water, health and development: an interdisciplinary evaluation.* London, Tri-Med Books

Feachem R G, Bradley D J, Garelick H, Mara D D (1983) *Sanitation and disease: health aspects of excreta and wastewater management.* Chichester, Wiley

Feachem R G, Graham W J, Timaeus I M (1989) Identifying health problems and health research priorities in developing countries. *Journal of Tropical Medicine and Hygiene* 92: 133–91

Feldman S (1987) Overpopulation as crisis: redirecting health care services in rural Bangladesh. *International Journal of Health Services* 17 (1): 113–31

Fendall R (1981) Primary health care: issues and constraints. *Third World Planning Review* 3: 387–401

Fendall R (1985) Myths and misconceptions in primary health care. *Third World Planning Review* 7 (4): 307–22

Fendall R (1987) The integration of vertical programmes into primary health care. *Third World Planning Review* 9 (3): 275–84

Ferguson A (1986) Women's health in a marginal area of Kenya. *Social Science and Medicine* 23 (1): 17–29

Ferguson A, Van Praag E, Absalom E O (1986) *Kibwezi health risk study.* Nairobi, Kenya Medical Research Institute

Fiedler J L A (1981) A review of the literature on access and utilization of medical care with special emphasis on rural primary care. *Social Science and Medicine* 15C: 129–42

Fincham R J (1985) *Food and nutrition in South Africa.* Paper No. 1, Carnegie Inquiry into Poverty and Development in Southern Africa. Cape Town, School of Economics, University of Cape Town

Findlay A, Findlay A (1987) *Population and development in the Third World.* London, Methuen

Foster G M (1983) An introduction to ethnomedicine. In: Bannerman R H, Burton J, Ch'en W C (1983) *Traditional medicine and health care coverage.* Geneva, WHO: 17–24

Foster G M (1987) Bureaucratic aspects of international health agencies. *Social Science and Medicine* **25** (9): 1039–48

Foster S, Drager N (1988) How community drug schemes may succeed. *World Health Forum* **9** (2): 200–6

Fosu G B (1986) Implications of mortality and morbidity for health care delivery in Ghana. *Sociology of Health and Illness* **8** (3): 252–77

Frank A G (1966) The development of underdevelopment. *Monthly Review* **18** (4), September: 17–31

Frank A G (1971) *Capitalism and underdevelopment in Latin America.* Harmondsworth, Middlesex, Penguin

Frank O, McNicoll G (1987) An interpretation of fertility and population policy in Kenya. *Population and Development Review* **13** (2): 209–43

Frankel S (1984) Peripheral health workers are central to primary health care: lesson from Papua New Guinea's aid posts. *Social Science and Medicine* **19** (3), 279–90

Freidson E (1970) *Profession of medicine.* New York, Dodd Mead

Freyhold, M. von (1979) *Ujamaa villages in Tanzania: analysis of a social experiment.* London, Heinemann

Fry J (1979) The place of primary care. In: *Trends in general practice.* London, Royal College of General Practitioners: 5–21

Garfield R M (1985) Health and the war against Nicaragua, 1981–84. *Journal of Public Health Policy* **6**: 116–31

Garfield R M (1989) War-related changes in health and health services in Nicaragua. *Social Science and Medicine* **28** (7): 669–76

Garfield R M, Taboada E (1984) Health services reforms in revolutionary Nicaragua. *American Journal of Public Health* **74** (10): 1138–44

Garner P (1989) The Bamako Initiative: financing health in Africa by selling drugs. *British Medical Journal* No 6694 **229** (29 July): 277–78

Gelfand M (1964) *Witch doctor: traditional medicine man of Rhodesia.* London, Harvill Press

Gesler W M (1984) *Health care in developing countries.* Washington, DC, Association of American Geographers

Girt J L (1973) Distance to general medical practice and its effects on revealed ill-health in a rural environment. *Canadian Geographer* **17**: 154–66

Gish O (1977) *Guidelines for health planners: the planning and management of health services in developing countries.* London, Tri-Med Books

Gish O (1979) The political economy of primary care and 'Health by the People': an historical exploration. *Social Science and Medicine* **13C**: 203–11

Gish O (1981) Health and family planning services in Bangladesh: a study in inequality. *International Journal of Health Services* **11** (2): 263–81

Gish O (1982) Selective primary health care: old wine in new bottles. *Social Science and Medicine* **16**: 1049–63

Good C M (1987a) *Ethnomedical systems in Africa: patterns of traditional medicine in rural and urban Kenya.* New York, Guilford Press

Good C M (1987b) Community health in tropical Africa: is medical pluralism a hindrance or a resource? In: Akhtar R (ed) *Health and disease in tropical Africa*. London, Harwood: 13–50

Good C M, Hunter J M, Katz S H, Katz S S (1979) The interface of dual systems of health care in the developing world: toward health policy initiatives in Africa. *Social Science and Medicine* **13D**: 141–54

Gosling D (1985) Thailand's bare-headed doctors. *Modern Asian Studies* **19** (4): 761–96

Gould P R, Leinbach T R (1966) An approach to the geographic assignment of hospital services. *Tijdschrift voor Economische en Sociale Geografie* **57**: 203–6

Grell G A C (ed) (1987) *The elderly in the Caribbean*. Kingston, Jamaica, Department of Medicine, University of West Indies

Gross P F (1972) Urban health disorders, spatial analysis and the economics of health facility location. *International Journal of Health Services* **2**: 63–84

Grosse R N, Harkavy O (1980) The role of health in development. *Social Science and Medicine* **14C**: 165–9

Guindo S, Jeannée E, Réveillon M, NDiaye B (1986) Soins de santé primaires en milieu urbain: l'exemple de Pikine. Paper presented at a Conference on Urbanization and Health in the Third World. Dakar, Senegal, ORSTOM

Habib O S, Vaughan J P (1986) The determinants of health services utilization in Southern Iraq: a household interview survey. *International Journal of Epidemiology* **15** (3): 359–403

Haines M R, Avery R C (1982) Differential infant and child mortality in Costa Rica: 1968–1973. *Population Studies* **36** (1): 31–43

Hakulinen T, Hansluwka H, Lopez A D, Nakada T (1986) Global and regional mortality patterns by cause of death in 1980. *International Journal of Epidemiology* **15** (2): 226–33

Halberstein R A (1985) Health implications of urbanization in the Third World. In: Jackson B E, Ugalde A (eds) *The impact of development and modern technologies in Third World health*. Studies in Third World Societies, No. 34. Williamsburg, VA, Department of Anthropology, College of William and Mary

Halpern D C, Garfield R (1982) Developments in health care in Nicaragua. *New England Journal of Medicine* **307** (6): 388–92

Hansluwka H, Lopez A D, Porapakkham Y, Prasartkul P (eds) (1986) *New developments in the analysis of mortality and causes of death*. Global Epidemiological Surveillance and Health Assessment. Bangkok, WHO and Institute for Population and Social Research, Mahidol University

Harpham T, Lusty T, Vaughan P (eds) (1988) *In the shadow of the city: community health and the urban poor*. Oxford, Oxford University Press

Harpham T, Vaughan P, Rifkin S (1985) *Health and the urban poor*. London, Evaluation and Planning Centre for Health Care, London School of Hygiene and Tropical Medicine

Harris N (1987) *The end of the Third World: newly industrializing countries and the decline of an ideology.* Harmondsworth, Middlesex, Penguin

Hart J T (1971) The inverse care law. *Lancet* i: 405–12

Hartmann B (1987) *Reproductive rights and wrongs: the global politics of population control and contraceptive choice.* New York, Harper and Row

Hartmann B, Standing H (1985) *Food, saris and sterilization: population control in Bangladesh.* London, Bangladesh Action Group

Hasan A (1988) Low-cost sanitation for a squatter community. *World Health Forum* **9** (3): 361–4

Haynes R M (1987) *The geography of health services in Britain.* London, Croom Helm

Haywood M A M (1988) Population control in Bangladesh: the antithesis of reproductive freedom. In MacKenzie F (ed) *Gender and processes in the Third World.* Discussion Paper No. 7. Ottawa, Department of Geography, Carlton University

Heggenhougen H K (1980) The utilization of traditional medicine – a Malaysian example. *Social Science and Medicine* **14B**: 39–44

Heggenhougen H K (1984) Will primary health care efforts be allowed to succeed? *Social Science and Medicine* **19** (3): 217–24

Heggenhougen H K, Vaughan P, Muhondwa E P Y, Rutabanzibwa-Ngaiza J (1987) *Community health workers: the Tanzanian experience.* Nairobi, Oxford University Press

Hellen J A (1981) Demographic change and public policy in Egypt and Nepal: some long-term implications for development planning. *Science and Public Policy*, August: 308–36

Hellen J A (1983) Primary health care and the epidemiological transition in Nepal. In: McGlashan N D, Blunden J R (eds) *Geographical aspects of health.* London, Academic Press: 285–318

Hellen J A (1986) Medical geography and the Third World. In Pacione M (ed) *Medical geography: progress and prospect.* London, Croom Helm: 284–332

Heller P S (1982) A model of the demand for medical and health services in Peninsular Malaysia. *Social Science and Medicine* **16**: 267–84

Henin R A, Korten A, Werner L H (1982) *Evaluation of birth histories: a case study of Kenya.* World Fertility Survey Scientific Reports, No. 36. London, WFS

Henkel R (1984) Distribution of health care services in Zambia since the 1880s with special reference to the role of the Christian missions and churches. Paper presented to an IGU Symposium on Health in the Tropics, April, University of Zambia, Lusaka

Herz B, Measham A R (1987) *The safe motherhood initiative: proposals for action.* World Bank Discussion Papers, No. 9. Washington, DC, World Bank

Higginbotham H N (1984) *Third World challenge to psychiatry: culture accommodation and mental health care.* Honolulu, East–West Center/University of Hawaii Press

Hill A G (ed) (1985) *Population health and nutrition in the Sahel.* London, Routledge and Kegan Paul

Hill A G, Roberts D F (eds) (1989) *Health interventions and mortality change in developing countries. Journal of Biosocial Science*, Suppl. No. 10

Hiller S, Jewell J (1983) *Health care and traditional medicine in China, 1800–1982.* New York, Routledge and Kegan Paul

Ho S C, Lun K C, Ng W K (1984) The role of Chinese traditional medical practice as a form of health care in Singapore: III: *Social Science and Medicine* **18** (9): 745–52

Ho T M (1988) The present problems and future needs of primary health care in Malaysia. *International Journal of Health Services* **18** (2): 281–91

Hollnsteiner M R (1979) The unwashed urban multitudes: water scarcity in slums and shanty towns. *Assignment Children* **45/46**: 79–92

Holmes E R, Holmes L D (1987) Western Polynesia's first home for the aged: are concept and culture compatible? *Journal of Cross-Cultural Gerontology* **2** (4), 359–75

Hou Z T (1986) Traditional Chinese medicine making its mark on the world. *Beijing Review* **29** (20), 19 May: 15–23

Hours B (1986) *L'état sorcier: santé publique et société au Cameroun.* Paris, Harmattan

Howe G M (ed) (1977) *A world geography of human diseases.* London, Academic Press

Howe G M (ed) (1986) *Global geocancerology.* Edinburgh, Churchill Livingston

Howe G M, Phillips D R (1983) Medical geography in the United Kingdom, 1945–1982 In: McGlashan N D, Blunden J R (eds) *Geographical aspects of health.* London, Academic Press: 33–52

Huang S M (1988) Transforming China's collective health care system: a village study. *Social Science and Medicine* **27** (9): 879–88

Hunt J (1957) The renaissance of general practice. *British Medical Journal* **1**: 1075–8 (Reprinted in 1972 in the *Journal of the Royal College of General Practitioners* **22**: Suppl. No. 4)

Hutt M S R, Burkitt D P (1986) *The geography of non-infectious disease.* Oxford, Oxford University Press

Hye H K M A (1988) Essential drugs for all. *World Health Forum* **9** (2): 214–17

Ikles C (1983) *Aging and adaptation: Chinese in Hong Kong and the United States.* Hamden, CT, Archon Books

Illich I (1976) *Limits to medicine.* London, Marion Boyars; 1977 Harmondsworth, Middlesex, Penguin

Ingram D R, Clarke D R, Murdie R A (1978) Distance and the decision to visit an emergency department. *Social Science and Medicine* **12D**: 55–62

Institute for Population and Social Research (1988) *Thailand: the morbidity and mortality differentials.* ASEAN Population Programme Phase III Country Study Report, IPSR Publication No. 119. Bangkok, Mahidol University

International Institute for Environment and Development (1983) *Health and habitat: the links between the health status of low income groups* and their housing conditions and the impact of government shelter policies on these. London, IIED

IPPF (1986) *Family planning in five continents*. London, IPPF

Iyun F (1983) Hospital service areas in Ibadan City. *Social Science and Medicine* **17** (9): 601–16

Iyun F (1989) Some observations on the spatial epidemiology of mental ill-health in Nigerian cities: a preliminary investigation of Ibadan mental clinics. In: Salem G, Jeanée E (eds) *Urbanisation et Santé dans le Tiers Monde*. Paris, ORSTOM: 61–73

Jackman M E (1972) Flying doctor services in Zambia. In McGlashan N D (ed) *Medical geography: techniques and field studies*. London, Methuen: 97–103

Jeffery R (1986) New patterns in health sector aid to India. *International Journal of Health Services* **16** (1), 121–39

Johnson N E, Nelson M R (1984) Housing quality and child mortality in the rural Philippines. *Journal of Biosocial Science* **16**, 531–40

Jones H R (1981) *A population geography*. London, Harper and Row

Joseph A, Abraham S, Bhattacharji S, Muliyil J, John K R, Ethirajan N, George K, Joseph K S (1988) Improving immunization coverage. *World Health Forum* **9** (3): 336–40

Joseph A E, Phillips D R (1984) *Accessibility and utilization: geographical perspectives on health care delivery*. London, Harper and Row

Joseph S C, Russell S S (1980) Is primary care the wave of the future? *Social Science and Medicine* **14C**: 137–44

Justice J (1987) The bureaucratic context of international health: a social scientist's view. *Social Science and Medicine* **25** (12): 1301–6

Kanji N (1989) Charging for drugs in Africa: UNICEF's "Bamako Initiative" *Health Policy and Planning* **4** (2): 110–120

Karalliedde L D, Senanayake N, Aluwihare A P R (1987) Young doctors' preferences in the Third World. *World Health Forum* **8** (4): 504–7

Kasteler J, Kane R L, Olsen D M, Thetford C (1976) Issues underlying the prevalence of 'doctor-shopping' behavior. *Journal of Health and Social Behavior* **17**: 328–39

Kendall C (1988) The implementation of a diarrheal disease control program in Honduras: is it 'selective primary health care' or 'integrated primary health care'? *Social Science and Medicine* **27** (1): 17–23

Kessler S, Favin M, Melendez D (1987) Speeding up child immunization. *World Health Forum* **8** (2): 216–20

Kikhela N, Bibeau G, Corin E (1981) Africa's two medical systems: options for planners. *World Health Forum* **2** (1): 96–9

Kim K G (1987) Environmental impacts of new town developments: the case of Gwachon New Town, Korea. In Phillips D R, Yeh A G O (eds) *New towns in East and Southeast Asia*. Hong Kong, Oxford University Press: 126–52

King M (ed) (1966) *Medical care in developing countries*. Nairobi, Oxford University Press

Kinsella K H (1988) *Aging in the Third World*. International Population

Report Series P–95, 79. Center for International Research, US Bureau of Census

Kitching G (1982) *Development and underdevelopment in historical perspective.* London, Methuen

Kleinman A (1980) *Patients and healers in the context of culture.* Berkeley, CA, University of California Press

Kleinman A, Kunstadter P, Alexander E R, Gale J L (eds) (1975) *Medicine in Chinese cultures.* National Institute of Health Publication 75-653. Washington, DC, US Department of Health, Education and Welfare

Knowles J H (1980) Health, population and development. *Social Science and Medicine* **14C**: 67–70

Kohn R, White K L (1976) *Health care: an international study.* Oxford, Oxford University Press

Koo J, Cowgill D O (1986) Health care of the aged in Korea. *Social Science and Medicine* **23** (12): 1347–52

Koumaré M (1983) Traditional medicine and psychiatry in Africa. In: Bannerman, R H, Burton J, Ch'en W C (eds) *Traditional medicine and health care coverage.* Geneva, WHO: 25–32

Koyano W, Inoue K, Shibata H (1987) Negative misconceptions about aging in Japanese adults. *Journal of Cross-Cultural Gerontology* **2** (2): 131–7

Kroeger A (1983) Anthropological and socio-medical health care research in developing countries. *Social Science and Medicine* **17** (3): 147–61

Kuang A K (1983) The Western Pacific Region. In: Bannerman R H, Burton J, Ch'en W C (eds) *Traditional medicine and health care coverage.* World Health Organisation: Geneva, 263–278

Lachenmann G (1982) *Primary health care and basic-needs orientation in developing countries.* Occasional Paper No. 69. Berlin, German Development Institute

Laforce F M, Henderson R H, Keja J (1987) The expanded programme on immunization. *World Health Forum* **8** (2): 208–15

Laloe F, Salem G, Bernard C (1986) Définition de zones à risques: dimensions geographiques de la couverture sanitaire à Pikine. Paper presented at a Conference on Urbanization and Health in the Third World. Dakar, Senegal, ORSTOM

Lasker J N (1981) Choosing among therapies: illness behavior in the Ivory Coast. *Social Science and Medicine* **15A**: 157–68

Last J M (ed) (1983) *A dictionary of epidemiology.* Oxford, Oxford University Press

Last J M (1987) *Public health and human ecology.* East Norfolk, CT, Appleton and Lange

Lavely W R (1984) The rural Chinese fertility transition: a report from Shifang Xian, Sichuan. *Population Studies* **38** (3): 365–84

Lawrence T L (1985) Health care facilities for the elderly in Japan. *International Journal of Health Services* **15** (4): 677–97

Learmonth A (1978) *Patterns of disease and hunger.* Newton Abbot, Devon, David and Charles

Learmonth A (1988) *Disease ecology: an introduction.* Oxford, Blackwell

Lee B T (1987) New towns in Malaysia: development and planning policies. In: Phillips D R, Yeh A G O (eds) *New towns in East and South-East Asia.* Hong Kong, Oxford University Press: 153–69

Lee R P L (1973) Population, housing and the availability of medical and health services in an industrializing Chinese community. *Journal of the Chinese University of Hong Kong* 1: 191–208

Lee R P L (1975) Interaction between Chinese and Western medicine in Hong Kong: modernization and professional inequality. In: Kleinman A, Kunstadter P, Alexander E R, Gale J L (eds) *Medicine in Chinese cultures.* National Institute of Health Publication 75–653. Washington, DC, US Department of Health, Education and Welfare: 219–40

Lee R P L (1980) Perceptions and uses of Chinese medicine among the Chinese in Hong Kong. *Culture, Medicine and Psychiatry* 4: 345–75

Lee S M C (1986) Dimensions of aging in Singapore. *Journal of Cross-Cultural Gerontology* 1 (3): 239–54

Leete R (1987) The post-demographic transition in East and South East Asia: similarities and contrasts with Europe. *Population Studies* 41 (2): 187–206

Leinbach T R (1988) Child survival in Indonesia. *Third World Planning Review* 10 (3): 255–69

Leng C H (1982) Health status and the development of health services in a colonial state: the case of British Malaya. *International Journal of Health Services* 12 (3): 397–417

Leslie C (1975) Pluralism and integration in the Indian and Chinese medical systems. In: Kleinman A, Kunstadter P, Alexander E R, Gale J L (eds) *Medicine in Chinese cultures.* National Institute of Health, Publication 75-653. Washington, D C, US Department of Health, Education and Welfare: 401–17

Leslie C (ed) (1976) *Asian medical system: a comparative study.* Berkeley, CA, University of California Press

Leslie J (1988) Women's work and child nutrition in the Third World. *World Development* 11, November: 1341–62

Lin T Y, Eisenberg L (1985) *Mental health planning for one billion people: a Chinese perspective.* Vancouver, University of British Columbia Press

Lindskog P (1987) *Why poor children stay sick.* Linköping Studies in Arts and Science, No. 16. Linköping, Sweden, Linköping University

Lindskog R U M, Lindskog P A (1988) Bacteriological contamination of water in rural areas: an intervention study from Malawi. *Journal of Tropical Medicine and Hygiene* 91: 1–7

Lindskog R U M, Lindskog P A, Wall S (1987) Water supply, sanitation and health education programmes in developing countries: problems of evaluation. *Scandinavian Journal of Social Medicine* 15: 123–30

Lipkin M (1982) Comments on selective primary health care. *Social Science and Medicine* 16, 1062–3

Lipton M (1977) *Why poor people stay poor.* London, Temple Smith

Lopez A (1989) La santé en tranisition à la Réunion de 1946 à 1986 *Annales de Géographie* **546**: 152–178
MacCormack C P (1984) Primary health care in Sierra Leone. *Social Science and Medicine* **19** (3): 199–208
McGlashan N D (1969) Measles, malnutrition and blindness in Luapula Province, Zambia. *Tropical and Geographical Medicine* **21**: 157–62
McGlashan N D (1982) *A West Indies geographic pathology survey.* Occasional Paper No. 12. Hobart, Department of Geography, University of Tasmania.
McGlashan N D, Blunden J R (eds) (1983) *Geographical aspects of health.* London, Academic Press
McKeown T (1965) *Medicine in modern society: medical planning based on evaluation of medical achievement.* London, Allen and Unwin
McKeown T (1976) *The modern rise of population.* London, Arnold
McKeown T (1985) Looking at disease in the light of human development. *World Health Forum* **6** (1): 70–5
McKeown T, Record R G (1962) Reasons for the decline of mortality in England and Wales during the 19th century. *Population Studies*, **16** (1): 94–122
McKinlay J B (1972) Some approaches and problems in the study of the use of services. *Journal of Health and Social Behavior* **13**: 115–52
McKinlay J B (1979) Epidemiological and political determinants of social policies regarding the public health. *Social Science and Medicine* **13A**: 541–58
Maclean U (1971) *Magical medicine: a Nigerian case-study.* Harmondsworth, Middlesex, Penguin
Maclean U, Bannerman R H (1982) Utilization of indigenous healers in national health delivery systems. *Social Science and Medicine* **16**: 1815–16
MacPherson S (1982) *Social policy in the Third World.* Brighton, Sussex, Wheatsheaf
MacPherson S (1987) Social security in developing countries. *Social Policy and Administration* **21** (1): 3–14
MacPherson S, Midgley J (1987) *Comparative social policy and the Third World.* Brighton, Sussex, Wheatsheaf; New York, St Martin's Press
Mahadev P D, Thangamani K (1984) Locational and accessibility constraints and planning for rural health services: a case study of Bellary District, India. *Indian Geographical Journal* **59** (1): 135–40
Maine D (1981) *Family planning: its impact on the health of women and children.* New York, Center for Population and Family Health, Columbia University
Manderson L (1987) Health services and the legitimation of the colonial state: British Malaya 1786–1941. *International Journal of Health Services* **17** (1): 91–112
Mangay-Maglacas A, Pizurki H (1981) *The traditional birth attendant in seven countries: case studies in utilization and training.* Geneva, WHO
Manoff R K (1985) *Social marketing: a new imperative for public health.* New York, Praeger

Manton K G, Myers G C, Andrews G R (1987) Morbidity and disability patterns in four developing nations: their implications for social and economic integration of the elderly. *Journal of Cross-Cultural Gerontology* 2 (2): 115–29

Maro P S (1987) Reducing inequalities in the distribution of health facilities in Tanzania. In: Akhtar R (ed) *Health and disease in tropical Africa*. London, Harwood: 415–25

Marshall L B (1985) Influences on the antenatal clinic attendance of central province women in Port Moresby, PNG. *Social Science and Medicine* 21 (3): 341–50

Massam B H (1975) *Location and space in social administration*. London, Edward Arnold

Massam B H (1980) *Spatial search*. Oxford, Pergamon Press

Massam B H (1987) Selected problems of health care policy making. In: Akhtar R (ed) *Health and disease in tropical Africa*. London, Harwood: 157–65

Massam B H (1988) *Evaluation and implementation: the location of health centres in Zambia. A study in consensus*. Occasional Paper No. 8. Exeter, Institute of Population Studies, University of Exeter

Massam B H, Akhtar R, Askew I (1986) Applying operations research to health planning: locating health centres in Zambia *Health Policy and Planning* 4: 326–334

Mechanic D (1968) *Medical sociology: a selective view*. New York, Free Press; London, Collier-Macmillan

Mechanic D (1979) Correlates of physician utilization. *Journal of Health and Social Behavior* 20: 387–96

Melrose D (1982) *Bitter pills: medicines and the Third World poor*. Oxford, Oxfam

Mesa-Lago C (1985) Health care in Costa Rica: boom and crisis. *Social Science and Medicine* 21 (1): 13–21

Meyer-Lie A (1987) The political abuse of medicine. *Social Science and Medicine* 25 (6): 645–8

Midgley J (1984) *Social security, inequality, and the Third World*. Chichester, Sussex, Wiley

Midgley J (1986) Industrialization and welfare: the case of the four little tigers. *Social Policy and Administration* 20 (3): 225–38

Minocha A A (1980) Medical pluralism and health services in India. *Social Science and Medicine* 14B: 217–23

Morgan J H (ed) (1983) *Third World medicine and social change*. Lanham, MD, University Press of America

Morley D (1973) *Paediatric priorities in the developing world*. London, Butterworths

Morley D, Lovel H (1986) *My name is today: an illustrated discussion of child health, society and poverty in less developed countries*. London, Macmillan

Morley D, Rhode J E, Williams G (eds) (1983) *Practising health for all*. Oxford, Oxford University Press

Morley D, Woodland M (1979) *See how they grow: monitoring child growth for appropriate health care in developing countries*. London, Macmillan

Morrill R L, Earickson R (1968) Hospital variation and patient travel distances. *Inquiry* 5: 26–33

Morrill R L, Earickson R (1969) Problems in modelling interaction: the case of hospital care. In: Cox K R, Golledge R G (eds) *Behavioral problems in geography: a symposium*. Research Studies No. 17. Northwestern University, Evanston, Illinois

Morrill R L, Earickson R, Rees P (1970) Factors influencing distance traveled to hospitals. *Economic Geography* 46: 161–71

Morrill R L, Kelley M B (1970) The simulation of hospital use and the estimation of location efficiency. *Geographical Analysis* 2: 283–300

Morris B (1986) Herbalism and divination in Southern Malawi. *Social Science and Medicine* 23 (4): 367–77

Moseley M J (1979) *Accessibility: the rural challenge*. London, Methuen

Muganzi Z (1989) The spatial distribution of health services in the urban centres of Kenya. In: Salem G, Jeanneé E (eds) *Urbanisation et santé dans le Tiers Monde*. Paris, ORSTOM: 235–55

Mull J D, Mull D S (1988) Mothers' concepts of childhood diarrhea in rural Pakistan: what ORT program planners should know. *Social Science and Medicine* 27 (1): 53–67

Mulvihill J L (1979) A locational study of primary health services in Guatemala City. *Professional Geographer* 31 (3): 299–305

Mundende D C (1984) Rural health needs in Zambia. Paper presented to an IGU Symposium on Health in the Tropics, April, Lusaka, University of Zambia

Musgrove P (1986) What should consumers in poor countries pay for publicly-provided health services? *Social Science and Medicine* 22 (3): 329–33

Mwabu G M (1986) Health care decisions at the household level: results of a rural health survey in Kenya. *Social Science and Medicine* 22 (3): 315–19

Mwabu G M, Mwangi W M (1986) Health financing in Kenya: a simulation of welfare effects of user fees. *Social Science and Medicine* 22 (7): 763–7

Myrdal G (1968) *Asian drama: an inquiry into the poverty of nations*. London, Allen Lane, Penguin Press

Naipaul S (1986) The illusion of the Third World. In: Naipaul S *An unfinished journey*. London, Sphere Books: 31–41

Narayan-Parker D (1988) Low-cost water and sanitation: tasks for all the people. *World Health Forum* 9 (3): 356–60

Navarro V (1974) The underdevelopment of health or the health of underdevelopment: an analysis of the distribution of human health resources in Latin America. *International Journal of Health Services* 4: 5–27

Neumann A K (1988) Anthropology and oral rehydration therapy. *Social Science and Medicine* 27 (1): 117–18

Neumann A K, Lauro P (1982) Ethnomedicine and biomedicine linking. *Social Science and Medicine* 16: 1817–24

Nordstrom C R (1988) Exploring pluralism: the many faces of Ayurveda. *Social Science and Medicine* 27 (5): 479–89

Nortman D L (1988) External funding for population programs in developing countries, 1982–85. *International Family Planning Perspectives* 14 (1): 2–8

Notestein F (1945) Population: the long view. In: Schultz T (ed) *Food for the world*. Chicago, IL, University of Chicago Press: 36–57

Nyanguru A C (1987) Residential care for the destitute elderly: a comparative study of two institutions in Zimbabwe. *Journal of Cross-Cultural Gerontology* **2** (4): 345–57

Oakley P (1989) *Community involvement in health development*. Geneva, WHO

Ojanuga D N, Lefcowitz M J (1982) Typology of health care consumers in Nigeria. *Social Science and Medicine* **16**: 1649–52

Okafor F C (1984) Accessibility to general hospitals in rural Bendel State, Nigeria. *Social Science and Medicine* **18** (8): 661–6

Okafor S I (1987) Inequalities in the distribution of health care facilities in Nigeria. In: Akhtar R (ed) *Health and disease in tropical Africa*. London, Harwood: 383–401

Omran A R (1971) The epidemiologic transition: a theory of the epidemiology of population change. *Milbank Memorial Quarterly* **49** (4), 1: 509–38

Omran A R (1977) Epidemiologic transition in the United States: the health factor in population change. *Population Bulletin* **32** (2)

Oni G A (1988) Child mortality in a Nigerian city: its levels and socioeconomic differentials. *Social Science and Medicine* **27** (6): 607–14

Oswald I H (1983) Are traditional healers the solution to the failures of primary health care in rural Nepal? *Social Science and Medicine* **17** (5): 255–7

Palmore E (1975) *The honorable elders: a cross-cultural analysis of aging in Japan*. Durham, NC, Duke University Press

Palmore E, Maeda D (1985) *The honorable elders revisited*. Durham, NC, Duke University Press

Parkin D M (ed) (1986) *Cancer occurrence in developing countries*. Scientific Publication No. 75. Lyon, International Agency for Research on Cancer

Parry W H (1979) *Communicable diseases*, 3rd edn. London, Hodder and Stoughton

Patel M (1980) Effects of the health service and environmental factors on infant mortality: the case of Sri Lanka. *Journal of Epidemiology and Community Health* **34**: 76–82

Patel M S (1987) Problems in the evaluation of alternative medicine. *Social Science and Medicine* **25** (6): 669–78

Patel S J (ed) (1983) Pharmaceuticals and health in the Third World. *World Development* **11** (3, special issue): 165–328

Paul B K (1983) A note on the hierarchy of health facilities in Bangladesh. *Social Science and Medicine* **17** (3): 189–91

Payne S M C (1987) Identifying and managing inappropriate hospital utilization: a policy synthesis. *Health Services Research* **22** (5): 709–69

Pebley A R, Millman S (1986) Birthspacing and child survival. *International Family Planning Perspectives* **12** (3): 71–9

Peretz S M (1983) Pharmaceuticals and the Third World: the problem from the suppliers' point of view. *World Development* **11** (3): 259–64

Pfleiderer B (1988) Permanence and change in Asian health care. *Social Science and Medicine* **27** (5): 415–16

Phillips D R (1981a) The planning of social service provision in the new towns of Hong Kong. *Planning and Administration* **8**: 8–23

Phillips D R (1981b) *Contemporary issues in the geography of health care.* Norwich, Norfolk, Geo Books

Phillips D R (1984) Medical services in new towns where mixed traditional and modern systems exist: the Hong Kong example. In: Boey Y M (ed) *High rise, high density living.* Singapore, Professional Centre: 223–30

Phillips D R (1986a) Primary health care in the Philippines: banking on the barangays? *Social Science and Medicine* **23** (10): 1105–17

Phillips D R (1986b) The demand for and utilisation of health services. In: Pacione M (ed) *Medical geography: progress and prospect.* London, Croom Helm: 200–47

Phillips D R (1986c) Urbanisation and health: the epidemiological transition in Hong Kong. In Palagiano C (ed) *Ambiente urbano et qualità della vita.* Perugia, Italy, Edizioni Rux: 287–99

Phillips D R (1987a) The Philippines: faltering new town policies but evidence of new towns in-town? In: Phillips D R, Yeh A G O (eds) *New towns in East and South-East Asia.* Hong Kong, Oxford University Press: 233–51

Phillips D R (1987b) Social services and community facilities in the new towns of Hong Kong. In: Phillips D R, Yeh A G O (eds) *New towns in East and South-East Asia.* Hong Kong, Oxford University Press: 82–106

Phillips D R (1988a) *The epidemiological transition in Hong Kong: changes in health and disease since the nineteenth century.* Occasional Papers and Monographs, No. 75. Hong Kong, Centre of Asian Studies, University of Hong Kong

Phillips D R (1988b) Accommodation for elderly persons in newly industrializing countries: the Hong Kong experience. *International Journal of Health Services* **18** (2): 255–79

Phillips D R, Vincent J, Blacksell S (1988) *Home from home? Private residential care for elderly people.* Community Care and Social Services Monographs: Research in Practice. Sheffield, University of Sheffield

Phillips D R, Yeh A G O (1983) Changing attitudes to housing provision: BLISS in the Philippines? *Geography* **68**: 37–40

Phillips D R, Yeh A G O (1987) *New towns in East and South-East Asia: planning and development.* Hong Kong, Oxford University Press

Picheral H (1989) Géographie de la transition épidémiologique *Annales de Géographie* **546**: 129–151

Pillsbury B L K (1982) Policy and evaluation perspectives on traditional practitioners in national health care systems. *Social Science and Medicine* **16**: 1825–34

Plath D (1972) Japan: the after years. In: Cowgill D O, Holmes L D (eds) *Aging and modernization.* New York, Appleton-Century-Crofts 133–50

Porapakkham Y (1982) Thailand case studies on sex differences in the utilization of health resources. Institute for Population and Social Research, Publication No. 59. Bangkok, Mahidol University

Porapakkham Y, Prasartkul P (1986) Causes of death: trends and differentials in Thailand. In: Hansluwka H, Lopez A D, Porapakkham Y, Prasartkul P (eds) *New developments in the analysis of mortality and causes of death*. Global Epidemiological Surveillance and Health Assessment. Bangkok, WHO and Institute for Population and Social Research, Mahidol University: 207–37

Prothero R M, Chapman M (eds) (1984) *Circulation in Third World countries*. London, Routledge and Kegan Paul

Pryer J, Crook N (1988) *Cities of hunger: urban malnutrition in developing countries*. Oxford, OXFAM

Pyle G F (1979) *Applied medical geography*. New York, Wiley

Quah S R (1981) Health policy and traditional medicine in Singapore. *Social Science and Medicine* 15A: 149–56

Queguiner F (1981) Evaluation of the traditional Arab technique of couching in the treatment of cataract in Mali. *Médicine Tropicale* 41: 535–40

Rakowski C A, Kastner G (1985) Difficulties involved in taking health services to the people: the example of a public health care center in a Caracas *barrio*. *Social Science and Medicine* 21 (1): 67–75

Ramachandran H, Shastri G S (1983) Movement for medical treatment: a study of contact patterns of a rural population. *Social Science and Medicine* 17 (3): 177–87

Ramesh A, Hyma B (1981) Traditional Indian medicine in practice in an Indian metropolitan city. *Social Science and Medicine* 15D: 69–81

Rashad H (1989) Oral rehydration therapy and its effects on child mortality in Egypt. In: Hill A G, Roberts D F (eds) *Health interventions and mortality change in developing countries. Journal of Biosocial Science*, Suppl. No. 10: 105–13

Rathwell T, Phillips D R (eds) (1986) *Health, race and ethnicity*. London, Croom Helm

Reforma M A (1977) The rural health practice program: an evaluation of the rural health service requirement for health professionals. *Philippine Journal of Public Administration* 21: 156–75

Reid J (1984) The role of maternal and child health clinics in education and prevention: a case study from Papua New Guinea. *Social Science and Medicine* 19 (3): 291–303

Ressler E M, Boothby N, Steinbock D J (1988) *Unaccompanied children: care and protection in wars, natural disasters and refugee movements*. Oxford, Oxford University Press

Rifkin S B (1985) *Health planning and community participation: case-studies in South-East Asia*. London, Croom Helm

Rifkin S B, Walt G (1986) Why health improves: defining the issues concerning 'Comprehensive Primary Health Care' and 'Selective Primary Health Care'. *Social Science and Medicine* 23 (6): 559–66

Rifkin S B, Walt G (1988) The debate on selective or comprehensive primary health care. *Social Science and Medicine* 26 (9): 877–8

Riphagen F E, de la Cueva O S, Koelb S (1988) A survey of family planning in the Philippines. *Journal of Biosocial Science* 20: 435–44

Rosenfield A (1986) Birthspacing and health: an overview. *International Family Planning Perspectives* 12 (3): 69–70

Rosenfield A, Wray J (1981) Conclusion. In: Maine D (ed) *Family planning: its impact on the health of women and children*. New York, Center for Population and Family Health, Columbia University: 49–50

Rosenstock I M (1960) What research on motivation suggests for public health. *American Journal of Public Health* 50: 295–302

Rosenthal M M (1987) *Health care in the People's Republic of China: moving towards modernization*. Westview Special Studies on China. Boulder, CO, Westview Press

Roundy R W (1985) Clean water provision in rural areas of less developed countries. *Social Science and Medicine* 20 (3): 293–300

Rossi-Espagnet A (1984) *Primary health care in urban areas: reaching the urban poor in developing countries*. Report by UNICEF and WHO. Geneva, WHO

Ruzicka L T (1986) The elusive paths of mortality transition. In: Hansluwka H, Lopez A D, Porapakkham Y, Prasartkul P (eds) *New developments in the analysis of mortality and causes of death*. Global Epidemiological Surveillance and Health Assessment. Bangkok, WHO and Institute for Population and Social Research, Mahidol University: 5–24

Ruzicka L T, Hansluwka H (1982) Mortality transition in South and East Asia: technology confronts poverty. *Population and Development Review* 8 (3): 567–88

Salem G (1989) Les fondements sociaux et spatiaux de la santé communautaire. In: Salem G, Jeanneé E (eds) *Urbanisation et santé dans le Tiers Monde*. Paris, ORSTOM: 257–63

Sanders D (1985) *The struggle for health: medicine and the politics of underdevelopment*. London, Macmillan

Sandler R H, Jones T C (eds) (1987) *Medical care of refugees*. Oxford, Oxford University Press

Scarpa A (1981) Pre-scientific medicines: their extent and value. *Social Science and Medicine* 15A: 317–26

Scarpaci J L (1988) Help-seeking behavior, use, and satisfaction among frequent primary care users in Santiago de Chile. *Journal of Health and Social Behavior* 29 (3): 199–213

Seers D (1969; new edn 1979) The meaning of development. In: Lehmann D (ed) *Development theory: four critical studies*. London, Frank Cass

Segall M, Vienonen M (1987) Haikko declaration on actions for primary health care. *Health Policy and Planning* 2 (3): 258–65

Sen A F (1981) *Poverty and famines: an essay on entitlement and deprivation*. Oxford, Oxford University Press (Clarendon Press)

Sène P (1983) The TBAs of Senegal. *World Health*, June: 22–5

Shepard D S, Sanoh L, Coffi E (1986) Cost-effectiveness of the expanded programme on immunization in the Ivory Coast: a preliminary assessment. *Social Science and Medicine* 22 (3): 369–77

Sidel V W, Sidel R (1979) Health care services as part of China's revolution and development. In: Maxwell N (ed) *China's road to development*. Oxford, Pergamon: 155–68

Silverman M, Lee P R (1982) *Prescriptions for death: the drugging of the Third World*. Berkeley, CA, University of California Press

Simmonds S, Vaughan P, Gunn S W (1983) *Refugee community health care*. Oxford, Oxford University Press
Simpson S H (1983) National health system and popular medicine: the case of Costa Rica. In: Morgan J H (ed) *Third World medicine and social change*. Lanham, MD, University press of America: 217–28
Sindiga I (1986) The persistence of high fertility in Kenya. *Social Science and Medicine* **20** (1): 71–84
Singapore Council of Social Service (1985) *A survey on homes for the elderly in Singapore*. Singapore, Council of Social Service
Singh K, Viegas O, Ratnam S S (1988) Fertility trends in Singapore. *Journal of Biosocial Science* **20**: 401–9
Sirikulchayanonta C (1989) A study of the use of model mothers as family planning motivators in a Thai rural village. *Journal of Population and Social Studies* **1** (2): 241–58
Smith D L, Bryant J H (1988) Building the infrastructure for primary health care: an overview of vertical and integrated approaches. *Social Science and Medicine* **26** (9): 909–17
Smith D M (1979) *Where the grass is greener: living in an unequal world*. Harmondsworth, Middlesex, Penguin
Smith G T (1987) The economics of essential drug programmes. *Social Science and Medicine* **25** (6): 621–4
Soeters R, Bannenberg W (1988) Computerized calculation of essential drug requirements. *Social Science and Medicine* **27** (9): 955–70
Soh, C T (1980) *Korea: a geomedical monograph*. Berlin, Springer-Verlag
Stanton B F, Clemens J D, Khair T, Khatun K, Jahan D A (1987) An educational intervention for altering water-sanitation behaviours to reduce childhood diarrhoea in urban Bangladesh: formulation, preparation and delivery of educational intervention. *Social Science and Medicine* **24** (3): 275–83
Starrs A (1987) *Preventing the tragedy of maternal deaths: a report on the International Safe Motherhood Conference, Nairobi, 1987*. Washington, DC, World Bank, with WHO and UNFPA
Stepan S (1983) Patterns of legislation concerning traditional medicine. In: Bannerman R H, Burton J, Ch'en W C (eds) *Traditional medicine and health care coverage*. Geneva WHO: 290–313
Stephen E H, Chamratrithirong A (1988) Contraceptive side effects among current users in Thailand. *International Family Planning Perspectives* **14** (1): 9–14
Stevenson D (1987) Inequalities in the distribution of health care facilities in Sierra Leone. In: Akhtar R (ed) *Health and disease in tropical Africa*. London, Harwood: 403–14
Stewart F (1985) *Basic needs in developing countries*. Baltimore, MD, Johns Hopkins University Press
Stimson R J (1983) Research design and methodological problems in the geography of health. In: McGlashan N D, Blunden J R (eds) *Geographical aspects of health*. London, Academic Press: 321–34
Stock R (1983) Distance and the utilization of health facilities in rural Nigeria. *Social Science and Medicine* **17** (9): 563–70
Stock R (1985) Drugs and underdevelopment: a case study of Kano State, Nigeria. In: Jackson B E, Ugalde A (eds) *The impact of development and modern technologies in Third World health*. Studies

in Third World Societies, No. 34. Williamsburg, VA, College of William and Mary: 115–39

Stock R (1986) 'Disease and development' or 'the underdevelopment of health': a critical review of geographical perspectives on African health problems. *Social Science and Medicine* **23** (7): 689–700

Stock R (1987) Understanding health care behavior: a model, together with evidence from Nigeria. In: Akhtar R (ed) *Health and disease in tropical Africa*. London, Harwood: 279–92

Stoker A, Jeffery R (1988) Pharmaceuticals and health policy: an Indian example. *Social Science and Medicine* **27** (5): 563–7

Strassburg M A (1982) The global eradication of smallpox. *American Journal of Infection Control* **19**, 53–9

Streefland P (1985) The frontier of modern Western medicine in Nepal. *Social Science and Medicine* **20** (11): 1151–9

Suchman E A (1964) Sociomedical variations among ethnic groups. *American Journal of Sociology* **70**: 319–31

Suchman E A (1966) Health orientation and medical care. *American Journal of Public Health* **56**: 97–105

Tata R J, Schultz R R (1988) World variation in human welfare: a new index of development status. *Annals of the Association of American Geographers* **78** (4): 580–93

Taylor C E, Sarma R S S, Parker R L, Reinke W A, Faruqee R (1983) *Child and maternal health services in rural India: the Narangwal experiment*, Vol. 2. Baltimore, MD, World Bank and Johns Hopkins University Press

Taylor D (1986) The pharmaceutical industry and health in the Third World. *Social Science and Medicine* **22** (11): 1141–9

Taylor P J, Carmichael C L (1980) Dental health and the application of geographical methodology. *Community Dentistry and Oral Epidemiology* **8**: 117–22

Thomlinson R (1965) *Population dynamics: causes and consequences of world demographic change*. New York, Random House

Tien H Y (1984) Induced fertility transition: impact of population planning and socio-economic change in the People's Republic of China. *Population Studies* **38** (3): 385–400

Timaeus I, Harpham T, Price M, Gilson L (1988) Health surveys in developing countries: the objectives and design of an international programme. *Social Science and Medicine* **27** (4): 359–68

Tipple A G, Hellen J A (1986) *Priorities for public utilities and housing improvements in Kumasi, Ghana: an empirical assessment based on six variables*. Seminar Paper No. 44. Newcastle-upon-Tyne, Department of Geography, University of Newcastle-upon-Tyne

Toye J (1987) *Dilemmas of development*. Oxford, Blackwell

Trowell H C, Burkitt D P (eds) (1981) *Western diseases: their emergence and prevention*. London, Edward Arnold

Trusswell A S (1985) Malnutrition in the Third World, Part I and Part II. *British Medical Journal* **291**, 24 August: 525–8; **291**, 31 August: 587–9

Tuckett D (ed) (1976) Becoming a patient. In: Tuckett D (ed) *An introduction to medical sociology*. London, Tavistock: 159–89

Tully B (1985) Clinical psychology and mental health services. *China Now*, No. 111: 17–18

Turshen M (1984) *The political ecology of disease in Tanzania.* New Brunswick, NJ, Rutgers University Press

Twumasi P A (1981) Colonialism and international health: a study in change in Ghana. *Social Science and Medicine* **15B**: 147–51

Twumasi P A, Freund P J (1985) Local politicization of primary health care as an investment for community development: a case study of community health workers in Zambia. *Social Science and Medicine* **20** (10): 1073–80

Ulin P R (1980) Introduction: traditional healers and primary health care in Africa. In: Ulin P R, Segall M H (eds) *Traditional health care delivery in contemporary Africa.* Foreign and Comparative Studies, African Series No. 35. Syracuse, NY, Maxwell School of Citizenship and Public Affairs, Syracuse University: 1–11

Ulin P R, Segall M H (eds) (1980) *Traditional health care delivery in contemporary Africa.* Foreign and Comparative Studies, African Series No. 35. Syracuse, NY, Maxwell School of Citizenship and Public Affairs, Syracuse University

UN (1986a) *Determinants of mortality change and differentials in developing countries.* Department of International Economic and Social Affairs, Population Studies No. 94. New York, UN

UN (1986b) *Consequences of mortality trends and differentials.* Department of International Economic and Social Affairs, Population Studies No. 95. New York, UN

Unger J P, Killingsworth J R (1986) Selective primary health care: a critical review of methods and results. *Social Science and Medicine* **22**(10): 1001–13

UNICEF (1986) *The state of the world's children, 1986.* Oxford, Oxford University Press

UNICEF (1987) *The state of the world's children, 1987.* Oxford, Oxford University Press

UNICEF (1988) *The state of the world's children, 1988.* Oxford, Oxford University Press

UNICEF (1989) *The state of the world's children, 1989.* Oxford, Oxford University Press

Unschuld P U (1985) *Medicine in China: a history of ideas.* Berkeley, CA, University of California Press

Veeder N (1975) Health services utilization models for human services planning. *Journal of the American Institute of Planners* **41**: 101–9

Vélimirovic B (1984) *Infectious diseases in Europe: a fresh look.* Copenhagen, WHO

Verhasselt Y (1985) Urbanization and health in the developing world. *Social Science and Medicine* **21**: 483

Verhasselt Y (1987) Agrarian projects and their consequences upon endemic diseases in developing countries – a review. In: Fricke W, Hinz E (eds) *Räumliche Persistenz und Diffusion von Krankheiten.* Heidelberg, Heidelberger Geographische Arbeiten, No. 83: 236–42

Vuori H (1982) The World Health Organization and traditional medicine. *Community Medicine* 4: 129–37

Waite G (1987) Public health in pre-colonial East-Central Africa. *Social Science and Medicine* 24 (3): 197–208

Walmsley D J (1978) The influence of distance on hospital usage in rural New South Wales. *Australian Journal of Social Issues* 13: 72–81

Walsh J A (1988) Selectivity within primary health care. *Social Science and Medicine* 26 (9): 899–902

Walsh J A, Warren K S (1979) Selective primary health care: an interim strategy for disease control in developing countries. *New England Journal of Medicine* 301 (18): 967–74 (Reproduced with additions in *Social Science and Medicine*, 1980, 14C: 145–63)

Walt G, Vaughan P (1981) *An introduction to the primary health care approach in developing countries*. Ross Institute of Tropical Hygiene, Publication No. 13. London, London School of Hygiene and Tropical Medicine

Wan T, Soifer J (1974) Determinants of physician utilization: a causal analysis. *Journal of Health and Social Behavior* 15: 100–12

Wang J (1988) China's medical and health services. *Beijing Review* 31 (29), 18–24 July: 14–18

Wang P (1983) Traditional Chinese medicine. In: Bannerman R H, Burton J, Ch'en W C (1983) *Traditional medicine and health care coverage*. Geneva, WHO: 68–75

Wang'ombe J K, Mwabu G M (1987) Economics of essential drugs schemes: the perspective of developing countries. *Social Science and Medicine* 25 (6): 625–30

Warren K S (1988) The evolution of selective primary health care. *Social Science and Medicine* 26 (9): 891–8

Warwick D P (1982) *Bitter pills: population policies and their implementation in developing countries*. Cambridge, Cambridge University Press

Way A A, Cross A R, Kumar S (1987) Family planning in Botswana, Kenya and Zimbabwe. *International Family Planning Perspectives* 13 (1): 7–11

Werner D (1977) *Where there is no doctor* (originally Donde no hay doctor). Palo Alto, CA, Hesperian Foundation; 1979, London, Macmillan

Werner D (1978) The village health worker: lackey or liberator? In: Skeet M, Elliott K (eds) *Health auxiliaries and the health team*. London, Croom Helm: 177–93

Werner D (1980) Health care and human dignity. *Contact*, Special series, No. 3: 91–105

White A (1977) *British official aid in the health sector*. Discussion Paper No. 107. Brighton, Sussex, Institute of Development Studies

WHO (1977) *The selection of essential drugs: report of the WHO expert committee*. Technical Report Series, No. 615. Geneva, WHO

WHO (1978a) *Alma Ata 1978: primary health care*. 'Health for All' Series, No. 1. Geneva, WHO

WHO (1978b) *The promotion and development of traditional medicine*. Technical Report Series, No. 622. Geneva, WHO

WHO (1979) *The selection of essential drugs: second report of the WHO expert committee.* Technical Report Series, No. 641. Geneva, WHO
WHO (1981) *Global strategy for health for all by the year 2000.* 'Health for ALL' Series, No. 3. Geneva, WHO
WHO (1985) *Health systems based on primary health care: 1985 digest.* Geneva, WHO
WHO (1986) *Intersectoral action for health.* Geneva, WHO
WHO (1987a) *The community health worker.* Geneva, WHO
WHO (1987b) *Evaluation of the strategy of health for all by the year 2000: seventh report on the world health situation,* Vol. 1, *Global review.* Geneva, WHO
WHO (1987c) Health for all: from words to deeds. *World Health Forum* 8 (2): 164–83
WHO (1987d) *Hospitals and health for all.* Report of a WHO Expert Committee on the role of Hospitals at the First Referral Level, Technical Report Series, No. 744. Geneva, WHO
WHO (1987e) EPI – success but no complacency. *World Health Forum* 8 (4): 551–2
WHO (1988) *Education for health: A manual on health education in primary health care.* Geneva, WHO
WHO (1989) *Strengthening the performance of community health workers in primary health care.* Technical Report Series, No. 780. Geneva, WHO
Williams C D, Jellife D B (1972) *Mother and child health: delivering the services.* Oxford, Oxford University Press
Williams P J (1989) Effects of measles immunization on child mortality in rural Gambia. In: Hill A G, Roberts D F (eds) *Health interventions and mortality change in developing countries. Journal of Biosocial Science,* Suppl. No. 10: 95–104
Williams P V A (1979) Primitive religion and healing. Totowa, NJ, Rowman and Littlefield; Cambridge, D S Brewer
Willms D G (1988) Dilemmas, trends and transformations in community health worker situations: Kenya's 'Nyamrerua' of Saradidi. *Environments* 19 (3): 101–11
Wilson R G, Ofosu-Amaah S, Belsey M A (1986) *Primary health care technologies at the family and community levels.* Report of an International Workshop held in Sri Lanka, 1985. Geneva, Aga Khan Foundation; New York, UNICEF
Wisner B (1988) GOBI versus PHC? Some dangers of selective primary health care. *Social Science and Medicine* 26 (9): 963–9
Wolf-Phillips L (1979) Why Third World? *Third World Quarterly* 1 (1): 105–14
Wolffers I (1988) Illness behaviour in Sri Lanka: results of a survey in two Sinhalese communities. *Social Science and Medicine* 27 (5): 545–52
Wolinsky F D, Coe R M, Miller D K, Prendergast J M, Creel M J, Chavez M N (1983) Health services utilization among the noninstitutionalized elderly. *Journal of Health and Social Behavior* 24: 325–37
Wolinsky F D, Marder W D (1983) Waiting to see the doctor: the impact of organizational structure on medical practice. *Medical Care* 21: 531–42

Wong E L, Popkin B M, Guilkey D K, Akin J S (1987) Accessibility, quality of care and prenatal care use in the Philippines. *Social Science and Medicine* **24** (11): 927–44

World Bank (1980) *Health: sector policy paper*. Washington, DC, World Bank

World Bank (1984) *World development report 1984* New York, Oxford University Press

World Bank (1988) *World development report 1988*. New York, Oxford University Press

Worsley P (1964) *The Third World*. London, Weidenfeld and Nicolson

Worsley P (1979) How many worlds? *Third World Quarterly* **1** (2): 100–7

Worsley P (1984) *The three worlds*. London, Weidenfeld and Nicolson

Worthington E B (ed) (1977) *Arid land irrigation in developing countries: environmental problems and effects*. Oxford, Pergamon Press

Yoder P S (ed) (1982) *African health and healing systems: proceedings of a symposium*. Los Angeles, CA, Crossroads Press and University of California

Zaidi S A (1985) The urban bias in health facilities in Pakistan. *Social Science and Medicine* **20** (5): 473–82

Zaidi S A (1986) Why medical students will not practice in rural areas: evidence from a survey. *Social Science and Medicine* **22** (5): 527–33

Zwi A, Ugalde A (1989) Towards an epidemiology of political violence in the Third World. *Social Science and Medicine* **28** (7): 633–42

Index